THE LOW-CARB COMPANION

Dr Austin Jeans

Dr Austin Jeans has asserted his moral right to be identified as the author of this work.

©Dr Austin Jeans 2016

All rights reserved. No part of this publication may be reproduced, stored in a retrieval system or transmitted, in any form or by any means, including electronic, mechanical, photocopying, recording or otherwise, without prior permission of the author.

www.thelowcarbcompanion.com
Follow Dr Jeans on Twitter @jeansdoc61

The information provided in this book is representative of the authors opinions and views. It is intended for educational, informational and reference purposes but is not a substitute for professional medical or healthcare advice, diagnosis or treatment specific to individual circumstances and locations. So far as the author is aware, the information given is correct and up to date as at March 2016. The author cannot be held responsible or liable for any outcomes arising directly or indirectly from the use, or misuse, of the information contained in this book.

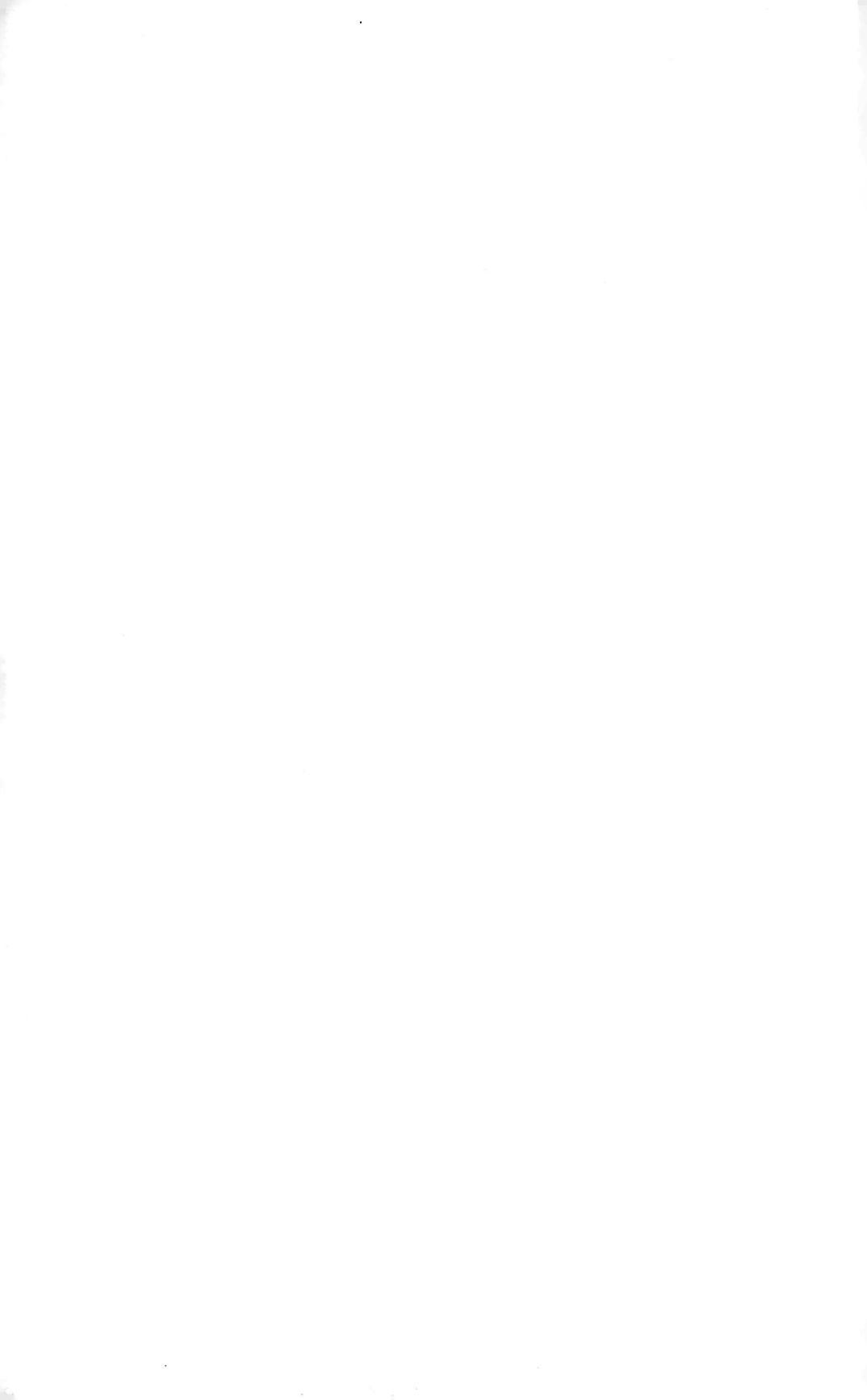

AUTHOR BIOGRAPHY

Dr Austin Jeans is a specialist sport, exercise and lifestyle medicine physician in Harare, Zimbabwe, where he has practised medicine for 30 years. He graduated in medicine from the Godfrey Huggins School of Medicine in Harare. After initially pursuing a medical career in the military and emergency medicine, he completed a postgraduate degree in Sports Medicine at the University of Cape Town.

He has been Zimbabwe's Chief Medical Officer to four Olympic teams, three Africa Games teams, National Cricket, Rugby, Judo and Hockey teams and consults for several National Sports Federations. He is a member of the Zimbabwe Olympic Committee's Medical Commission and sits on World Rugby's Developing Nations Medical Subcommittee.

He is currently the Medical Director of the Rolf Valley Sports Medicine Centre, the Innovate High Performance Centre and the Low-Carb Companion Lifestyle Program. He has written many public information media articles and has given numerous lectures on topics relating the low-carb, high-fat lifestyle to weight loss, improved health outcomes and sports performance. He is an active age-group athlete in triathlon, swimming and eco-adventure racing.

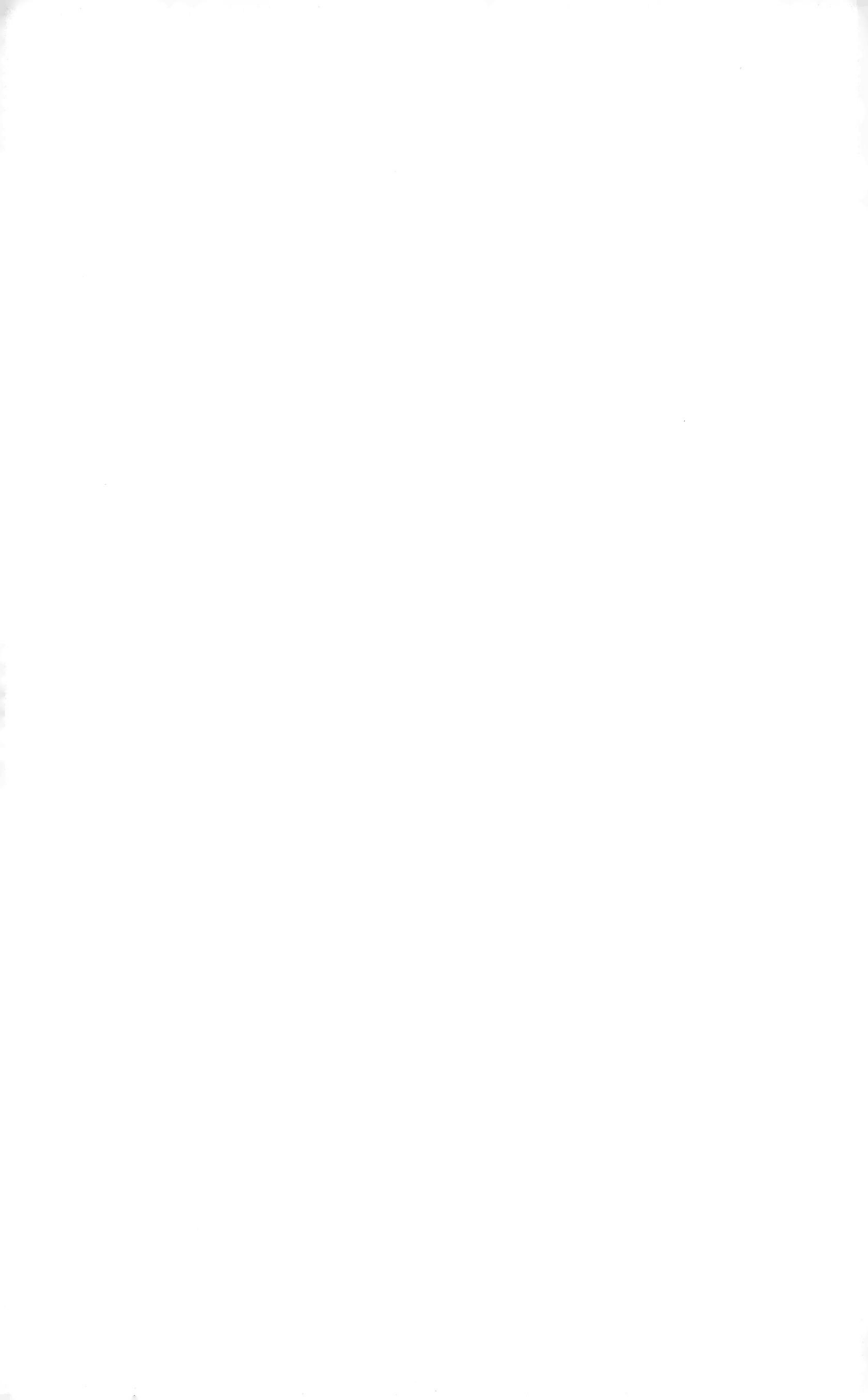

For Debi, Michael, Phillip & Rachel

In memorium Brian

TABLE of CONTENTS

PAGE

Foreword		xv
i.	Introduction	15
ii.	A Personal Journey	18
iii.	Consensus Versus Influence	21
iv.	Self-Assessments	27
v.	Health Targets For Body Measurements And Blood Tests	32

Part 1: THE KNOWLEDGE COMPANION

SECTION 1: FOOD, FAT & METABOLISM

1.	Low-Carbohydrate Nutrition – The Overview	36
2.	Why We Eat What We Eat	40
3.	Carbohydrate Intolerance And Insulin Resistance: The Metabolic Basis Of Obesity	78
4.	Heavy Weight or Healthy Weight - Belly Fat and Obesity	86
5.	Cholesterol, Saturated Fat, Sugar and Heart Disease	94

SECTION TWO: THE DIET

6.	Low-Carb, High-Fat Nutritional Guidelines	122
7.	Low-Carb Nutrition – Getting Started	138

SECTION THREE: SPECIAL POPULATIONS

8.	Low-Carb For Babies, Children, Teens & Pregnant Mums	152
9.	Low-Carb Nutrition and Diabetes	162
10.	Low-Carb Nutrition and Cancer	186
11.	Low-Carb Nutrition and the Athlete	192

PAGE

SECTION FOUR: QUESTIONS AND ANSWERS

12.	The 'Top 40' Most Frequently Asked Low-Carb Questions	206
13.	In Search Of Greater Low-Carb Knowledge	222
14.	Glossary Of Terms and Abbreviations	228

Part 2: THE FOOD COMPANION

1.	Broths & Soups	253
2.	Eggs	271
3.	Fish	287
4.	Poultry	299
5.	Beef	319
6.	Lamb	337
7.	Pork	345
8.	Sides, Salads & Vegetables	353
9.	Salad Dressings, Sauces, Dips, Marinades & Rubs	371
10.	Bread	393
11.	Pizza, Quiches & Pasta	401
12.	Pancakes & Muffins	413
13.	Cupcakes, Cakes & Cookies	421
14.	Desserts	433
15.	Smoothies & Shakes	441
16.	Snacks & Miscellaneous	447
17.	Conversion Charts & Oven Temperatures	461

APPENDICES

Acknowledgements	467
List Of Works Cited	468
Index	486

TOOLS, TABLES AND FIGURES

SELF ASSESSMENT TOOLS   PAGE

Food Questionnaire   28
Health Questionnaire   29
Diet-Health Wheel   30
Sugar-Addiction Screening Questionnaire   31

TABLES

TABLE 1	Your Body Measurements	32
TABLE 2	Your Health Targets for Blood Tests	33
TABLE 3	Fatty Acid Profiles of Food Oils	59
TABLE 4	Fat Content of Real Foods	61
TABLE 5	Smoking Points of Fats / Oils	62
TABLE 6	Sources of Vitamins and Minerals	68
TABLE 7	A Nutritional Comparison of Processed Foods (sugar & flour) vs. a Low-Cost Basket of Real Food in Providing Essential Macronutrients, Vitamins and Minerals	70
TABLE 8	Percentage of Male Adult Recommended Daily Allowance (RDI) or Adequate Intake (AI) Provided by 100g Lean Meat or Vegetarian Sources	72
TABLE 9	Effects of Diet on Heart Disease Risk Factors	101
TABLE 10	Know Your Numbers That Count and What They Mean	116
TABLE 11	The Yes List	126
TABLE 12	The No List	128
TABLE 13	The Sometimes List	130
TABLE 14	The 25 Grams of Carb List	132
TABLE 15	Macronutrient Content of Real vs. Processed Foods	134
TABLE 16	Macronutrient Composition on Nuts & Nut Butters	135

TABLES   PAGE

TABLE 17	The Many Names for Sugar Added to Processed Foods	142
TABLE 18	Easy Low-Carb Substitution Options	143
TABLE 19	Insulin Responses of Common Foods	182
TABLE 20	% Insulinogenic Calories in Common Foods	184

FIGURES

FIG 1	Diet and Metabolic Health	38
FIG 2	The Changing Human Diet From Ancient Hunter-Gatherer to Modern Day	42
FIG 3	The Fate of Carbs in the Body	45
FIG 4	The Fate of Carbs in the Body	45
FIG 5	Glycaemic Index, The Effects of High and Low GI Foods	47
FIG 6	Human Sugar Consumption	51
FIG 7	Wheat Intake, Coronary Heart Disease and Body Weight	52
FIG 8	Fats and their Major Dietary Sources	56
FIG 9	A Triglyceride	57
FIG 10	Increased Production of Omega-6 Vegetable Oils for Human Consumption 1920-2000	60
FIG 11	The Nine Essential Amino Acids Humans Require from Dietary Proteins	67
FIG 12	The Physiology of Carbohydrate Intolerance and Insulin Resistance	80
FIG 13	The Inter-Relationships between Carb Intolerance and Diet in Diseases of Lifestyle	82
FIG 14	Sites Of Fat Accumulation In The Body	87
FIG 15	The Biochemical Difference between Fat and Cholesterol	96
FIG 16	Lipoprotein 'Taxi-cabs' for Cholesterol & Triglycerides	100
FIG 17	Insulin, Insulin Resistance and the Development of Type 2 Diabetes	166

FOREWORD

by Professor Tim Noakes

....

The joy of being an educator is that amongst one's students are so many who are quite remarkable in who they are, what they stand for, and how they influence the world in unique ways. So it is that each of these outstanding students enriches one's own life in very special ways. And now that I am old(er), I have the added joy that some of those extraordinary students have raised children who are themselves bursting with promise. And so the endless cycle of renewal is sustained. Austin Jeans, the author of this book, is one of my most special students with just such a vibrant family.

He is one of the most engaging, most passionate, most committed, most positive, most selfless, most inquisitive, most intellectually combative, and most exhausting of all the students I have ever been privileged to teach; in short, he is one of the most dynamic and one of the very best. Austin truly lives his life in a state of perpetual overdrive. The only people who can possibly stay with him are those in his immediate family: his equally supercharged and indefatigable wife, Debi, and now their children. Theirs is a family that embraces life as if each millisecond will be its last.

That Austin is like me, also a Zimbabwean, gives me even more pleasure. For whilst life circumstances saw my parents leave Zimbabwe more than 60 years ago when I was just 5 years old, Austin and his family have dedicated themselves to the service of its people because they wish to influence the future of that country. Now, with his first book, Austin introduces his nation's people to the low-carbohydrate, healthy-fat (LCHF) eating phenomenon.

As he tells it, Austin's introduction to the LCHF eating plan was very similar to mine. There is one big difference: Austin is a much better athlete than I am with real competence in running, swimming and triathlon. He also has the build of the elite endurance athlete - 70kg lean, rangy and muscular with a small 31-inch waist. But at age 48, after decades of doing as I had done - eating the 'healthy', 'prudent', and 'balanced' high-carbohydrate, low-fat (HCLF) diet based on generous daily helpings of cereals and grains - as we had been taught by the United States Department of Agriculture and as I, in my supreme stupidity, had passed on to him - Austin finally realised that all was not well with his own health. He had gained 4kg of unwanted fat that encased his muscular body and which despite heroic efforts to exercise more and eat less, stubbornly persisted. Wisely, he asked the important questions: Why is this happening to me when I have all the knowledge and all the discipline to stay lean and healthy? Surely this cannot be because in my middle age I have suddenly become slothful and gluttonous?

Fortunately, at the correct moment his prepared mind came upon my description of how reading the book, *The New Atkins for a New You*, had changed my life. That book had shown me that for 33 long years I had been eating the wrong foods and giving the wrong dietary advice to my students, including Austin. The similarities between our two mid-life experiences are striking; both our fathers had developed type 2 diabetes mellitus indicating that Austin and I have both likely inherited a common genetic condition - insulin resistance or what he terms carbohydrate intolerance - perhaps the most common medical condition in the world. It is in those with carbohydrate intolerance that the high-carbohydrate diet produces its most lethal long-term effects, including obesity, diabetes and perhaps also dementia and cancer.

Predictably then, when Austin stopped fuelling his genetic condition with the one foodstuff, carbohydrate, for which his body is intolerant, he began to heal, just as I had. His weight rapidly returned to a lean and muscular 70kg, and he

Foreword

began to run, cycle and swim with the same vigour that he had 20 years earlier. His blood markers also showed that he was healthier.

As a practising sports medicine physician, the next question he faced was then more obvious: What if I prescribe this eating plan for my patients suffering from the same condition as I have? He began a 12-month experimental intervention where he treated patients with the carbohydrate intolerance (insulin resistance) syndrome - comprising obesity, type 2 diabetes, high blood pressure and gout - with the LCHF diet. The results were sufficiently encouraging and he then felt the responsibility to share his experiences more widely.

Austin wrote this book because, like me, he believes that the condition of carbohydrate intolerance is the missing link that no doctors are taught at medical school. Our personal experiences have taught us that carbohydrate intolerance cannot be cured by expensive life-long medications that do nothing more than ineffectively treat its symptoms. Rather, if we wish to reverse the current obesity/diabetes epidemic that is spreading, uncontrolled, across the globe, we have to understand that the root cause is a high-carbohydrate diet in those with carbohydrate intolerance. It really is that simple. No more, no less. Not rocket science.

What strikes me about his book is just how good and complete it is. It covers complex topics in depth, yet it is academically sound and easy to follow because it is so well written. It includes a detailed section of the science explaining why carbohydrates harm those with carbohydrate intolerance, and conversely, why the LCHF eating plan works so well for those with that condition. The section describing what constitutes healthy fats is particularly excellent, as are the sections that explain why those of us with insulin resistance/carbohydrate intolerance become obese. He clearly spells out why carbohydrate and sugar in the diet, not dietary fat and cholesterol, cause heart disease.

From this background of hard science, the next, more practical, section details how to get started on the LCHF eating lifestyle. He then moves on to the specific needs of special populations including pregnant mothers, diabetics, cancer patients and athletes.

The second half of the book provides all the recipes one needs to begin this new journey to better health.

My final conclusion is that the book is as good an introduction to the LCHF lifestyle as has been published anywhere in the world. What an achievement for Zimbabwe and its leading sports physician and educator! With this book, Austin introduces the LCHF eating plan to the heart of Africa. And beyond.

It is a key moment in the battle to raise the awareness of Africa to the damaging health consequences of high-carbohydrate diets for those with carbohydrate intolerance.

Austin is not the only world-class Zimbabwean who has grown to love the LCHF way of eating. In the 1980s, I advised Zimbabwean ex-pat, Paula Newby-Fraser, to consider eating more fat during her training for the 242km Ironman Triathlon, which is usually considered to be the toughest one-day sporting event in the world. She followed my advice, and after her retirement - having won the Hawaiian Ironman World Championship a record 8 times, as well as a total of 28 Ironman Triathlons, thereby earning the title of the Greatest Triathlete (either gender) of the Millennium - she told me that that my advice was the single most important contributor to her remarkable Ironman record.

More recently, another Zimbabwean ex-pat, Wallabies rugby star, former Wallabies captain and outstanding player at the 2015 Rugby World Cup, David Pocock, changed to the LCHF diet with obviously great results. Both he and Paula became the best in the world at their particular disciplines.

Foreword

I owe a great deal of gratitude to my own personal Zimbabwean heritage; this is something I have only come to appreciate later in life. I was fortunate to be raised by parents in Harare in the early 1950s on a high-quality farm produce diet comprising eggs, dairy produce, meat and offal from animals raised in pristine pastures. It was only when I moved to Cape Town and became 'clever' and 'educated', did the wheels of my health fall off; I began to eat an unhealthy high-carbohydrate diet, which is typical of big-city living.

I'm so proud that through this book and the work of my student Austin Jeans, I have made a small contribution to the future health of all Zimbabweans.

The future of our good health begins in these pages.

Professor Tim Noakes OMS, MD, DSc
Emeritus Professor – University of Cape Town

'The mainstream dietary advice that we are currently giving to the world has simply not worked. Instead it is the opinion of the speakers at this convention that this incorrect nutritional advice is the immediate cause of the global obesity and diabetes epidemics.

This advice has failed because it completely ignores the history of why and how human nutrition has developed over the past three million years. More importantly, it refuses to acknowledge the presence of insulin resistance (carbohydrate intolerance) as the single most prevalent biological state in modern humans.

Persons with insulin resistance are at an increased risk of developing a wide range of chronic medical conditions if they ingest a high carbohydrate diet for any length of time (decades)'.

Speakers' Consensus Statement at the Low-Carb High-Fat Health Summit, Cape Town, February 2015

INTRODUCTION

'When the student is ready, the teacher will appear'.
Chinese Proverb

....

Whether you are a medical professional, a dietician, a patient or someone seeking guidance in the 'Enlightened New World' of lower-carbohydrate, higher-fat nutrition, this book is designed to provide you with the necessary tools to make a transition towards a healthier way of life. Once armed with the facts surrounding the various aspects, benefits and features of low-carb, high-fat nutrition, you will be able to implement a lifestyle change with confidence. *The Low-Carb Companion* has been written in order to share these facts.

Part One of this book is the *Knowledge Companion*. This section is dedicated to expanding your knowledge about low-carb nutrition and understanding its importance. Once you understand how a low-carb, high-fat diet works scientifically and systematically in the body to maintain a healthy weight and to prevent obesity and diseases of lifestyle such as diabetes, heart disease, cancer and to enhance athletic performance, you will be able to see how beneficial low-carb habits can be. I have laid this section out in an easy-to-read format with 'Key Points' for quick review and have included simple charts and graphs for your rapid digestion.

A former professor of medicine once taught me that 'The secret to knowledge is not necessarily having all the required information in one's head, but knowing where to find it'. I have also highlighted some well-researched and well-documented references in order to satisfy what I am sure will be your growing curiosity regarding the information supported in this book. The *Knowledge Companion* also contains a Frequently Asked Questions section with answers to guide you, as well as a comprehensive Glossary of Terms to help explain the terms used. The Self-Assessment section is a fun way to get started. Find out where you rate in the Diet Health Wheel and you will then have an idea of what areas in your lifestyle need to be addressed.

Part Two of this book is the *Food Companion*. This section is devoted to delicious and healthy low-carb recipes that will boost your knowledge and your ability to implement the recommended diet. It includes everything from soups and snacks to main meals, desserts, low-carb bread and even ice cream! These recipes have been collected, collated, and tested in our home, over the past three years. Many of my friends, patients and family have enjoyed the novel excitement that low-carb food preparation brings to the kitchen.

My personal and professional experience of this lifestyle change has clearly shown me the importance of being equipped with the correct resources in this program. *The Low-Carb Companion* is here to negotiate your low-carb journey in a clear, concise and comprehensive manner that will lead the way to a healthier lifestyle.

Introduction

A PERSONAL JOURNEY

'When the facts change, I change my mind. What do you do'?
Lord Keynes

As a medical doctor specialising in sport and exercise medicine, I have been involved in the lifestyle aspects of medicine for over 25 years. However, my personal and professional journey into the renewed science of low-carb nutrition began relatively recently. I have been an active athlete my entire life and have engaged in a variety of sports and activities since school age. The majority of that exercise time was spent as a swimmer, a triathlete, a fitness instructor and an indoor cycling instructor. As such, I consumed a high-carb diet as we were advised to do at that time, and I encouraged my patients and students to do the same. I smugly maintained a 70kg frame and a trim 31-inch waist from the age of 18, and I believed all was in order.

But wait! When I reached age 48, my life included a significant amount of stress, an intense physical training regime, and a predominantly high-carb diet. I began to fatten up around the belly and gained 4kg in two years to my great dismay. My health markers (blood cholesterol levels indices and blood sugar levels) were quickly heading in the wrong direction. I had even begun to take a low dose statin drug for elevated cholesterol. Needless to say, I was not at all impressed with these developments given my supposed 'exemplary healthy lifestyle'! I reflected on my late father who had developed type 2 diabetes and coronary heart disease as a result of an unhealthy diet that included a lot of alcohol, tobacco and very little exercise. He had also fattened in his middle-age years. I had always believed that we could avoid these diseases of lifestyle with regular exercise and a healthy high-carb, low-fat balanced diet, and indeed, I was leading my patients in that same direction.

Well, it wasn't working. Anthropologist Claude Levi Strauss once said, 'The wise man is not the man who gives the right answers, he is the one who asks the right questions'. I then asked my first important question: 'Why is this happening to me'?

The Transformation

My search for answers began fortuitously when I read a career biography written by one of my most respected medical professors, South African Professor Tim Noakes, Emeritus Professor of Exercise and Sports Science at the University of Cape Town. He is also a friend, a colleague and a mentor. I had the privilege of doing my post-graduate training in sports medicine under his inspirational tutelage 25 years ago. His book, written in 2012, *Challenging Beliefs*, revealed his own personal experience with weight gain and diabetes, which led to his critical review of the science behind low-carb nutrition. The 2010 book, *A New Atkins for a New You*, written by three prominent nutrition scientists, Drs Eric Westman, Stephen Phinney and Jeff Volek, inspired him. These books inspired me and provided insight into my own developing carbohydrate intolerance, and subsequently the need for a low-carb, high-fat lifestyle transformation that I adhere to today. Another significant influence on my rapidly expanding personal knowledge was the 2007 book, *The Diet Delusion*, by Gary Taubes. This is one of the most comprehensive reviews of the science behind obesity on the market. These books, along with many others that are listed on page 222, were beacons in my journey and quest for knowledge and I can highly recommend them all. My own positive experience with low-carb nutrition returned me to my ideal weight of 70kg in three months. My body fat fell from 17% to 10%, and my waist (and my wardrobe!) returned to the 31 inches I was accustomed to. My health biomarkers like HbA1c (blood sugars) and blood triglycerides (fats) showed significant improvements and, best of all, my athletic performances in running and triathlon over the past two years have been reminiscent of my 30s! In 2012, my team at the Centre for Sport and Exercise Medicine began a low-carb, high-fat intervention trial program for overweight patients. These patients volunteered to participate in a twelve month supervised nutritional remodeling program. The results of the program were positive for many of the participants and inspiring for us as a medical team. This prompted the birth of the Lifestyle Medicine Program that is specifically targeted at patients who are overweight or suffer from obesity, type 2 diabetes and hypertension issues. We continue to promote low-carb, high-fat nutrition as a lifestyle medical intervention through clinical programs and educational forums. *The Low-Carb Companion* is a direct result of this program and the participants and patients who have requested more user-friendly information.

Introduction

CONSENSUS VERSUS INFLUENCE

'Never in the field of human progress has anything been achieved by unanimous consent and those who are enlightened before the others are condemned to pursue that light despite the others'.
Christopher Columbus

....

South African heart transplant pioneer, Professor Chris Barnard, wrote to the effect that he had 'saved the lives of 150 people through heart transplantations' but that if he had 'cared about preventative medicine earlier' he 'would have saved 150 million people'.

It would be naïve of me to suggest that consensus on the benefits of low-carbohydrate, higher-fat nutrition has been reached amongst my colleagues in the medical profession, or the allied dieticians and nutritionists from either the perspective of patient care or as advice for the population at large. Opinions vary widely on this topic through to the greater horizons of Public Health authorities, political decision makers and the Agro-Food industry.

I am one, however, who is convinced that a low-carb, high-fat lifestyle is the way forward for most people as the primary preventative tool and a key medical intervention strategy for the most pressing diseases of lifestyle that include obesity, metabolic syndrome, type 2 diabetes, heart disease and many cancers. The ancient Roman satirist Aulus Flaccus Persius claimed, 'Confront disease at its first stage'. Thankfully, I am not alone in this view and stand amongst the enlightened giants of our age who continue to 'beat the drum' in research, educational, medical and nutritional practice on broad fronts all over the world. To mention a few of these enlightened medical and scientific giants: Gary Taubes (USA), Prof Tim Noakes (South Africa), Drs Eric Westman, Steve Phinney, Jeff Volek, Robert Lustig, Prof Mary Enig, Peter Attia (USA), Dr Jason Fung (Canada), Dr Aseem Malhotra and Zoe Harcombe (UK). We owe our respect and our global gratitude to these and to the many other men and women of, not only our time, but also to those who went before them. This is best epitomised in a comment attributed to Isaac Newton that 'If I have seen further than others, it is by standing upon the shoulders of giants'.

The problem facing 'the enlightened' and indeed all of us, is that if we are to wait for consensus amongst all the nutrition scientists, doctors and dieticians of the world on low-carb nutrition, then we might wait 10 to 20 years or longer! What will happen to the epidemics of obesity and type 2 diabetes in that time given their dramatic rise in the past 35 years? History is littered with tragic examples of how slow the medical fraternity and public health custodians can be to adopt major changes in health interventions or advice based on the intuitive research of enlightened individuals. As Winston Churchill once put it, 'He occasionally stumbled over the truth, but hastily picked himself up and hurried on as if nothing had happened'.

There are three historical examples that illustrate these concerns.

1. The first is provided by the story of scurvy (a disease caused by vitamin C deficiency) and Scottish naval surgeon, James Lind who, in 1753, documented that scurvy could be prevented and cured in sailors by drinking citrus fruit juice on long voyages. It took 42 years between the discovery of his clearly described and experimentally proven treatment, and its actual introduction in 1795 by the English naval authorities of the day, unnecessarily costing the health and lives of thousands of English seamen. Then, and even today,

Introduction

it appears to be one of the most idiotic episodes in the history of medical science and practice.

2. The second lesson occurred in Hungary between 1844-1849 when a young obstetrician, Dr Ignaz Semmelweis, discovered that doctors were responsible for the spread of puerperal sepsis (childbed fever), a condition that killed many young women after childbirth. Semmelweis showed that the condition was simply prevented when doctors washed their hands between tending patients, and therefore concluded that the disease was spread by a lack of basic medical hygiene (we now know that puerperal sepsis is caused by a bacterial agent). This ran contra to the theory of the day that the disease was caused by 'a mysterious contagion in polluted air'. Despite his discovery, his advice to wash their hands was ignored by his medical colleagues for decades and indeed until long after his death, leading to the continued and unnecessary deaths of hundreds of thousands of young women. Semmelweis wrote, 'When I look back upon the past, I can only dispel the sadness which falls upon me by gazing into that happy future when the infection will be banished...The conviction that such a time must inevitably sooner or later arrive will cheer my dying hour'.

3. The third illustration occurred in the response to the discovery that smoking was the foremost risk factor for lung cancer. Up until 1950, smoking, believe it or not, had been advertised as a healthy and enjoyable habit, but by then medical observers were questioning why rates of lung cancer had soared. The significant findings of Richard Doll and Austin Bradford Hill in 1956, in the *British Doctors' Study*, strongly indicated a causative relationship between smoking and lung cancer. How long did it take the authorities to institute anti-tobacco legislation? It took 22 years, when in 1972 the British government increased sales tax on cigarettes in Britain.

Changing the world of nutrition as it stands today presents even greater challenges, as there are just so many competing interests:

1. The Medical Scientific community, whose bedrock of 'certainty' on nutritional issues is cemented by over 50 years of research that promotes more dogma than science.

2. The Medical Profession, whose primary role in the world today seems increasingly based on treating the disease rather than the patient, focusing on the use of drugs ahead of preventative medicine.

3. The mega Agricultural and Food industries, whose existence, to a large extent, hinges upon feeding the world with grains and processed carbohydrate foods.

4. The Political and Economic forces, that drive countries, and that promote and support economics linked to agriculture and industry.

5. The so-called 'Big Pharma', the world's major drug producing companies whose main aim is to profit from a predominantly pharmaceutical approach to treating disease.

6. The Public, who is left confused by the scientific and medical debates, indoctrinated by the Public Health authorities, captivated by the offerings of the food industry and content to take the medicines prescribed by their doctor and produced by the pharmaceutical industry.

In the words of Wendell Berry, 'People are fed by the food industry which pays no attention to health and are treated by the health industry which pays no attention to food'.

So what is to be done? The reality is that those who are enlightened now bear the burden of sharing information, in the hope that they are able to convince those who are ready to listen, of the benefits of low-carb nutrition. We are all challenged to define and to work in our 'circles of influence',

Introduction

a concept prescribed by author Stephen Covey in *The Seven Habits of Highly Effective People*. As Tim Noakes writes in *Challenging Beliefs*, 'If civil society is not going to save us, our only hope is that we act as individuals to liberate ourselves'. The supply of information regarding the health benefits of low-carb nutrition is increasing, as is the number of people exposed to this information in the public and medical arena. At some point in the not-too-distant future, a critical mass of people will cause a major shift in thinking followed by landmark public health policy changes.

Until that time, to quote 18th century surgeon John Jones in olde English, 'Thus men of more enlighten'd genius and more intrepid spirit must compose themselves to the risque of public censure, and the contempt of their jealous contemporaries, in order to lead ignorant and prejudic'd minds into more happy and successful methods'.

THE DIFFICULT QUESTIONS

> 'The known is finite, the unknown is infinite; intellectually we stand on an island in the middle of an illimitable ocean of inexplicability. Our business in every generation is to reclaim a little more land'.
> Thomas Huxley

Moving forward will not be without controversy, but knowing this is to be forearmed. In addition to spreading the word as enlightened doctors, dieticians, patients or concerned members of the public, we should also be enquiring, if not demanding, of our colleagues, medical advisors and policy-makers that they supply evidence supporting the out-dated dietary practices they purport.

This inquiry will beg the following difficult questions:

a. Why low-fat, high-carb diets continue to be prescribed despite their proven ineffectiveness in long term weight management and other diseases of lifestyle?

b. Why the existing *U.S. Dietary Guidelines for Americans* (USDGA) that promote low-fat, high-carb nutrition continue to be recommended worldwide at the population level as a 'healthy balanced diet' when the greatest increases in population rates of obesity and diabetes have occurred on this diet since 1980?

c. Why is fat still the 'bad guy', when the published population food data show carbohydrate intake over the past 30 years to be the only macronutrient that has significantly increased in the human diet?

d. Why do low-fat, high-carb diets continue to be prescribed for people with cardiovascular disease, when all recent review studies can find no evidence to link dietary fat intake to increased risks of heart disease?

e. Why women of any age, or men over 50 years of age, without clinical heart disease, should be prescribed statin drugs for mild to moderately elevated cholesterol, given that elevated cholesterol is a weak risk factor for heart disease and that statins prevent heart attacks in less than 1% of patients?

f. Why people living with type 2 diabetes are still conventionally advised to follow diets that allow up to 150g of carbohydrate, when the disease itself is a direct metabolic result of severe carbohydrate intolerance causing insulin resistance?

Introduction

SELF-ASSESSMENTS

'This above all, to thine own self be true'.
William Shakespeare

....

Food and Health Questionnaires
Diet-Health Wheel
Sugar Addiction Questionnaire
Health Targets for Body Measurements
and Blood Tests

FOOD AND HEALTH QUESTIONNAIRES

This questionnaire-based assessment of diet related to health is a great tool to get started with. Answer YES or NO to the list of questions. Give yourself a score of 1 point for each YES answer. For each YES answer, use a pencil to shade in the appropriate section on your Diet-Health Wheel.

	YES = 1 pt	NO = 0 pt
FOOD QUESTIONS		
On a daily basis do you eat or drink the following?		
Bread		
Rice, pasta or potatoes		
Foods labelled 'Low Fat'		
Cereals		
Fruit		
Sugared sweets, desserts		
Honey, Agave or fructose		
Fruit juice		
Soft drinks / colas / carbonated drinks – normal or lite		
Sugar added to tea, coffee or other hot beverage		
Beer		
Vegetable oils eg sunflower, canola, soybean, margarine in cooking or dressings		
Score		

Introduction

	YES = 1 pt	NO = 0 pt
HEALTH QUESTIONS		
Do you currently suffer from?		
Overweight or obesity		
Belly fat (fat around your middle)		
Sugar cravings		
Fear of fat in fatty foods		
Metabolic syndrome (pre-diabetes)		
Type 2 Diabetes (or a family history of diabetes)		
High blood pressure		
High total cholesterol with low HDL ('good cholesterol')		
Elevated blood triglycerides (fats)		
Elevated blood sugar		
Elevated fasting insulin		
Are you taking statins?		
Score		
TOTAL SCORE		

How did you fare?

SCORE:

0 = Optimal diet related to health profile. Well done!

1 – 5 = You need help. Start looking at low-carb nutrition as a plan for you.

> 6 = You need a lot of help. Consider seeing your doctor and start low-carb nutrition.

The Low-Carb Companion

Shade in the YES answers on your Diet – Health Wheel.
At the end of this exercise, you will see if your Wheel shows a SHINING HEALTH profile or a SHADOWY HEALTH profile.

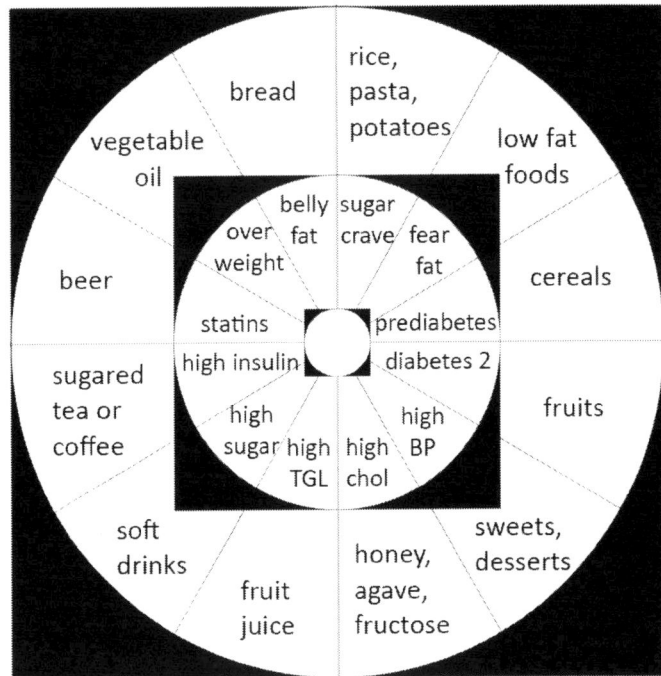

BP = blood pressure
Chol = cholesterol
TGL = triglycerides

© Dr A K Jeans: The Low-carb Companion 2015

For a final 'fill in' of your wheel: if you smoke and/or do little physical exercise, then shade in the middle section. The 'HEALTH SHADOW' may become complete!
From a Diet-Health perspective, the more white spaces in your wheel the better, the more shaded, well that's not so great. You can view the wheel as representative of the potential state of your arteries. The more shaded the wheel, the more dysfunctional they are likely to be or to become. Reading this book will help you to make choices that can improve your ateries and your bodily health, both now and in the future.
Hopefully, your Self-Assessment Questionnaire score and personal Diet-Health Wheel have now focused your attention! Read on to learn more about improving your diet and health in the future.

Introduction

SUGAR AND CARB ADDICTION SCREENING QUESTIONNAIRE

Are you addicted to sugar and carbs?
* Note: sweet carbs = sugar, sweets, chocolate, cake, biscuits, desserts, soft drinks

	Do you:	Yes / No
1.	Eat sweet carbs until uncomfortably full?	
2.	Feel very hungry within 2 – 3 hours of eating a main meal?	
3.	Eat lots of sweet carbs even when not hungry?	
4.	Feel guilty, self-loathing or depressed after eating sweet carbs?	
5.	Tend to eat sweet carbs when lonely, depressed or upset?	
6.	Find that you need more and more sweet carbs to feel better?	
7.	Tend towards binge-eating on sweet carbs?	
8.	Have a hard time stopping once you start eating sweet carbs?	
9.	Find it hard to cut back on eating sweet carbs?	
10.	Feel that your eating habits impact negatively on your work, social or physical abilities?	
11.	Fail to stick to your own resolutions to eat healthier?	
12.	Have cravings for sweet carbs after eating a main meal?	
13.	Secretly eat sweet carbs and hide the 'evidence' from others?	
14.	Feel foggy-headed in between eating sweet carbs?	
15.	Have irresistible thoughts about sweet carbs on a daily basis?	

(Adapted with permission from Karen Thomson)

If you answered YES to 5 or more questions, then you are likely to be a sugar and carb addict.

HEALTH TARGETS FOR BODY MEASUREMENTS AND BLOOD TESTS

Table 1: Your Measurements & Health Targets for Biometric Data

Biometric Data	Units	Target (Female)	Target (Male)
Weight	kg		
Height	m		
Waist circumference (measured at the umbilicus / bellybutton)	cm	< 88	< 102
Hip circumference (measured at widest buttock width)	cm		
Mid upper arm circumference Right or Left	cm		
Mid upper thigh circumference Right or Left	cm		
Blood pressure	mmHg	< 120/80	< 120/80
Body Mass Index BMI (weight/height^2)	kg/m^2	< 24	< 24
Waist : Height ratio		< 0.5	< 0.5
Waist : Hip ratio		< 0.85	< 0.92

Table 2: Your Health Targets for Blood Tests

Blood Results	Units	Target (Female)	Target (Male)
Blood sugar (fasted)	mmol/l	< 5	< 5
Glycolated Haemoglobin (HbA1c)	%	< 5.4	< 5.4
Fasting insulin*	µIU/mL	< 6	< 6
Total cholesterol	mmol/l	< 7	< 6.2
LDL cholesterol	mmol/l	< 5.5	< 5.0
HDL cholesterol	mmol/l	> 1.2	> 1.2
Apolipoprotein B	g/L	< 0.9	< 0.9
Triglycerides (TGL)	mmol/l	< 1.2	< 1.2
Total cholesterol : HDL ratio		< 4.5	< 4.5
TGL : HDL ratio		< 1.0	< 1.0
Liver function test Gamma-glutamyl transferase (GGT)	IU/L	< 12	< 12

Single fasting insulin samples can have a coefficient of variation of 25-50%.

The Low-Carb Companion

SECTION 1:

FOOD, FAT & METABOLISM

Chapter 1
LOW-CARBOHYDRATE NUTRITION – THE OVERVIEW

'That which seems to be the height of absurdity in one generation often becomes the height of wisdom in another'.
John Stuart Mill

Traditionally, we have been taught that consuming excessive fat in our diet is the predominant nutritional reason behind weight problems and diseases of lifestyle like obesity, coronary heart disease, high blood pressure, diabetes and cancer. However, published nutritional research has challenged this forty-year-old belief and has promoted a key shift in our understanding. The evidence indicates that the underlying cause of weight gain, especially 'belly fat', along with associated diseases of lifestyle like diabetes, heart disease, high blood pressure and certain cancers, starts with the development of progressive carbohydrate intolerance. This intolerance, in turn, leads to an increased insulin resistance.

Carbohydrate intolerance is a condition that exists in our genetic make-up and is provoked by the quantity of refined carbohydrate and sugar in our diet.

The result of such a diet, for a carbohydrate-intolerant person, is the stimulation of excessive insulin levels in the body. Increased insulin levels cause an increased conversion of sugar to fat in the liver. Carbohydrate-intolerant individuals who eat a highly-refined carb diet end up with increasingly full fat cells, but are not able to utilise their fat stores effectivley to fuel bodily processes, including muscle work in exercise. The body's cells, without sufficient long-term fat fuel for energy, rely on short-term sugar fuel and are thereby consistently 'starved'. This energy starvation causes the brain to stimulate hunger and fatigue, which manifest as lethargy and food cravings, and ultimately increased weight gain. A vicious cycle.

How do you know if you may be carbohydrate-intolerant? Some indicators are as follows:

- If you have close relatives who are overweight
- If you have struggled with weight for most of your life and are now very overweight
- If you have a tendency to accumulate excess weight around your middle ('belly fat')
- If you have gained a significant amount of weight with age, after menopause, pregnancy or stress
- If you have had blood tests indicating that you are pre-diabetic or have type 2 diabetes

Studies on the traditional low-fat and low-calorie dieting approach show poor long-term results in terms of sustainable weight loss because eating fat is actually not the fundamental problem. Evidence shows that eating sugar and refined carbohydrates plays the greater role in making us fat! Conventional low-fat and low-calorie diets, even when combined with exercise, are more likely to result in hunger, fatigue and the rapid regain of lost weight.

Figure 1: Diet and Metabolic Health

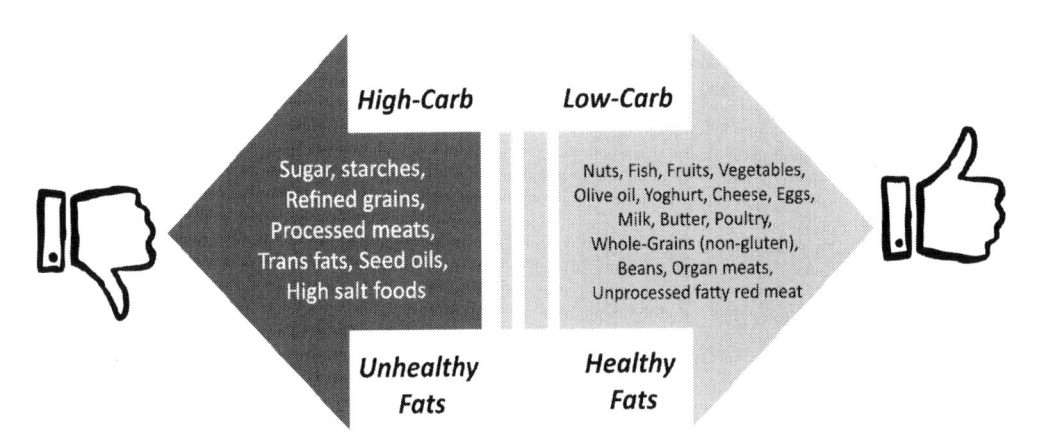

High-Carb	Low-Carb
Sugar, starches, Refined grains, Processed meats, Trans fats, Seed oils, High salt foods	Nuts, Fish, Fruits, Vegetables, Olive oil, Yoghurt, Cheese, Eggs, Milk, Butter, Poultry, Whole-Grains (non-gluten), Beans, Organ meats, Unprocessed fatty red meat
Unhealthy Fats	Healthy Fats

Adopting an eating program that eliminates sugar and refined carbs and includes a higher, healthy fat intake results in positive metabolic changes with the following direct health benefits:

- Reduced blood sugar and insulin levels
- Increased utilisation of fat stores by the body
- Reduced appetite and increased energy levels
- Sustainable weight loss
- Reduced risk factors for diabetes, heart disease and cancer
- Measured improvements in people with type 2 diabetes and high blood pressure

A low-carb diet is a nutritional program for life, as you are never 'cured' of carbohydrate intolerance. Principally we have to control the effects of our intolerance to carbohydrates principally by avoiding refined carbs and concentrating on eating real food food, including fruits and vegetables, as well as adopting a higher intake of healthy fats.

Chapter 1 - The Low-Carb Nutrition Overview

> **Key points : Low-carb overview**
> 1. Carbohydrate intolerance is the key to understanding the metabolic basis for weight gain and obesity.
> 2. In the face of a high-carb diet, carbohydrate intolerance leads to insulin resistance.
> 3. Low-carb, higher, healthy-fat nutrition is the way to achieve improved health and a healthy weight.

You need to get (metabolically) healthy to lose weight .... not lose weight to get healthy!

Chapter 2
WHY WE EAT WHAT WE EAT

'Food is an important part of a balanced diet'.
Fran Lebowitz

WHY FOOD?

We eat food to obtain important nutrients in the form of:
- Macronutrients
  - Carbohydrates
  - Fats
  - Proteins
- Micronutrients
  - Vitamins
  - Minerals
  - Phytochemicals

The main biological roles of nutrients:
- Macronutrients
  - Carbohydrates provide energy and fibre.
  - Fats provide energy, insulation and cell structure.
  - Proteins are essential for tissue structure, energy, body fluids and blood function.

- Micronutrients
  - ➢ Vitamins, minerals and phytochemicals are vital for multiple biochemical and hormonal processes that are essential to life.
- Food also plays an important role in body temperature regulation and psychological comfort. Think of 'comfort eating'.

The Points to Ponder

- The primary building blocks for human tissues are protein and fat.
- Carnivorous (i.e. predominantly meat and fat-eating) human populations do not develop vitamin deficiencies.
- If you eat a diet with 0% fat ⟶ you DIE
- If you eat a diet with 0% protein ⟶ you DIE
- If you eat a diet with 0% carb ⟶ you LIVE!

Key point : Why we eat what we eat
Carbohydrate is not an essential macronutrient in the human diet.

Our Ancestors' Diet

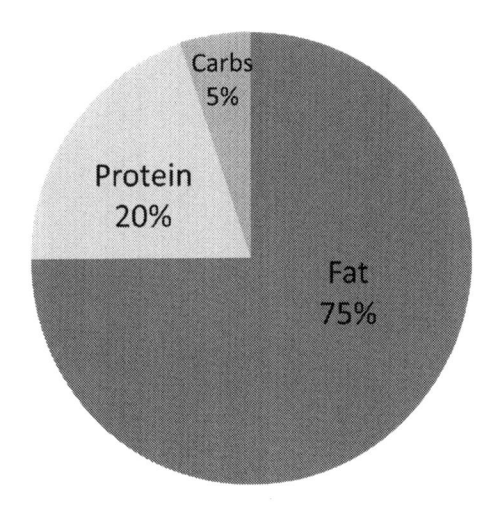

- Carbs 5%
- Protein 20%
- Fat 75%

Figure 2: The changing human diet from ancient hunter-gatherer to modern day

USDGA recommended diet 1977 - present

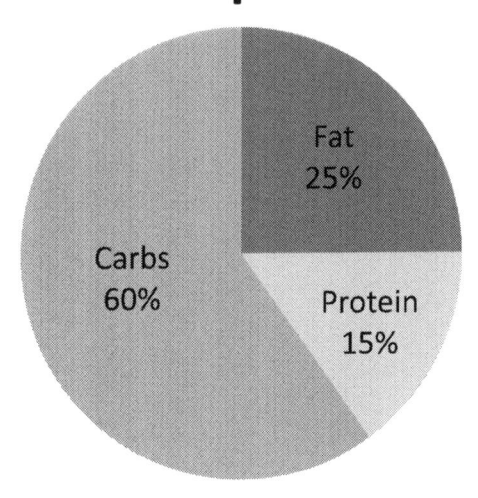

- Fat 25%
- Carbs 60%
- Protein 15%

Source: *Grain Brain* by **Dr David Perlmutter**

Chapter 2 - Why We Eat What We Eat

CARBOHYDRATES

'Nature made sugar hard to get; man made it easy'.
Dr Robert Lustig

....

Carbohydrates (carbs) can be classified as:
- Sugars
- Starches
- Fibre

Carbs Quick Fact guide:
- All sugars and starches are carbs.
- All carbs are made of sugars.
- All carbs end up as sugars in the body (except for fibre, which is an indigestible carb).
- Some carbs digest *rapidly* to sugar, and others digest *slowly*.
- Carbs have low energy density (containing only 4 calories per gram).
- There are no vitamins and minerals in sugar.

> Of all the macronutrients, carbohydrates have increased significantly in the human diet over time.

Over the last 35 years, the Public Health guidelines advised us to eat a 'healthy' low-fat, high-carb diet. Our evolutionary ancestors most likely obtained less than 5% of their total calories from carbs, compared to the modern day where the official dietary guidelines encourage us to eat 60% of our daily calories from carbohydrate-rich foods.

The main carbs in a 'high-carb' diet come from:
- Sugar (sucrose or high fructose corn syrup) taken 'neat' or added to foods
- Grains, e.g. wheat, rice, maize (corn), oats
- Processed cereals
- Bread
- Starchy vegetables (potatoes)
- Non-starchy vegetables (beetroots, beans, peas, carrots)
- Sweet fruits (bananas, grapes, melons)
- Confectionary (sweets, candy, chocolate)
- Sugar sweetened beverages and fruit juices

> Humans are consuming up to 70kg of sugar per person per year. This is five to ten times of what our great-great grandparents were eating 100 years ago!

Chapter 2 - Why We Eat What We Eat

Figure 3: The Fate of Carbs in the Body

What happens to carbs?

Carbohydrates
⬇
Digestion
⬇
Simple Sugars
Glucose   Fructose

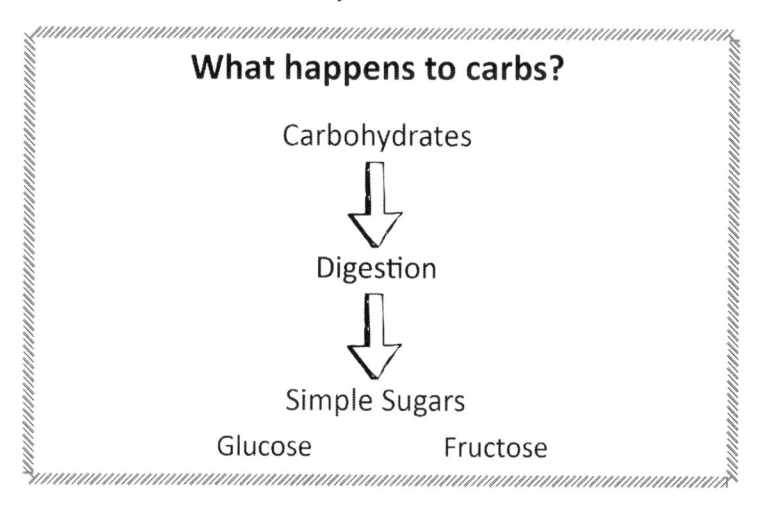

Figure 4: The Fate of Sugar in the Body

The two most common sugars added to food are sucrose (table sugar) and high fructose corn syrup (HFCS). HFCS is chemically similar to sucrose but is cheaper, sweeter and worse for your health.

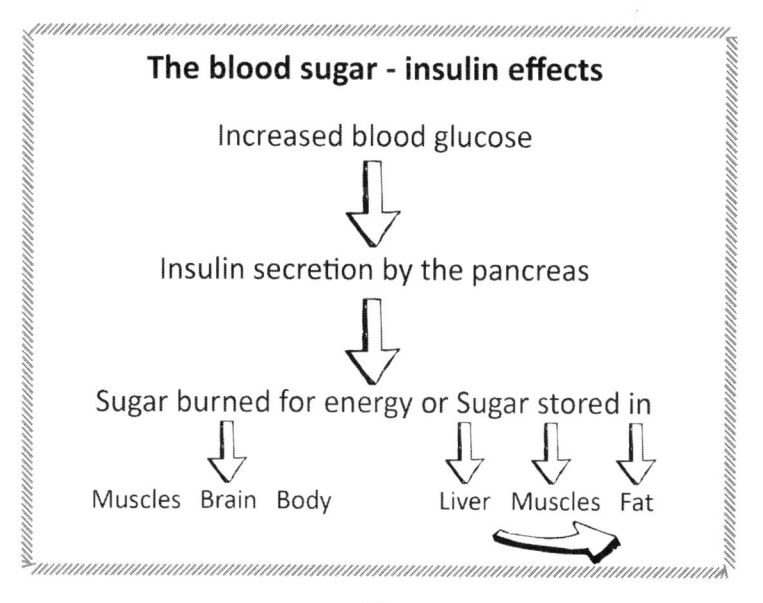

The blood sugar - insulin effects

Increased blood glucose
⬇
Insulin secretion by the pancreas
⬇
Sugar burned for energy or Sugar stored in
⬇   ⬇   ⬇   ⬇
Muscles Brain Body   Liver Muscles Fat

Figures 3 and 4 show the process of carbohydrate breakdown via digestion into simple sugars. Glucose, which is the most common simple sugar, comes from grains and constitutes half of the sugars in sucrose and high fructose corn syrup. It also elevates blood sugar levels that then stimulate production of the hormone insulin from the pancreas. Insulin controls the partitioning of all 'fuels' in the body. After ingesting carbohydrate, elevated blood glucose levels are either used for energy or stored in the muscles and the liver as glycogen (a storage form of sugar). Excess sugar (glucose) is converted to fat in the liver and stored in body fat stores. Fructose cannot be used for energy production nor can it be stored and therefore, it is almost entirely converted to fat in the liver.

Glycaemic index (GI)

Not all carbs are treated equally in the body. The GI of a foodstuff is a comparative measure of the rate at which the carbohydrate-containing food raises the level of blood sugar. Pure glucose has a GI of 100. The more refined the carb, the higher the GI, which will influence the insulin response.

HIGH GI FOODS	**LOW GI FOODS**
= 'Unhealthy'	= 'Healthier'
Refined flour	Nuts
Bread	Dairy
Sugar	Meat
Refined cereal	Fish
Refined maize meal	Eggs
Pasta	Pasta
White rice	Wholegrains (oats, wild rice)
Potatoes	Unrefined maize
Fruits (bananas, grapes)	Vegetables
	Fruits (berries, citrus)

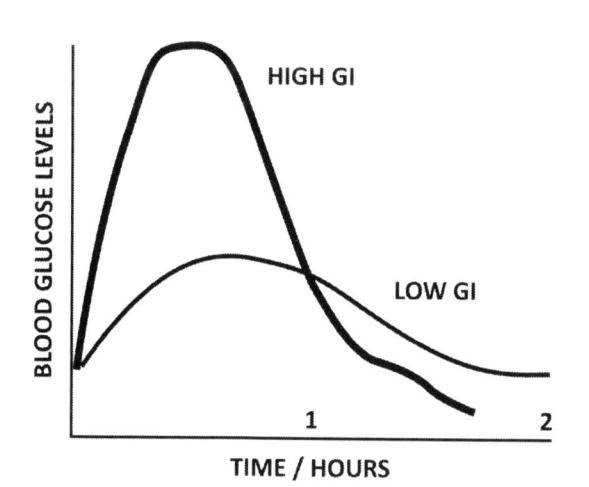

Figure 5 : Glycaemic Index, The Effects of High and Low GI Foods

The Two Main Reasons Why Refined Carbs are Fattening:

1. Refined carbs excessively stimulate appetite.
- Carbs fill us up quickly, but are expended quickly because of their low-energy density. They directly stimulate the brain and thereby trigger hunger and cravings.

2. Refined carbs directly stimulate elevated insulin levels and promote insulin resistance.
- Spiking blood sugar levels stimulate increased insulin release from the pancreas.
- A surge in insulin release promotes fat production in the liver, fat storage and reduced fat utilisation for energy in the body.
- Carbs that cause the biggest surge in blood sugar and insulin are refined wheat and grain foods such as bread, cereals, 'liquid carbs' like sugar sweetened beverages and fruit juices, sugars, confectionary and highly-refined starches like white rice and maize meal.

- Sugars like high fructose corn syrup (HFCS) lead to high fructose levels that are converted almost exclusively to fat by the liver under the control of insulin (80% of fructose is converted to fat compared to only 20% of glucose).

> **Foods that reduce the GI and insulin response to carb ingestion:**
>
> - Acidic foods (vinegar)
> - Fermented foods (fermented soy, fermented dairy, pickled foodstuffs)
> - High fibre foods

These act as 'nutritional antidotes' to reduce blood sugar spikes and elevated insulin levels.

Fibre is indigestible carbohydrate, which does not contribute to blood sugar or provide energy. It is found naturally as intact fibre in foods and classified as:

- **Soluble fibre** (found in grains, nuts, fruit skins and vegetables) which speeds food through the intestines.
- **Insoluble fibre** (found in beans, oats and some fruits and vegetables) which tends to slow the rate of food digestion and absorption.

It also occurs as **Isolated fibre**, which is chemically synthesised, isolated or extracted from certain plant foods and added to processed food to boost fibre intake. Fibre does not contribute to blood sugar or provide energy.

> When reading food labels, a useful practical guide to identify healthier grain choices is to look for a ratio of total carbohydrate : dietary fibre of < 10:1 (as grams/serving) (Mozaffarian, D. 2016).

Chapter 2 - Why We Eat What We Eat

SUGAR

- In the USA, it is estimated that of the 600,000 available processed food products, over 80% of them contain added sugar.
- Sucrose and high fructose corn syrup are the most common sugars added to processed food (sucrose = 50% glucose: 50% fructose, HFCS = 45% glucose: 55% fructose).
- Carbonated drinks contain over 10 teaspoons of sugar per 330ml can.
- Fruit juices are often worse as they contain large amounts of sugar per serving.

Sugar can be highly ADDICTIVE:
- In neuroscience research done on rats by NM Avena, sugar fulfils the following four behavioural criteria that classify a substance as being addictive:
    1. Bingeing
    2. Withdrawal
    3. Craving
    4. Cross-sensitisation
- Highly processed foods that may share characteristics with drugs of abuse appear to be particularly associated with food addiction.
- Research shows some of the most addictive foods to be pizza, milk chocolate, chips, cookies, bread, carbonated drinks, doughnuts, pasta, cake, 'French' fries and ice-cream (Gearhardt, Schulte).
- According to a 2011 study in *Frontiers of Psychiatry*, 10% of underweight people, 6.3% of normal weight people, 14% of overweight people and 37.5% of obese people can be diagnosed with food addiction (Meule).
- The food industry scientists are continuously researching ways to increase the addictive effects of processed food. The relative amounts of sugar, salt and other additives are manipulated to reach their 'bliss point', and increase the desire and craving for more (Moss in *Salt Sugar Fat*).

The TOXIC effects of sugar:
- High blood sugar levels have been shown to exert toxic effects on cells in the body through a process called GLYCATION.
- Glycation involves glucose and fructose molecules 'sticking' to, and thereby damaging, cell proteins.
- Damaged proteins are dysfunctional and cause cells to dramatically increase their production of free radicals and advanced glycation end products (AGEs). This leads to the destruction of tissues (including damage to fats, other proteins and DNA), inflammation and blood vessel disease in the heart and brain.
- High levels of glycation are associated with ageing, diabetes, vascular and coronary heart disease, eye cataracts, kidney disease and declining brain cognitive conditions like Alzheimer's.
- Glycated blood haemoglobin (HbA1c) is a blood test utilised as a measure of glycation damaged protein in the body. The test is used to evaluate levels of carbohydrate intolerance, to monitor blood sugar control in diabetics and to determine a predictive index of future heart disease, diabetes, stroke and brain atrophy.
- Fructose increases the rate of glycation 10 fold!
- High fructose consumption is associated with increased risks of insulin resistance, impaired glucose tolerance, obesity, elevated blood fats (triglycerides), hyperuricaemia (high uric acid) and high blood pressure.

A high and potentially toxic fructose load in the body is caused by a high intake of sucrose (sugar) or high fructose corn syrup (Lustig).

Figure 6: Human Sugar Consumption

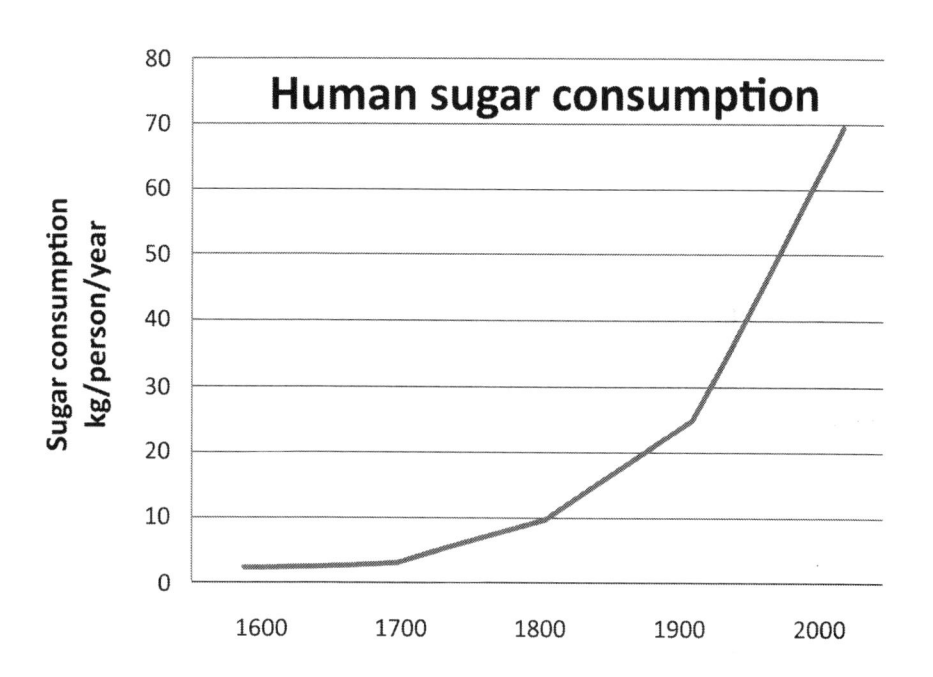

Human sugar consumption (kg/person/year) from 1600 to 2000, rising from about 2 kg/person/year in 1600 to approximately 70 kg/person/year by 2000.

Sugar, from a global health perspective, could be considered a WMD (a weapon of mass destruction)!

Figure 7: Wheat Intake, Coronary Heart Disease and Body Weight

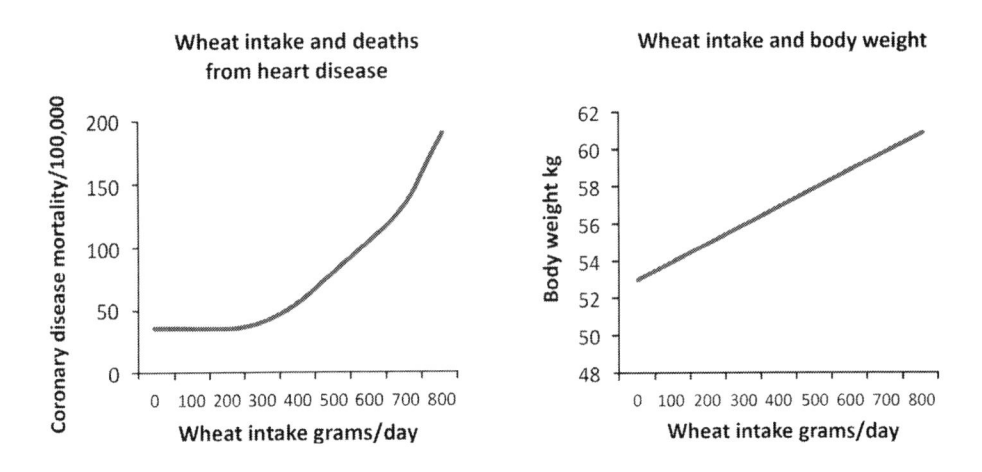

Wheat intake and deaths from heart disease

Wheat intake and body weight

The two graphs show correlations* between wheat intake and coronary disease and wheat intake and body weight.
(Sourced from the China Study data reworked by Denise Minger)

The findings:
1. A significant correlation exists between wheat (flour) intake and deaths from coronary heart disease.
2. Wheat intake is the strongest predictor of body weight of any dietary variable.

Although this data shows an association between wheat intake and heart disease and body weight, it does not prove causation.

Key points : Carbs
1. Humans are consuming too many carbs and too much sugar.
2. Not all carbs are treated equally by the body.
3. Two carbonated soft drinks contain over 20 teaspoons of sugar.
4. Carbs and sugar are fattening and addictive!
5. Fructose may be the most 'toxic' sugar.

FAT

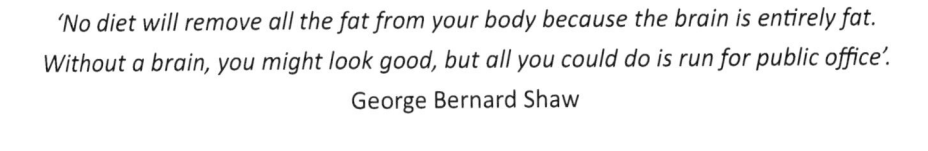

'No diet will remove all the fat from your body because the brain is entirely fat. Without a brain, you might look good, but all you could do is run for public office'.
George Bernard Shaw

For most people, the word 'fat' is just a bad word. Fat has been demonised by the nutritional establishment for decades and falsely accused of being the main culprit responsible for obesity and coronary heart disease.

However, fats are, in fact, the most important fuel for human energy and are the key to both healthy weight loss and weight maintenance.

Fat Facts

- Fat as a macronutrient is an essential component of healthy body structure and function.
- For over two million years, our ancestors consumed a diet with more than 60% of calories from fat.
- Fats are made of different fatty acids.
- Fatty acids form TRIGLYCERIDES in the body that are stored in body fat stores.
- Fatty acids are used as fuel in cellular energy production.
- Your brain is 70% fat.
- Vitamins A, D, E and K need dietary fat for their absorption and are stored in body fat.
- Fat insulates tissues and forms 50% of all cell membrane structure.
- Fat plays an important role in the healthy function of the immune system.

- Fats are classified into three types: saturated, monounsaturated and polyunsaturated.
- Fat in foods is usually a mix of all three types with a predominance of one, as shown in Table 4. Three good examples of this are red meat, lard and olive oil. Although we tend to consider red meat as a source of saturated fat, in reality a porterhouse steak is 51% monounsaturated, 45% saturated and 4% polyunsaturated fats; lard (pork fat) is 48% monounsaturated, 40% saturated and 12% polyunsaturated; olive oil (considered a monounsaturated fat) has nine times the saturated fat of pork!
- Fats can also be classified according to their carbon chain length as short chain, medium chain or long chain fatty acids. Each has differing metabolic effects in the body.
- **All naturally occurring fats can be considered healthy, but man-made fats (margarine, seed oils and trans-fats) are dangerously unhealthy.**
- Dietary fats provide the essential omega-3 and omega-6 polyunsaturated fatty acids that cannot be produced in the body.
- The fat content in food strongly influences the taste and palatability of that food.
- Fat is a 'super-fuel' for the brain and muscles; it has nine calories of energy per gram.
- Fats do not stimulate appetite in the brain. They do not provoke insulin secretion and their energy density promotes satiety for hours after eating.
- Under severe carb restriction, the body will enter 'nutritional ketosis', a safe and natural state of supplying fuel for energy to the brain and muscles through KETONE BODIES derived from fat.
- Eating fat does not make you fat unless it is combined with a high-refined carb intake.
- Low-fat foods are generally sugared (i.e. high in carbs) to make up for flavour and calories.

Figure 8: Fats and their Major Dietary Sources:

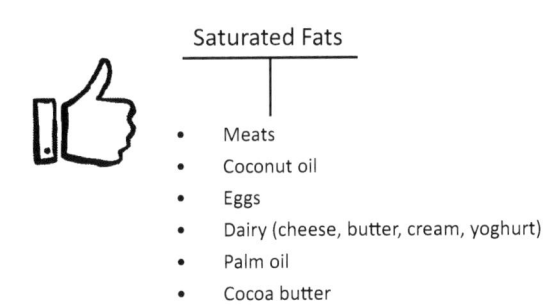

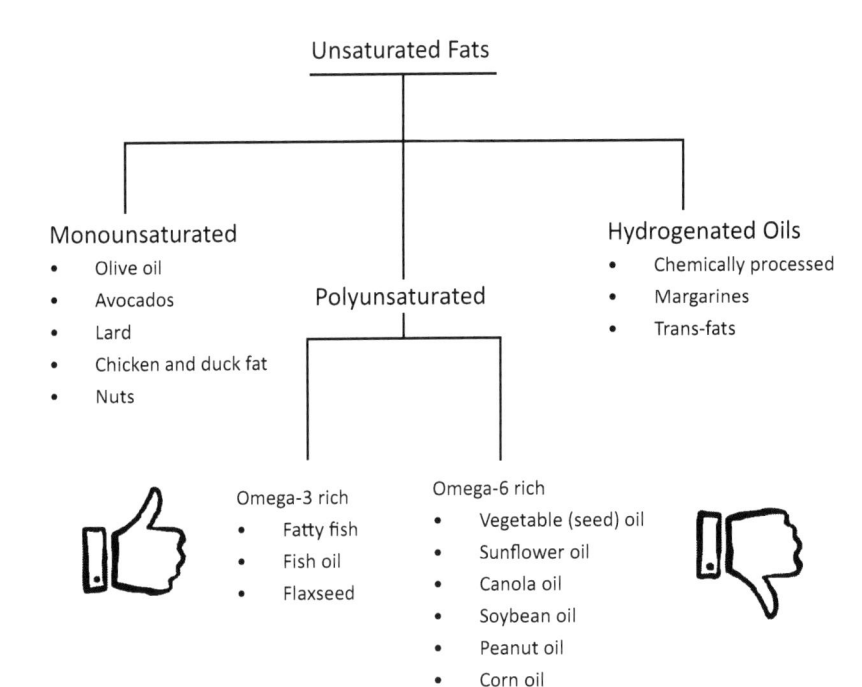

Saturated Fats
- Meats
- Coconut oil
- Eggs
- Dairy (cheese, butter, cream, yoghurt)
- Palm oil
- Cocoa butter

Unsaturated Fats

Monounsaturated
- Olive oil
- Avocados
- Lard
- Chicken and duck fat
- Nuts

Polyunsaturated

Omega-3 rich
- Fatty fish
- Fish oil
- Flaxseed

Omega-6 rich
- Vegetable (seed) oil
- Sunflower oil
- Canola oil
- Soybean oil
- Peanut oil
- Corn oil
- Safflower oil
- Cottonseed oil

Hydrogenated Oils
- Chemically processed
- Margarines
- Trans-fats

Chapter 2 - Why We Eat What We Eat

Saturated Fat - Useful Facts

- Saturated fats are the most stable fats, chemically resistant to oxidation.
- Fat in breast milk is mostly saturated and constitutes 54% of the total energy.
- Dietary saturated fat has very little correlation to blood fat (triglyceride) levels; refined carbs have a much more profound effect on blood triglyceride levels.
- Saturated fats comprise 50% of every cell membrane in the body.
- Saturated fats make up lung surfactant that enables breathing.
- Heart muscle preferentially uses saturated fats for sustainable energy.
- Medium-chain saturated fatty acids found in coconut oil are absorbed directly for energy and have infection fighting properties.
- Saturated fats and dietary cholesterol, which are both lipid substances, occur together in food sources like eggs, meat and dairy.
- **According to recent, major review research studies, saturated fat is not associated with an increased risk of heart disease. See Chapter 5.**
- Credible published research findings also show that heart disease risk factors improve on a low-carb, higher-fat nutrition program.

Figure 9: A Triglyceride

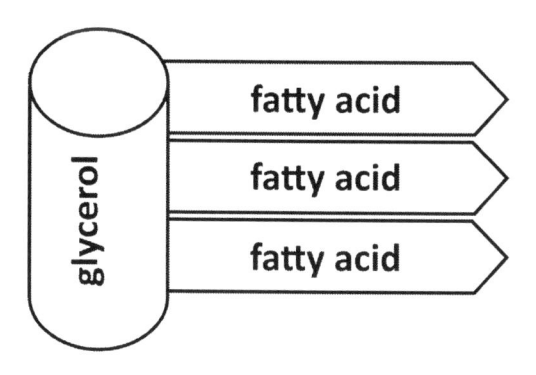

Monounsaturated Fat - Useful Facts
- This is the second most stable group of fats and oils.
- They tend to be liquid at room temperature and turn solid in the fridge.
- The best-known monounsaturated fat is oleic acid, which is the main component of olive oil and is also found in nuts and avocados.

Polyunsaturated Fat - Useful Facts
- Polyunsaturated fats are the most chemically unstable fats, reactive to heat, light and oxygen.
- Essential OMEGA-3 and OMEGA-6 fatty acids are polyunsaturated fats that are vital for health and have to be obtained from the diet.
- Research shows that the ratio of omega-3 to omega-6 intake in our diet is an important factor determining health.
- The optimal dietary omega-3:omega-6 ratio is 1:1, and even up to 1:4 is acceptable.
- Excessive intakes of omega-6 fatty acids occur in diets rich in grains, seed oils, margarine and trans-fats. Omega-6 fatty acids also come from grain-fed meat, poultry and eggs.
- The modern low-fat, high-carb diet is excessively high in omega-6 (ratios 1:14 up to 1:25).
- High intakes of omega-6 from polyunsaturated oils are associated with inflammation in the body and increased risks of heart disease, diabetes and cancer.
- Higher intakes of omega-3 fats from fatty fish and pasture-fed meat, poultry and eggs are associated with reduced inflammation and reduced heart disease.
- Polyunsaturated fats, especially when used as unrefined cooking oils, are relatively unstable at high cooking temperatures and produce toxic chemicals when they reach the smoking point.

Table 3: Fatty Acid Profiles of Food Oils

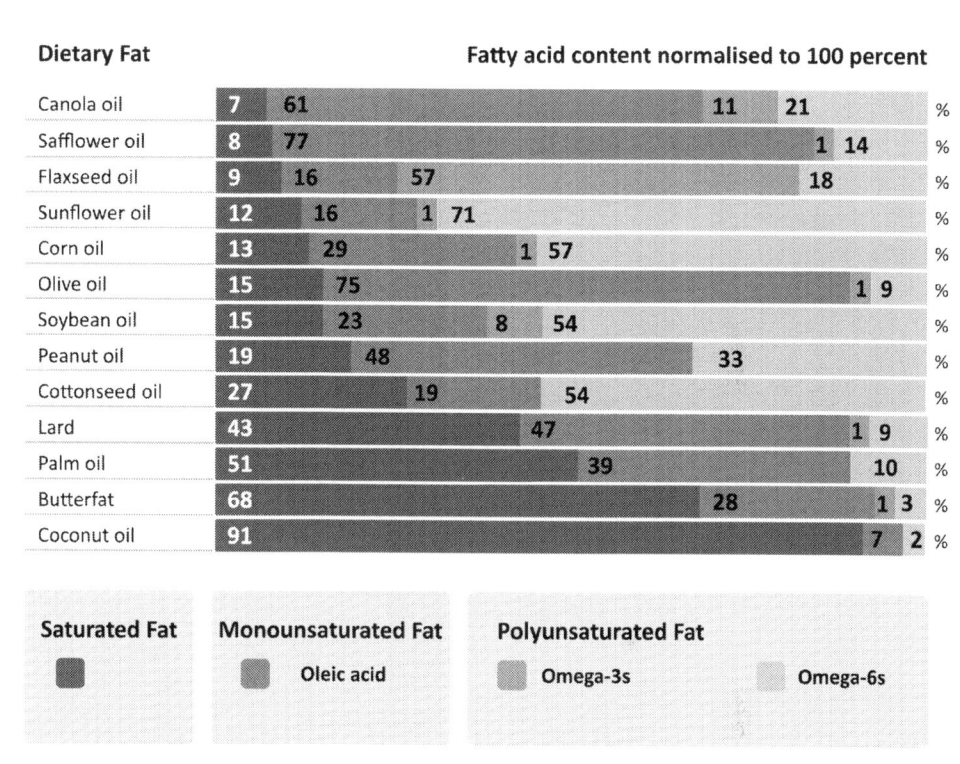

Dietary Fat	Saturated	Monounsaturated (Oleic)	Omega-3	Omega-6	
Canola oil	7	61	11	21	%
Safflower oil	8	77	1	14	%
Flaxseed oil	9	16	57	18	%
Sunflower oil	12	16	1	71	%
Corn oil	13	29	1	57	%
Olive oil	15	75	1	9	%
Soybean oil	15	23	8	54	%
Peanut oil	19	48		33	%
Cottonseed oil	27	19		54	%
Lard	43	47	1	9	%
Palm oil	51	39		10	%
Butterfat	68	28	1	3	%
Coconut oil	91		7	2	%

Saturated Fat

Monounsaturated Fat — Oleic acid

Polyunsaturated Fat — Omega-3s, Omega-6s

Source: POS Pilot Plant Corporation

a. Milk from cows: pasture-fed vs. corn and soy-fed

Amount of pasture in the dairy diet	Omega-3 (mg/g)	Omega-6 (mg/g)
ALL pasture	16.6	16.6
2/3 pasture	13.5	31.4
1/3 pasture	8.2	42.7

b. Ratio of Omega-3: Omega-6 Fatty Acids in Foods 1960 – 2000

Food	1960	2000	Increase since 1960
Butter	1:2	1:6	3x
Pork	1:4	1:12	3x
Beef	1:4	1:16	4x
Eggs	1:2	1:30	15x

Figure 10: Increased Production of Omega-6 Vegetable Oils for Human Consumption 1920-2000

(kg per person per year)

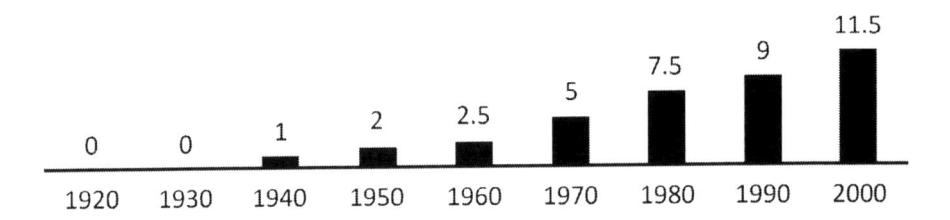

1920	1930	1940	1950	1960	1970	1980	1990	2000
0	0	1	2	2.5	5	7.5	9	11.5

Table 4: Fat Content of 'Real Foods'

Food	Total fat %	Saturated %	Monounsaturated %	Polyunsaturated %
Chicken (skinless)	2.5	35	**45**	20
Milk	3.4	**65**	30	5
Salmon (pink)	3.5	17	26	**40**
Pork chop	4	40	**47**	13
Liver (chicken)	4.8	**33**	25	27
Eggs	10	31	**38**	16
Mackerel	14	27	**45**	28
Beef steak	15	45	**51**	4
Avocado	15	14	**67**	13
Cheese (Cheddar)	33	**64**	28	2.7
Goose	33	31	**57**	12
Cream	37	**62**	29	3.8
Butter	75	**51**	21	3
Olive oil	100	14	**72**	14
Coconut oil	100	**91**	6	3
Lard	100	40	**48**	12

Note:

- *The predominant fat (shown in **bold**) in meat, lard (pork fat) and eggs is monounsaturated, so we should refrain from referring to these foods as 'saturated fats'.*
- *Real foods listed in the table offer both unsaturated (mainly monounsaturated) and saturated fat predominance options, providing a model for a balance of fat intake.*
- *Full cream milk is only 3.4% fat so there is little point in consuming 'fat reduced' milk, like 2% or fat free.*

Table 5 : Smoking Points of Fats / Oils

Oil / Fat	Smoking point (Celsius)
Canola Oil - Unrefined	107°C
Flaxseed oil – Unrefined	107°C
Safflower Oil - Unrefined	107°C
Sunflower Oil - Unrefined	107°C
Corn Oil - Unrefined	160°C
Peanut Oil - Unrefined	160°C
Olive Oil - Extra Virgin	160°C
Safflower Oil - Semi-refined	160°C
Sesame oil - Unrefined	177°C
Coconut oil extra virgin	**177°C**
Butter	**177°C**
Vegetable shortening	182°C
Lard	**188°C**
Macadamia nut oil	**199°C**
Olive Oil - High Quality, Extra Virgin	**206°C**
Olive Oil - Virgin	**215°C**

Chapter 2 - Why We Eat What We Eat

Oil / Fat	Smoking point (Celsius)
Cottonseed oil	216°C
Grapeseed oil	216°C
Coconut Oil - Refined	**232°C**
Corn Oil - Refined	232°C
Peanut Oil - Refined	232°C
Safflower Oil - Refined	232°C
Sunflower Oil - Refined	232°C
Soybean oil - Refined	238°C
Canola Oil – Semi refined	240°C
Olive Oil - Extra Light	**242°C**
Canola Oil - Refined	243°C
Ghee (clarified butter)	**252°C**
Rice bran oil	254°C
Avocado Oil	**271°C**

Notes:

*1. The healthiest oils, shown **in bold**, for high-temperature cooking (over 190°C) are the following:*
a. *High temperatures and deep frying - Avocado oil, Ghee, Olive oil (extra light), Coconut oil (refined/neutral)*
b. *Moderate to high temperatures, quick frying – Olive oil (Virgin/Extra virgin), Macadamia nut oil, Lard, Butter, Coconut oil (extra virgin)*

2. Canola oil is made from GMO (genetically modified) rapeseeds using a highly unnatural industrial processing method that involves high heat, deodorization and the toxic solvent, hexane. Significant amounts of trans-fats are formed in this process (often not reflected on product labelling). It is therefore not recommended as a healthy oil.

> **Key Points: Fat**
> 1. All naturally occurring fats are considered healthy.
> 2. Saturated fats do not cause obesity or heart disease.
> 3. Man-made trans-fats, margarines and vegetable oils are highly inflammatory and very unhealthy.
> 4. Higher-fat, low-carb diets produce effective weight loss and improve heart disease risk factors.
> 5. Heat-stable fats with high smoking points are the best for cooking

'Eat Fat Get Thin'

Chapter 2 - Why We Eat What We Eat

PROTEIN

'Tongue, aagh I don't eat anything that comes out of an animal's mouth, I'd rather eat eggs'!
Anon

....

Proteins are the building blocks of body tissues and are essential to good health. Proteins occur with fat in many foodstuffs like meat, fish, eggs, dairy, nuts and are also found in vegetables. An adequate protein intake is required in order to acquire essential amino acids, to preserve lean body mass and to achieve satiety after eating.

Protein Facts
- Protein is a component of every cell, tissue and organ in your body.
- All growth and repair processes require an adequate protein intake.
- Digesting and metabolising protein consumes about 25% of its energy value (more than twice the energy needed for processing either carbs or fats).
- Proteins are made of strings of up to 20 AMINO ACIDS.
- When we digest proteins, we break them down and absorb the amino acids.
- Nine specific amino acids are deemed ESSENTIAL, as the body cannot make them.
- A protein food source that contains all nine essential amino acids is called a COMPLETE PROTEIN. (see Figure 11)
- Animal based proteins (i.e. meat and dairy) are complete proteins.
- No individual vegetable source is a complete protein, therefore vegetarians have to mix vegetable protein foods to achieve adequate essential amino acid intake*.

*Note - there is academic debate about whether quinoa and amaranth may be considered complete protein sources.

- The human liver will convert amino acids into glucose for fuel when carbs are restricted, a process called GLUCONEOGENESIS. Evidence shows that up to 200g of glucose per day can be produced from protein sources, which is more than an adequate amount to meet the limited glucose requirements of the brain, eye lens and red blood cells.

- **Healthy low-carb, high-fat nutrition includes a moderate protein intake and is NOT A HIGH-PROTEIN DIET.**

- Dietary Reference Intakes support a wide range of protein intake from 10% - 35% of calories. Only diets above this intake are truly 'high protein'.
- Moderate protein intake is measured as approximately a palm-sized portion per meal.
- Moderate protein intake does not put any abnormal stress on normal functioning kidneys and it does not promote calcium loss from bones.
- Protein is a significant appetite suppressant and assists in hunger control.
- Proteins, especially lean animal protein, stimulate approximately half the insulin response of carbs.
- An adequate protein intake is required to reduce lean muscle mass loss during periods of weight loss.
- Excessive protein intakes are associated with fat storage and weight gain in individuals.

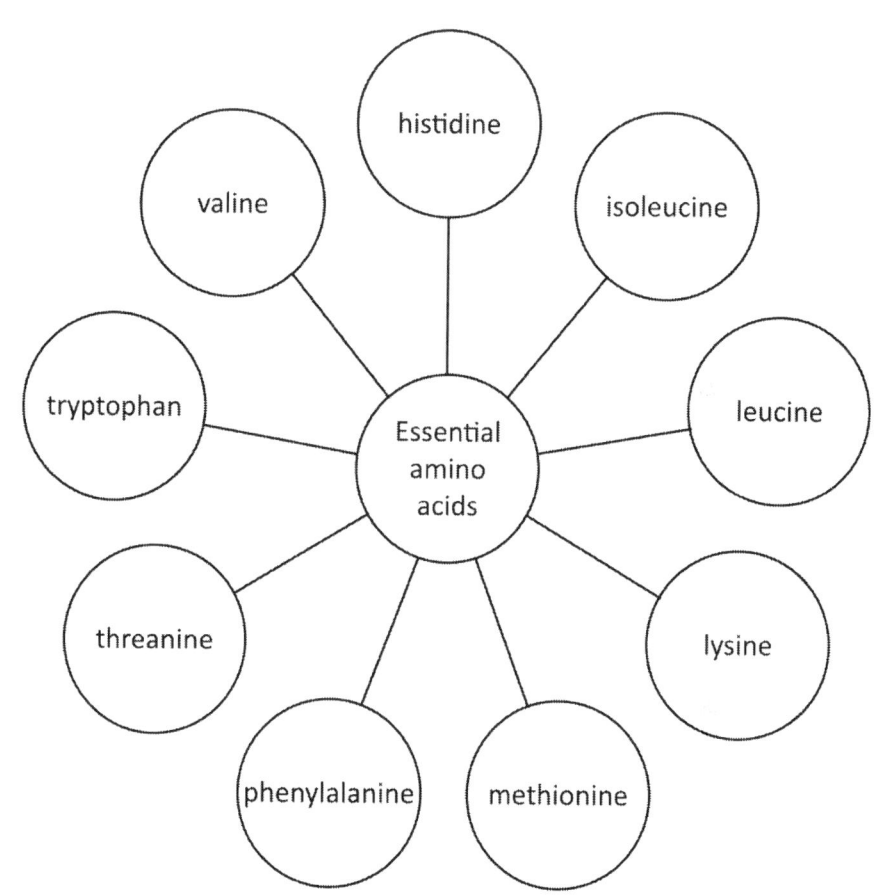

Figure 11: The Nine Essential Amino Acids Humans Require From Dietary Protein

- histidine
- isoleucine
- leucine
- lysine
- methionine
- phenylalanine
- threanine
- tryptophan
- valine

Essential amino acids

Key Points: Protein
1. Meat, fish and dairy are complete proteins.
2. Low-carb, high-fat nutrition is not a high protein diet.

VITAMINS and MINERALS

'By the proper intakes of vitamins and other nutrients and by following a few other healthful practices from youth or middle age on, you can, I believe, extend your life and years of well-being by twenty-five or even thirty-five years'.
Linus Pauling

....

When it comes to micronutrients in our diet, there are three common nutritional myths.

Myth 1: We need to eat a certain number of fruits and vegetables daily in order to take in adequate amounts of micronutrients in the form of vitamins and minerals.

Fact 1: Table 6 shows that of the 13 most important vitamins required for good health, **11 of them are best obtained from animal product sources** rather than plant foods; the same holds true for the required minerals.

Table 6: Sources of Vitamins and Minerals

FAT SOLUBLE VITAMINS	BEST SOURCES
Vitamin A	Liver, dairy, fish oils
Vitamin D	Oily fish
Vitamin E	Seeds, nuts, oils, meat
Vitamin K1 and K2	K2 in animal foods, K1 in avocados and green leafy vegetables

Chapter 2 - Why We Eat What We Eat

WATER SOLUBLE VITAMINS	BEST SOURCES
Vitamin B1	Pork, liver, wholegrains
Vitamin B2	Dairy
Vitamin B3	Meat, cereals
Vitamin B5	Liver, eggs
Vitamin B6	Meat, fish, potatoes
Vitamin B12	Animal products only Biotin Liver, eggs, cereals, yeast
Folate	Liver
Vitamin C	Fruits and vegetables *(especially guavas and peppers)*
MINERALS	
Calcium	Dairy, tinned fish, eggs
Iron	Red meat, liver, fish and shellfish, dark green vegetables
Chromium	Eggs, beef, cheese, liver
Iodine	Fish, kelp
Selenium	Organ meats, fish and shellfish
Zinc	Oysters, liver, meat, cheese, fish
Magnesium	Nuts and wholegrains
Manganese	Nuts and wholegrains
Potassium	Fruits and vegetables, animal products

Myth 2: Processed foods are nutritionally balanced because they are fortified with vitamins.

Fact 2: Processed food from grains contains very little micronutrients as the processing strips away those parts of the grain that contain the vitamins and minerals (along with most of the protein and fibre). Food manufacturers therefore 'fortify' processed foods by adding back trace amounts of vitamins to give the illusion of healthy food. See the comparative table below.

Table 7: A Nutritional Comparison of Processed Food (Sugar and Flour) vs. a Low-Cost Basket of Real Food in Providing Essential Macronutrients, Vitamins and Minerals

Nutrient	Processed Food, Sugar and Flour	Real Foods	Main source from real food basket*
Calories	1100kcal	1100kcal	Eggs
Carbs	250g	62g	Oats
Protein	17g	95g	Sardines
Fat	2g	57g	Eggs
	(% RDA / AI)	(% RDA / AI)	
Vitamin A	0%	1400%**	Liver and spinach
Vitamin D	0%	115%	Sardines, eggs and milk
Vitamin E	7%	105%	Seeds, sardines
Vitamin K	8%	800%	Spinach, sardines
Vitamin B1 (Thiamin)	17%	110%	Liver, seeds
Vitamin B2 (Riboflavin)	0%	270%	Liver, eggs

Chapter 2 - Why We Eat What We Eat

Nutrient	Processed Food, Sugar and Flour	Real Foods	Main source from real food basket*
Vitamin B3 (Niacin)	14%	110%	Liver, sardines
Vitamin B5 (Pantethine)	14%	200%	Liver, eggs
Vitamin B6 (Pyridoxine)	0%	110%	Liver, seeds, sardines
Vitamin B12 (Cobalamin)	0%	1125%	Liver, sardines
Folate (Folic acid)	11%	260%	Liver, eggs
Biotin	0%	600%	Liver, eggs
Vitamin C (Ascorbic acid)	0%	130%	Broccoli, spinach
Calcium	3%	100%	Sardines, milk
Magnesium	9%	120%	Cocoa, spinach
Phosphorous	26%	275%	Sardines, eggs
Copper	22%	275%	Cocoa, liver, seeds
Iron	11%	140%	Liver, spinach
Manganese	52%	200%	Oats, spinach
Selenium	100%	360%	Sardines, eggs
Zinc	9%	100%	Liver, eggs

% RDA / AI = percentage of recommended daily allowance or adequate intake

*The real food basket above contains nine foodstuffs: oats, milk, liver, broccoli, spinach, cocoa, sardines, eggs, and sunflower seeds.

**Half of the vitamin A comes from the spinach, which will be poorly absorbed and therefore the actual uptake would be much less than the % RDA shown.

(Table adapted from *The Obesity Epidemic* by Zoe Harcombe)

Myth 3: A vegetarian diet is easily balanced to supply all the required vitamins and minerals.

Fact 3: Vegetarians cannot get Vitamin B12 from plant sources. Pure vegans have to take a supplement unless they consume milk or eggs; they are also at high risk of Vitamin D deficiency (especially in sunlight-deficient parts of the world) and calcium deficiency as these vitamins and minerals are not plentiful in plant sources. See the table below.

Table 8: Percentage of Male Adult Recommended Daily Intake (RDI) or Adequate Intake (AI) Provided by 100g Lean Red Meat or Vegetarian Protein Sources

	RDA/AI for male 31-50yr	Beef %	Lamb %	Egg %	Cheddar Cheese %	Baked beans %	Walnuts %
Protein	64g	36	34	21	40	7	23
Long-chain omega-3 fat	160mg	50	53	111	55	0	0
Thiamin	1.2mg	3	8	8	3	4	28
Riboflavin	1.3mg	25	15	31	39	0	14
Niacin	16mg	31	70	0	<1	5	9
Vitamin B6	1.3mg	23	43	5	6	8	33
Vitamin B12	2.4µg	79	71	58	35	0	0
Pantothenic acid	6mg	12	13	34	7	<1	11

Chapter 2 - Why We Eat What We Eat

	RDA/AI for male 31-50yr	Beef %	Lamb %	Egg %	Cheddar Cheese %	Baked beans %	Walnuts %
Vitamin A	900µg	<1	<1	25	43	<1	<1
Vitamin E	10mg	7	5	22	40	1	26
Phosphorus	1000mg	22	23	20	47	8	37
Zinc	14mg	3	31	9	26	4	18
Iron	8mg	24	25	26	3	20	31
Magnesium	420mg	6	6	2	7	6	36
Selenium	70µg	29	21	37	15	5	3
Sodium	920mg	6	7	13	72	23	<1
Potassium	3800mg	9	9	3	2	6	12

Getting the recommended daily allowance of vitamins and minerals

In her informative book, *The Obesity Epidemic*, Zoe Harcombe calculates that the RDAs can be obtained from just five nutritious foods without the need for large amounts of fruit and vegetables:

Normal diet:

- Liver 100g
- Sardines (or other oily fish) 200g
- Whole milk 200ml
- Sunflower seeds 100g
- Broccoli 200g

Vegan diet:

- Mushrooms 2.25kg (raw, sunshine grown) and vegetable oil
- Porridge oats 175g
- Oriental radishes 100g
- Sunflower seeds 25g
- Spinach 200g and Vegetable oil
- Vitamin B12 supplement

Interesting facts regarding vitamins

- The term 'vitamine' was coined by Polish-born biochemist, Casimir Funk, in 1912 (the 'e' was later dropped).
- The presence of vitamins in food that were necessary for human health was hypothesised in observations by early 20th century medical researchers of diseases such as beriberi, pellagra, rickets and scurvy. These diseases occurred in populations as they consumed an increased intake of refined sugar, white flour and white rice. Nutritionists at the time wrote that the 'chronic diseases of civilisation could be attributed to the extensive use of vitamin-poor white flour and to the inordinate use of vitamin-less sugar'.
- Scurvy (Vitamin C deficiency) occurs in populations, like the sailors of old, who changed their diet on board ship to one high in refined

carbohydrates, as well as one that was deficient in fresh fruit and vegetables.
- Carnivorous populations like the Inuit (Canadian Eskimos) do not get scurvy; it has been shown that some Inuit populations get Vitamin C from eating whale's skin.
- Type 2 diabetes and Metabolic Syndrome are associated with reduced circulating levels of Vitamin C by up to 30%; high blood sugar levels reduce cellular Vitamin C uptake and reduce Vitamin C reabsorption in the kidneys.
- It is possible that high blood sugar and insulin may therefore increase the body's requirement for Vitamin C.
- Vitamin A from animal sources is in a pure form called retinol; plant sources of Vitamin A are in the form of carotene, which must be converted to retinol at a relatively poor conversion rate of 6:1. Children make the conversion poorly, as do people on a low-fat diet who often secrete inadequate bile salts that are required to absorb fat. Diabetics and people with low thyroid function cannot convert plant carotene to retinol.
- Vitamin D is found naturally in oily fish and we also synthesise it in our skin from cholesterol upon exposure to sunlight. Vitamin D operates in the body like a hormone and is important for bone health, immune function, and mental health. Vitamin D3 is currently being studied for its role in cancer prevention and in slowing down early cancer growth.
- Vitamin E is a powerful antioxidant, anti-clotting agent and keeps skin and blood vessels healthy.
- Vitamin K is essential for a healthy gut biome. It comes in two forms (K1 and K2). K2 comes from animal sources and is thought to play an important role in healthy hearts and arteries.
- Vitamins B2 and B3 play important roles in carbohydrate fuelled ATP energy metabolism.
- Vitamins function better when absorbed from real food sources rather than supplements.

Key points: Vitamins and Minerals
1. The best sources of most micronutrients are animal foods.
2. Vegans face challenges in obtaining specific micronutrients.
3. There is little evidence to support a requirement for large amounts of fruit and vegetables to obtain micronutrients.

Chapter 2 - Why We Eat What We Eat

Chapter 3
CARBOHYDRATE INTOLERANCE AND INSULIN RESISTANCE: THE METABOLIC BASIS OF OBESITY

'Genes load the gun, lifestyle pulls the trigger'.
Anon

....

What is carbohydrate intolerance?
Carbohydrate intolerance describes a state of reduced carbohydrate tolerance to which susceptible people have a genetic predisposition. It leads to the development of progressive insulin resistance in affected individuals who eat carbohydrates, especially sugar and refined carbs, in excess of their tolerance.

What is insulin resistance?
Insulin resistance is a state in which cells of the body, primarily in the liver and muscles, become increasingly insensitive and resistant to the normal effects of insulin. This resistance induces even higher levels of insulin secretion by the pancreas to compensate. A useful analogy is that of hearing impairment, whereby exposure to very loud noise induces deafness and thereafter we need to turn the volume of sounds up and up in order to hear them 'normally'.

Insulin resistance is a direct result of the following:
- Frequent intake of sugar and refined carbs
- Persistently elevated blood insulin levels
- Fat deposition in the liver

Chapter 3 - Carbohydrate Intolerance and Insulin Resistance

The following physiological effects of insulin resistance are:
- Elevated blood insulin levels
- Reduced sugar (glucose) uptake by liver and muscle cells for storage and energy
- Elevated blood sugar levels
- Increased conversion of sugar to fat in the liver
- Fatty infiltration of the liver
- Increased storage of body fat (lipogenesis), especially in the belly
- Inhibition of fat release (lipolysis) from fat stores

An understanding of carbohydrate intolerance and insulin resistance reveals that the metabolic basis of obesity is an interaction between:
- Our genetic makeup - it is estimated that up to 75% of people carry the genes for carbohydrate intolerance
- What we eat rather than how much we eat
- The control of appetite
- The hormones that regulate fuel partitioning in the body

This is a more accurate view of the problem, as opposed to the old model of 'calories in versus calories out', which blamed obesity simply on an excessive calorie intake and a lack of exercise.

Triggers that 'switch on' the genes for carbohydrate intolerance include the following:
- Age
- A diet high in sugar and refined carbs
- Physical inactivity
- Prolonged stress (especially in men)
- Menopause
- Pregnancy

The effects of increasing insulin resistance include the following:
- Inflammation
- Fatness (especially belly fat) leading to obesity
- Metabolic syndrome
- Type 2 Diabetes
- High blood pressure
- Heart disease
- Cancer
- Gout
- Alzheimer's

Figure 12 : The Physiology of Carbohydrate Intolerance and Insulin Resistance

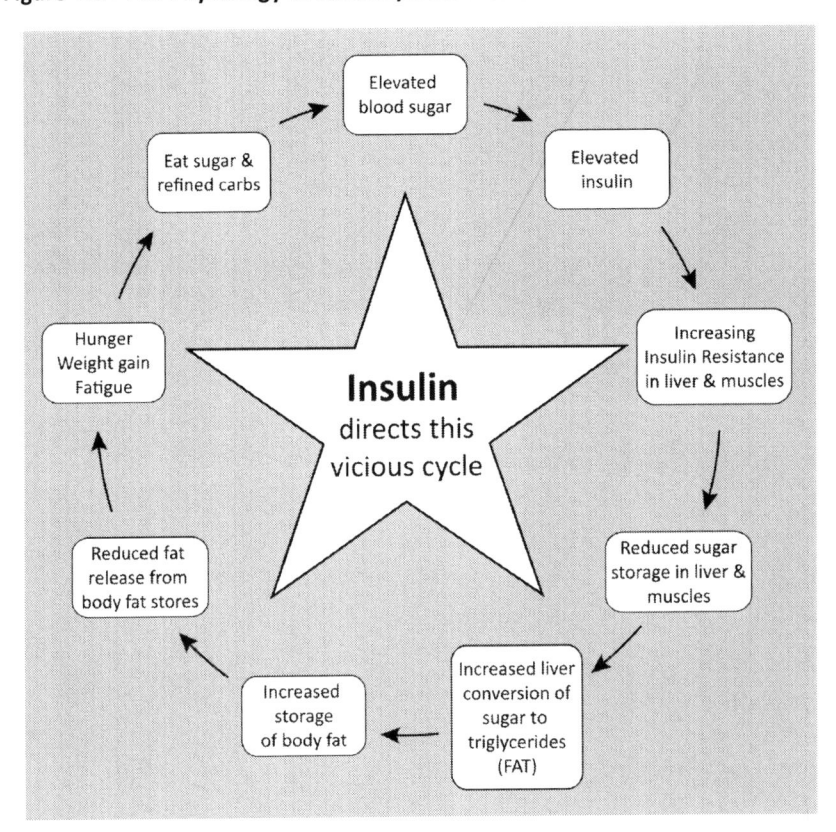

Chapter 3 - Carbohydrate Intolerance and Insulin Resistance

You are not what you eat....
you are what you store from what
you eat

Why are obese people hungry and tired all the time?

- Not because they are gluttonous and lazy!
- It is because the metabolic cycle of high-carb intake, insulin resistance and elevated insulin levels blocks the release of sustainable fuel from fat stores and creates a state of 'cellular starvation'.
- The consequences of this condition:
  - ➢ Increased stimulation of appetite that leads to HUNGER
  - ➢ A brain-mediated sense of FATIGUE to reduce activity levels in order to conserve energy
  - ➢ A compensatory reduction in resting energy expenditure (basal metabolic rate)

> - Generally, obese people suffer an increased appetite and a lack of energy for exercise as a CONSEQUENCE of their metabolic problem, not as the root cause!
> - The common belief that obese people are morbidly fat because they are 'gluttonous and lazy' is not scientifically supported; they are, in fact, metabolically ill and their obesity, hunger and fatigue are all markers of their disordered metabolic state.

- This is a powerful viewpoint shift and one that all who advise significantly overweight people need to appreciate.

CARBOHYDRATE INTOLERANCE and DIET - THE INTER-RELATIONSHIPS TO DISEASES OF LIFESTYLE

'Healing is a matter of time, but it is sometimes also a matter of opportunity'.
Hippocrates

All that you have learnt so far can be summarised in the organogram below showing the inter-related processes of genetics, carb intolerance, diet, insulin resistance and inflammation, which lead to the evolution of diseases of lifestyle.

Figure 13: The Inter-Relationships Between Carb Intolerance and Diet in Diseases of Lifestyle

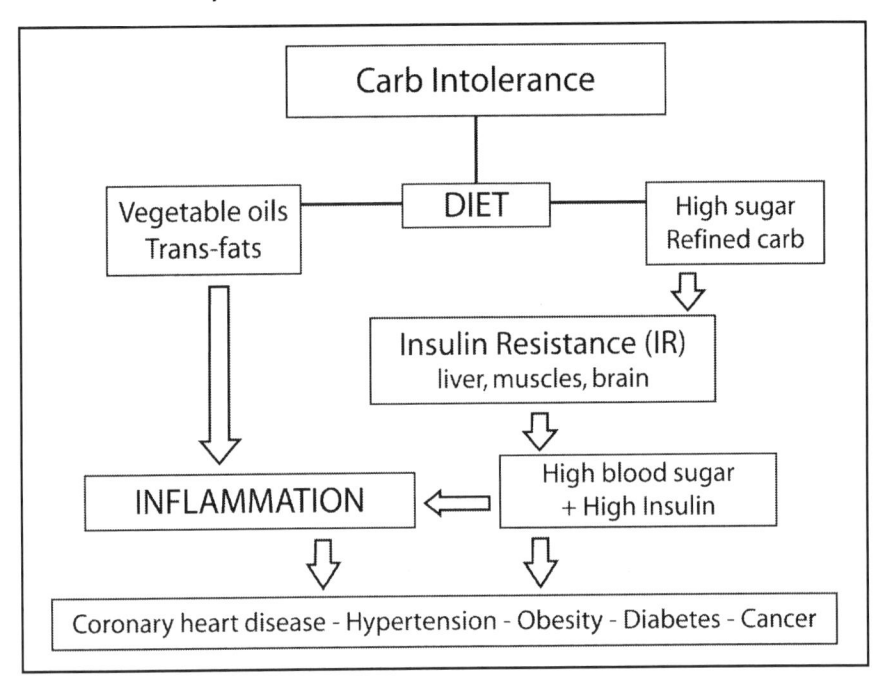

```
                    Carb Intolerance
                          |
  Vegetable oils  ——   DIET   ——  High sugar
  Trans-fats                       Refined carb
        |                              ⇩
        |                   Insulin Resistance (IR)
        |                    liver, muscles, brain
        |                              ⇩
        ⇩                     High blood sugar
  INFLAMMATION   ⇐           + High Insulin
        ⇩                              ⇩
  Coronary heart disease - Hypertension - Obesity - Diabetes - Cancer
```

Chapter 3 - Carbohydrate Intolerance and Insulin Resistance

The concepts are neatly summed up in these 7 simple messages promoted by *The Noakes Foundation* in South Africa:

1. Insulin resistance is the most common medical condition present in a majority of the world's populations.
2. Those with insulin resistance who eat high-carbohydrate diets develop persistently elevated blood insulin concentrations.
3. Persistently elevated blood insulin concentrations (hyperinsulinaemia) over many years are the direct cause of many of the chronic medical maladies that currently plague modern societies.
4. Obesity is a disorder of abnormal fat accumulation driven by hyperinsulinaemia in those people with insulin resistance who eat more carbohydrate than their insulin-resistant bodies can handle.
5. Obesity cannot occur without an associated dysfunction of the brain appestat that determines when we are hungry and regulates how much we eat.
6. Dysfunction of the appestat is caused by the addictive, highly-processed, industrial diet that has become the global norm since the release of the 1977 Dietary Guidelines. These guidelines demonized real foods as being 'unhealthy', and paved the way for the current global epidemics of obesity and type 2 diabetes.
7. The reversal of these conditions requires that we promote the consumption of real foods that do not cause hyperinsulinaemia and appestat dysfunction.

(Source: www.noakesfoundation.org)

The research consensus is that hyperinsulinaemia precedes hyperglycemia by up to 24 years; perhaps an opportunity exists therein for early detection? Given the close relationship between insulin resistance and hyperinsulinaemia, we can assume that most of the people who are insulin resistant are also hyperinsulinaemic (Crofts et al.).

Key Points: Carbohydrate intolerance
1. Carbohydrate intolerance leads to increasing insulin resistance.
2. Carbohydrate intolerance and insulin resistance form the metabolic basis for obesity.
3. Carb intolerance explains why obese people are often hungry and tired.
4. Genetics and lifestyle triggers play a role in carb intolerance.
5. Insulin levels provoked by sugar and carb intake create a fatty liver and weight gain.
6. Carbohydrate intolerance and insulin resistance are strongly associated with diseases of lifestyle.

Chapter 3 - Carbohydrate Intolerance and Insulin Resistance

Chapter 4
HEAVY WEIGHT OR HEALTHY WEIGHT - BELLY FAT AND OBESITY

'Illnesses do not come upon us out of the blue. They are developed from small daily sins against nature. When enough sins have accumulated, illnesses will suddenly appear'.
Hippocrates

....

Belly Fat Facts

- Obesity rates have tripled in countries like the USA since 1980.
- Globally, childhood obesity rates have increased at an alarming rate.
- Rising obesity rates in these populations follow closely on increased overall carbohydrate consumption (including increased consumption of sugars) and a decline in dietary fat intake.
- World Health Organisation data indicate that the average UK citizen consumes 38 kg of sugar per year; statistics from the Flour Advisory Bureau record that per capita flour consumption reached 74 kg in 2008/9. This means that sugar and flour represent 50%-65% of the average diet.
- Fat deposited around the abdominal organs is officially called visceral fat, but 'belly fat' is also a good term.
- Belly fat is a cardinal feature of the carb-intolerant person who eats a highly refined high-carb diet.
- Visceral fat acts like an endocrine organ that secretes many pro-hormone, hormone and pro-inflammatory substances that cause

inflammation in fat stores and arteries, and that also aggravate insulin resistance.
- Hormones, like oestrogen and prolactin, released from visceral fat increase breast cancer risk in women and produce gynaecomastia ('man boobs') in obese men.
- Visceral fat releases inflammatory signals, abnormal cytokines or cell to cell hormone signal molecules like leptin, resistin and tumour necrosis factor. All of these have significant metabolic and inflammatory effects on the body. As a result, diminished quantities of the protective cytokines like adiponectin (which reduces heart disease and diabetes risk) are produced.
- Belly fat is significantly associated with the accumulation of fat in the liver (called steatosis) which can cause non-alcoholic fatty liver disease (NAFLD) and lead to long-term liver damage.
- In most cases, obesity is a marker of severe metabolic dysfunction (metabolic syndrome), which needs to be reversed in order to 'cure' the obesity.
- 80% of people with type 2 diabetes are obese.

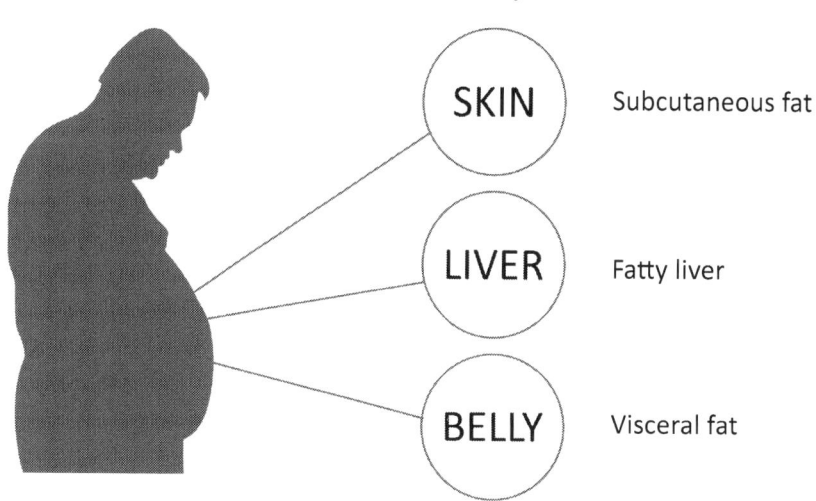

Figure 14 : Sites Of Fat Accumulation In The Body

SKIN — Subcutaneous fat

LIVER — Fatty liver

BELLY — Visceral fat

Six ways to know you have too much belly fat:
1. Your jeans are too tight!
2. The scale shows 5kg or more of weight gain, mostly in the belly
3. Your waist measurement exceeds
   - 102cm (40 inches) in men
   - 88cm (35 inches) in women
4. Your BMI (Body Mass Index) calculated as your weight (kg) divided by the your height (m) squared
   - is over 25 kg/m² = overweight
   - is over 30 kg/m² = obese
5. Your waist: hip ratio (waist circumference divided by hip circumference)
   - is greater than 0.92 in men
   - is greater than 0.85 in women
6. Your waist: height ratio (waist circumference divided by height) exceeds 0.5

Waist circumference is a powerful predictor of:
- Metabolic syndrome (pre-diabetes)
- Type 2 diabetes
- Heart disease
- High blood pressure
- Cancer - significantly increased risks for cancers of the breast and colon
- Dementia & Alzheimer's
- Overall mortality

Belly fat is the 2nd highest risk factor for cancer after smoking.

The failure of conventional dieting to cure obesity

- Traditional diets to 'lose weight' have been modelled on either a low-fat diet or a diet low in calories.
- A low-fat diet means you are, by definition, on a high-carb diet.

Lowering the fat content of foodstuffs is achieved by adding sugar and carbs to increase taste and energy.
- Major review studies of the effectiveness of low-fat and low-calorie dieting over the long term uniformly show failure in 95 – 98% of cases.
- Measured over 24 months, people who lose weight on low-fat and low-calorie diets will regain 98% of the weight that they lost in the initial 6 months, and 66% will regain even more weight than when they started.
- **The principal reasons for failure:**
  - Low-fat diets and low-calorie diets induce appetite stimulation and eventually irresistible hunger, which drives people to eat.
  - Low-fat and low-calorie diets ignore the influence of what we eat on our metabolism. Eating more carbs aggravates the vicious metabolic cycle of carb intolerance, insulin resistance, fat storage and weight gain.
  - Low-calorie diets create a compensatory reduction in resting energy expenditure (basal metabolic rate).

A question that is often asked is why some populations, like those in Southeast Asia, who eat a predominantly 'high-carb diet' do not exhibit significant obesity rates and other diseases of lifestyle?

The answer is that these populations are generally living and eating at a subsistence level that means that in addition to relatively high levels of physical activity, their dietary practices are characterised by the following:
- Low in calories
- Low in sugar
- Predominantly small amounts of unrefined carbohydrates
- Not based on significant wheat consumption
- Not having significant processed foods

Such people do not have dietary induced insulin resistance issues and therefore no significant IR associated diseases of lifestyle.

The failure of EXERCISE to curb or cure obesity

For decades, we have been advised to 'eat less and exercise more' in order to lose weight.

- The theory is that if one subscribes to the oversimplified 'calories in vs. calories out' model, then exercise is the obvious way to burn more calories.
- Research has shown that exercise is a very poor intervention for weight loss.
- Overweight people, who exercise regularly but do not address the nutritional fundamentals in a meaningful way, will be lucky to lose any more than 1.5kg with moderate levels of exercise, and will not lose more than 3kg with intense exercise over a 24 month period!

Why does exercise fail to deliver on weight loss? Two main reasons:
1. Exercise is a powerful stimulant of appetite and therefore, after exercise, people feel HUNGRY; most people will eat the same or often a greater amount of calories than they 'burned' during the exercise bout; if they resort to eating carbs and they are carb-intolerant, the fattening process carries on.
2. Exercising individuals often reduce their overall daily activity levels.

As Albert Einstein once said, *'Insanity is doing the same thing over and over again and expecting a different result'!* This certainly describes the low-fat diet and exercise weight loss plan.

The 'cure' for obesity and belly fat

- The number one intervention that provides effective weight loss in the short to medium term, and effective weight maintenance in the long term is a LOW-CARB, HIGH-FAT nutrition program. A LIFESTYLE change for LIFE!

- Low-carb, high-fat nutrition provides food satiety, reduces appetite, breaks the high blood sugar-insulin-fattening cycle and reduces daily calorie intake.
- In most published quality trials, low-carb programs have proven to be more effective in measured weight loss than low-fat diets. Patient compliance with low-carb nutrition was equal to and, in some studies better than, those on low-fat diets (Brehm BJ).
- The important point is that if you are a carb-intolerant person who is overweight, there is no short-term diet that will solve your weight problem. A commitment to a lifestyle change and to a nutrition program that is carb-restricted and high in healthy fats is required.
- As Dr Dariush Mozaffarian stated in a recent 2015 review article, 'Diet-related priorities to reduce obesity and type 2 diabetes worldwide should include reductions in consumption of starchy and sugary foods and their marketing by industry; increasing consumption of fruits, vegetables, nuts, yoghurt, fish, healthy vegetable oils, and whole grains; and identification of the effects of maternal–foetal interactions, the microbiome and sleep on metabolic health'.
- Exercise amplifies the effectiveness of a low-carb program and thereby increases the insulin sensitivity of muscle tissue.
- Exercise is a highly recommended component of a healthy lifestyle and is associated with the maintenance of functional capacity and longevity.

The Role of Leptin Resistance in Obesity

- In 1994, a new hormone called leptin, which is intricately involved in fat metabolism, was discovered in fat cells.
- Leptin influences all other hormones and the part of the brain (the hypothalamus) responsible for stimulating hunger.
- Leptin has an oversight role on our energy stores. After we eat and our fat is stored, leptin is released from fat cells and signals the brain that we are full and reduces appetite.

- A high-refined carb intake leads to high blood sugar and has inflammatory effects on the brain. The increasing insulin resistance creates LEPTIN RESISTANCE where the brain becomes 'deaf' to the leptin signal, and we continue to eat.
- Belly fat obesity results in the production of excessive amounts of leptin that act as a pro-inflammatory molecule and contributes to an inflammatory environment in the body and associated disorders.
- Leptin resistance is also aggravated by poor sleep patterns.

Overweight Children

Childhood and adolescent obesity rates are increasing worldwide as the result of the combined effect of poor eating habits and decreased levels of physical activity. Type 2 diabetes and hypertension in children are associated with rising childhood obesity, an unheard of condition in children 30 years ago. Recent research by Gow, Sondike and others does show that low-carb nutrition (carbs restricted to <60g/day) is effective for weight loss in overweight children and adolescents without causing negative health outcomes.

Nutritional strategies to combat obesity in children

- Talk to children about the benefits of real food for healthy minds and bodies.
- Involve them in the weekly shopping choices.
- Read food labels to look for hidden added sugar that is often disguised under aliases. (see page 142)
- Remove all cereals, other refined carbs and junk food options from the household.
- Actively discourage sweetened drinks and fruit juices; up to one-third of total sugar in their diet currently originates from sweetened beverages.

- Teach and encourage them to prepare healthy low-carb food options including baking and making 'treats'; they make great 'chefs', just show them and provide the ingredients.
- Start an organic herb and veggie patch in your garden and involve children in the growing, harvesting and use of your home-grown produce.
- Make food fun both in preparation and eating.
- Eat the 'low-carb way' as a family and provide an effective role model.
- Give children choices within the low-carb options.
- Position healthy food and snack options at the front of the fridge.

> **Key Points: Belly Fat and Obesity**
> 1. Belly fat (central visceral fat) is a cardinal feature of carbohydrate intolerance and insulin resistance.
> 2. Leptin resistance plays a role in weight gain.
> 3. Belly fat increases the risks of diseases of lifestyle.
> 4. Exercise and low-fat dieting are generally not successful for sustainable weight loss.
> 5. Low-carb nutrition works in obese children.

Chapter 5
CHOLESTEROL, SATURATED FAT, SUGAR AND HEART DISEASE

'For every complicated problem there is a solution that is simple, direct, understandable and wrong'.
HL Mencken

Cholesterol and Coronary Heart Disease: A Flawed Hypothesis?

In the 1950s and 1960s, flawed research and conclusions based chiefly on the Seven Countries Study done by Ancel Keys, an American physiologist and researcher specialising in diet and heart disease, set in motion the DIET-HEART HYPOTHESIS that still exists today but more as dogma than science!

Essentially, Keys's studies found associations between saturated fat intake, blood cholesterol levels and deaths from heart disease in a few 'cherry-picked' countries. This created the theory that dietary fat influenced cholesterol levels leading to arteriosclerosis and heart attacks. Modern day reviews of available research strongly question this dogma; the hypothesis, however, prevails in mainstream medical practice and has spawned a multibillion-dollar statin drug industry.

Chapter 5 - Cholesterol, Saturated Fat, Sugar and Heart Disease

Let's review the salient points relevant to today's understanding of the issues.

The Relationship between Cholesterol and Saturated Fat:

- Saturated fat and cholesterol are not the same thing!
- Biochemically, cholesterol is a sterol which is not the same as a fat (see Figure 15).
- Cholesterol and fat share common dietary sources like eggs, meat, organ meats and dairy.
- Cholesterol is secreted in bile so that fat digestion can take place in the intestine.
- Both cholesterol and fats are 'lipids', which means they don't dissolve in water or blood; they therefore require a special transport system in the body.
- Cholesterol and fat share the lipoprotein body transport system in the bloodstream which means they are both transported through the blood in the same 'taxi-cabs'.

The Lipoproteins:
- These 'taxi-cabs' are known as very low density lipoproteins (VLDL), low density lipoproteins (LDL) and high density lipoproteins (HDL).
- When the liver manufactures a lot of fats (triglycerides) from carbs, then it secretes these fats inside VLDL.
- LDL is not cholesterol, but is formed from VLDL, and transports cholesterol along with fats (triglycerides) from the liver to the body's cells as well as to the brain.
- 70% of the body's circulating cholesterol is carried in LDL.

- LDL occurs as different sized particles broadly classified as large LDL or small dense LDL; people with predominantly large LDL are classified as *LDL Pattern A* and those with predominantly small dense LDL as *LDL Pattern B*.
- LDL levels are regulated by cell receptors, especially in the liver, which can take up more or less LDL as and when required in order to maintain LDL levels.
- People with Familial Hypercholesterolaemia (FH) have a deficiency of these liver LDL receptors resulting in very elevated LDL cholesterol levels up to 5x normal.
- The liver also ineffectively removes small dense LDL from the circulation resulting in accumulation of small dense LDL in people with *LDL Pattern B*.
- 80% of men and women who show a triglyceride : HDL ratio of greater than 3.8 will predictably have *LDL Pattern B* with a predominance of small dense LDL (Hanak et al.).
- HDL transports cholesterol from the body tissues back to the liver and is also an antioxidant.

Figure 15: The Biochemical Difference Between Fat and Cholesterol

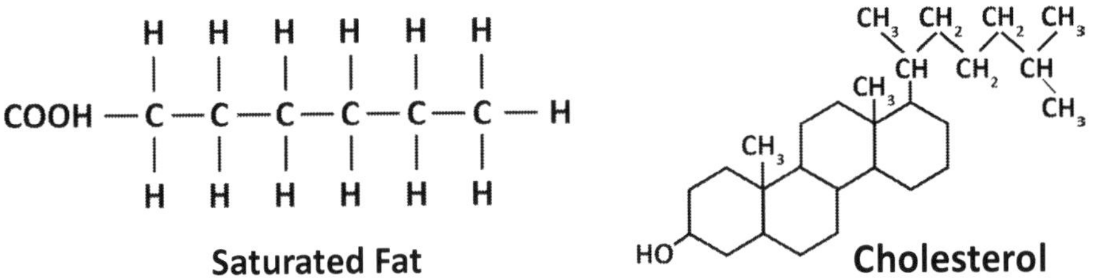

Saturated Fat

Cholesterol

Cholesterol is ESSENTIAL to life!!!

Its huge biological value can be gauged by the following facts:
- 90% of the body's cholesterol is found in all the cell membranes of the body.

Chapter 5 - Cholesterol, Saturated Fat, Sugar and Heart Disease

- 25% is found in the brain and nerve tissue; one-fifth of the brain's weight is cholesterol.
- Cholesterol
  - facilitates the growth of brain neural connections and is a component of all neuron sheaths, a critical brain nutrient and neuronal fuel.
  - acts as a powerful antioxidant in the brain protecting brain cells from free radical damage.
  - is used in all cellular repair.
  - forms the steroid hormones of the body, e.g. testosterone and oestrogen.
  - is converted in the skin by sunlight into Vitamin D (important for bone health, weight, mental and immune function).
  - is made into bile, which we need to digest and absorb essential fats and Vitamins A,D,E,K.
  - is a vital cog in the normal function of the immune system.

The Sources of Cholesterol in the body

- Dietary cholesterol intake contributes minimally to blood cholesterol levels.
- We absorb less than half of the cholesterol available in the gut from food and bile.
- Liver and cell production accounts for more than 85% of bodily cholesterol.
- The body has a feedback capacity to modulate cholesterol production, i.e. if more cholesterol is available in the diet, then the liver production is reduced, and vice versa.
- Saturated fat intake has very little effect on blood cholesterol levels in most people, but saturated fat is a diverse class of compounds, with different implications for lipid profiles depending on the type of fatty acids the fats contain.
- Eating saturated fat can decrease small-dense LDL and increase large

bouyant LDL. The saturated fatty acid, palmitate, raises levels of LDL whilst stearate, does not. Stearate and laurate reduce the total cholesterol : HDL ratio (DiNicolantonio et al., 2015).

The key recommendation from the 2010 Dietary Guidelines to limit consumption of dietary cholesterol to 300 mg per day is not included in the recently released 2015 edition. The 2015 Dietary Guidelines go on to say 'More research is needed regarding the dose-response relationship between dietary cholesterol and blood cholesterol levels. Adequate evidence is not available for a quantitative limit for dietary cholesterol specific to the Dietary Guidelines.

The Scientific Report of the 2015 Dietary Guidelines Advisory Committee (DGAC Report) released in February 2015 actually stated that the 'available evidence shows no appreciable relationship between consumption of dietary cholesterol and serum cholesterol, consistent with the conclusions of the AHA/ACC report. Cholesterol is not a nutrient of concern for overconsumption'.

My interpretation is that the current evidence does not support dietary cholesterol as a risk factor for heart disease!

The modern understanding of lipids and heart disease risk
- There is no such thing as 'good' or 'bad' cholesterol - cholesterol is cholesterol!
- Total blood cholesterol is a weak predictor of future heart disease.
- More than half of all heart attacks occur in people with normal blood cholesterol levels.
- Increased heart attack risk is associated with
    - An increase in the number of small dense LDL particles*.
    - Low levels of HDL.
    - Elevated levels of blood triglycerides (fats).

Chapter 5 - Cholesterol, Saturated Fat, Sugar and Heart Disease

- Glycation and oxidation of LDL causing oxidised (damaged) LDL particles.

*People with mostly small dense LDL particles have a 3x greater risk of heart disease compared to those with mostly large LDL particles.

How useful are blood cholesterol tests in predicting heart disease risk?

The 2015 Academy of Nutrition and Dietetics Comments on the Scientific Report of the 2015 Dietary Guidelines Advisory Committee highlights the findings in a 2010 Institute of Medicine (IOM) report on the use of biomarkers as surrogates for disease outcomes, which examined LDL and HDL as case studies and came to the following conclusions:

- *That LDL and HDL were not suitable for use as surrogates for the impact of diet on heart disease.*
- *Lowering LDL-C does not always correlate with improved patient outcomes.*
- *Published drug trials show evidence of an 'increase in cardiovascular events and death where the drug therapy 'successfully' decreased LDL-C levels and increased HDL-C.*
- *There is 'demonstration of a disconnect between lipoprotein modulation therapies {such as statin drugs} and the expected improvements in cardiovascular disease outcomes'.*
- *Data supports use of LDL as a surrogate endpoint for some cardiovascular outcomes for statin drug interventions, but not for all cardiovascular outcomes or other cardiovascular interventions, foods, or supplements.*
- *Current data does not support use of HDL as a surrogate endpoint.*

The effects of diet on lipids

- A low-fat, HIGH-CARB diet is associated with
  - Smaller dense LDL particles

- Lower HDL
- Raised blood triglycerides (by increasing liver production from carbs)
- Increased oxidised LDL particles

• A LOW-CARB, high-fat diet is associated with*
  - Larger less-dense (bouyant) LDL particles
  - Raised HDL
  - Lower blood triglycerides
  - Reduced oxidised LDL particles

YES read this carefully!!! A high-carb (low-fat) diet increases heart disease risk factors .... A low-carb (high-fat) diet reduces them.

* some people experience elevation in total blood cholesterol levels on a low-carb program, but little net effect on their ratio of total cholesterol : HDL (as HDL rises too), see page 211 for more on this issue.

Figure 16: Lipoprotein 'Taxi-cabs' for Cholesterol & Triglycerides

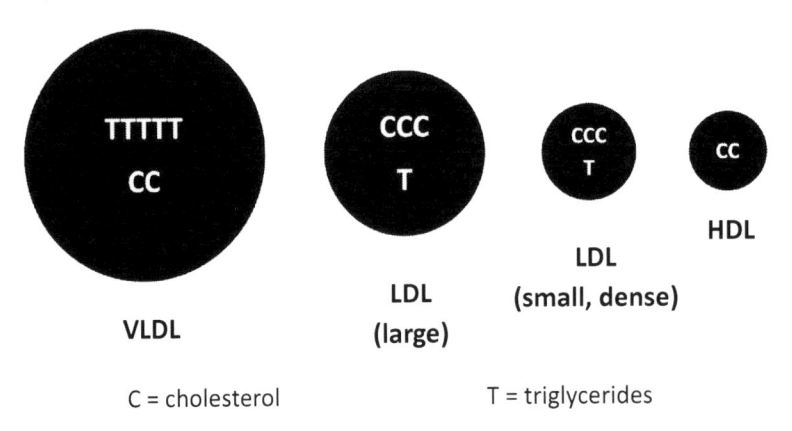

VLDL (TTTTT CC)
LDL (large) (CCC T)
LDL (small, dense) (CCC T)
HDL (CC)

C = cholesterol   T = triglycerides

There are also other lipoproteins 'taxi-cabs' called IDL and Chylomicrons

Chapter 5 - Cholesterol, Saturated Fat, Sugar and Heart Disease

Table 9: Effects of Diet on Heart Disease Risk Factors

	HIGH-CARB DIET Low fat	LOW-CARB DIET High fat
Total cholesterol	may ↓	may ↑ or nil change
LDL cholesterol	may ↓	may ↑ or nil change
LDL particle size & no.	small, many (●●●●●●●●●●●●●)	large, few (○○○)
HDL cholesterol	↓	↑
Triglycerides	↑	↓
RISK OF HEART DISEASE	↑	↓
	👎	👍

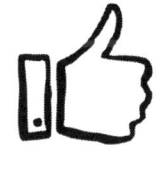

> 'One of the main functions of the liver is to make cholesterol, not because your liver wants you dead, but because life isn't possible without cholesterol'.
> Lierre Keith, *The Vegetarian Myth*

High versus Low Cholesterol – some of the surprising facts:
- HIGH CHOLESTEROL is associated with
    - Reduced rates of cancer
    - Reduced risk of death from heart disease in women
    - Reduced risk of non-cancer, non-cardiovascular death in women
    - Reduced rates of infections

- VERY LOW CHOLESTEROL is associated with
    - Increased risk of death from suicide and violent behaviour
    - Increased risk of haemorrhagic stroke
    - Increased risk of cancer
    - Increased risk of death in men of all ages and women over 50 yrs. through cancer, liver diseases and mental conditions

Cholesterol, heart disease and overall mortality
- **Under 50 yrs. of age:**
    - A very low blood cholesterol slightly improves longevity, but overall, the cholesterol level doesn't make that much difference to your risk of death.
    - The exception is some of the 1 in 500 people with the hereditary disorder of Familial Hypercholesterolaemia. These people have cholesterol levels in excess of 15mmol/L (3-5x 'normal') with an associated increased risk of premature heart disease.

- **Over 50 yrs. of age:**
    - The association between raised cholesterol levels and heart disease disappears.
    - If your cholesterol level starts falling, according to the 30-year follow-up data from the Framingham Heart Study, you have an increased overall risk of death and specifically from a heart attack! (Anderson, et al.)
    - A low cholesterol level is associated with a significantly increased

overall mortality, ie the older you are the more risky it is to have low cholesterol.

Coronary artery disease (CAD)

CAD is not a simple 'plumbing blockage problem', but a multifactorial process associated with ARTERIAL INFLAMMATION, for which the major risk factors are:
- Diabetes
- Smoking
- Age
- High blood pressure (high BP)
- Atherogenic dyslipidaemia (AD) in the form of increased numbers of oxidised small dense LDL particles, elevated blood triglycerides and low HDL levels
- Metabolic syndrome (pre-diabetes) = belly fat + elevated blood sugar + elevated insulin + high BP + AD
- Dietary
  - high sugar (fructose and glucose) and refined carbohydrate intake
  - high intake of vegetable oils and trans-fats
- Elevated blood glucose and insulin

The Inflammatory Hypothesis of CAD
- High blood sugar (glucose), insulin, fructose and AGEs cause progressive endothelial damage and stimulate inflammation in the artery wall.
- Increased free radicals associated with the inflammatory reaction oxidise LDL particles (especially small dense LDL with a high polyunsaturated triglyceride content).
- Oxidised (damaged) LDL particles penetrate the artery wall (endothelium).
- Inflammatory cytokines that attract white blood cells (monocytes) are released.

- The monocytes convert to macrophages and ingest the oxidised LDL particles forming foam cells.
- Foam cells accumulate beneath the artery endothelium forming 'fatty streaks', which are the start of atherosclerosis (plaque).
- Smooth muscle proliferation occurs in the arterial wall (insulin stimulates this)!
- Atherosclerotic plaques may grow to cause progressive coronary artery obstruction or rupture. This provokes clot formation in the artery and can lead to a heart attack (myocardial infarction).

Statins
- Statin drugs are widely used to reduce cholesterol levels in people with 'elevated cholesterol'.
- The statin industry is worth billions of dollars a year.
- Statins are proven to reduce the risk of coronary heart events in people who have had a previous heart attack or have proven coronary artery disease (called secondary prevention).
- Statins HAVE NOT BEEN SHOWN TO SIGNIFICANTLY REDUCE CORONARY HEART EVENTS IN PEOPLE WITHOUT PRE-EXISTING DISEASE (primary prevention).
- Although statins are effective at reducing cholesterol levels, their published benefit in reducing cardiovascular outcomes may well have been amplified through statistical manipulation (Diamond & Ravnskov).
- Statin therapy prevents 1 serious cardiovascular event (e.g. heart attack) per 140 low-risk people treated for five years and does not reduce all-cause mortality or serious illness in a low-risk population (Abramson).
- Side effects associated with statin use occur in up to 20% of patients and range from minor and reversible to serious and irreversible; the risk increases with the dose of drugs.
- Notable side effects include diabetes, muscle pain, amnesia (short-term memory loss), dementia (in the elderly), polyneuropathy,

rhabdomyolysis, raised liver enzymes, an increased incidence of acute and chronic kidney disease and non-melanoma skin cancer (Acharya et al., Mascitelli et al.).
- Recent research by Okuyama et al., showed evidence that statins may even worsen heart disease through mechanisms which:
  - ➤ actually promote coronary artery calcification (atherosclerosis)
  - ➤ act as mitochondrial toxins impairing muscle function in the heart and blood vessels
  - ➤ aggravate or incite congestive heart failure

Effects of low-carb nutrition on total cholesterol

We know that dietary cholesterol does not make a significant difference to blood cholesterol levels. Elevated blood cholesterol levels reflect the overproduction of cholesterol by the liver, not cholesterol that is being absorbed from our food. Most people who eat a low-carb, high-fat diet do not experience an increase in their total blood cholesterol and see positive improvements in their other risk markers for heart disease (like increased HDL and reduced triglycerides). Some people experience a transient increase in blood cholesterol that declines to normal levels after 4-6 weeks. This is believed to reflect the release of stored cholesterol from fat stores.

In a small number of people, an 'outlier' response of very elevated total cholesterol levels, but with improved heart risk biomarkers is described; these cases are still being investigated and no one yet has all the answers for this subgroup. If blood testing indicates you are one of these 'outliers', then the following measures need to be considered in formulating a plan of action with your doctor:
1. Further tests of LDL particle size and number (NMR TEST or APO B TEST) may need to be conducted to ascertain whether the cholesterol is being carried in large LDL (= low risk) or small dense LDL (= higher risk).
2. The ratio of total cholesterol:HDL may need to be considered. If it is less than 4.5, then the risk of heart disease is reduced.

3. Reducing the total saturated fat intake (animal and coconut fats) and substituting monounsaturated fats (olive oil, avocados) may reduce total cholesterol levels.
4. Introducing small amounts of unrefined carbs back into the diet may also reduce total cholesterol levels.
5. Statin therapy (at low doses, initially) could be considered.

Saturated Fat and Coronary Heart Disease: Another Flawed Hypothesis?

Some of the recent compelling evidence discrediting the notion that eating saturated fat causes or increases your risk of having a heart attack is listed below.

> To summarise: THERE IS NO DEFINITIVE EVIDENCE THAT SATURATED FAT IN THE DIET CAUSES CORONARY ARTERY DISEASE OR THAT REDUCING SATURATED FAT IN THE DIET REDUCES CORONARY ARTERY DISEASE.

Here are 20 of the more recent published research articles on the subject with their relevant findings:

1. 2015, Mozaffarian D., Diverging global trends in heart disease and type 2 diabetes: the role of carbohydrates and saturated fats (SFAs).

> *Finding*: 'To summarise, these lines of evidence—no influence on apolipoprotein B, reductions in triglyceride rich lipoproteins and lipoprotein (a), no relation of overall intake with coronary heart disease, and no observed cardiovascular harm for most major food sources—provide powerful and consistent evidence for absence of appreciable harms of SFAs. The overall evidence suggests that total SFAs are mostly neutral for health—neither a major nutrient of concern, nor a health-promoting priority for increased intake'.

Chapter 5 - Cholesterol, Saturated Fat, Sugar and Heart Disease

2.   2015, Mozaffarian D., Ludwig D. 'The 2015 US Dietary Guidelines Lifting the Ban on Total Dietary Fat'. Viewpoint

Finding: 'The limit on total fat presents an obstacle to sensible change, promoting harmful low-fat foods, undermining attempts to limit intakes of refined starch and added sugar, and discouraging the restaurant and food industry from providing products higher in healthful fats. It is time for the US Department of Agriculture and Department of Health and Human Services to develop the proper signage, public health messages, and other educational efforts to help people understand that limiting total fat does not produce any meaningful health benefits and that increasing healthful fats, including more than 35% of calories, has documented health benefits. Based on the strengths of accumulated new scientific evidence and consistent with the new DGAC report, a restructuring of national nutritional policy is warranted to move away from total fat reduction and toward healthy food choices, including those higher in healthful fats'.

3.   2015, Harcombe Z., Baker JS., Cooper SM., et al. 'Evidence from randomised controlled trials did not support the introduction of dietary fat guidelines in 1977 and 1983: a systematic review and meta-analysis'.

Finding: 'It is a widely held view that reductions in cholesterol are healthful per se. The original RCTs did not find any relationship between dietary fat intake and deaths from CHD or all-causes, despite significant reductions in cholesterol levels in the intervention and control groups. This undermines the role of serum cholesterol levels as an intermediary to the development of CHD and contravenes the theory that reducing dietary fat generally and saturated fat particularly potentiates a reduction in CHD'.

4.   2015, Puaschitz NG., Strand E., Norekvål TM., et al. 'Dietary intake of saturated fat is not associated with risk of coronary events or mortality in patients with established coronary artery disease'.

Finding: 'There was no association between dietary intake of saturated fatty acids and incident coronary events or mortality in patients with established coronary artery disease CAD '.

5.   2014, Cambridge University review by Chowdhury R., Warnakula S., Kunutsor S., et al. 'Association of Dietary, Circulating, and Supplement Fatty Acids With Coronary Risk: A Systematic Review and Meta-analysis'. The meta-analysis of 76 studies found no basis for guidelines that advise increased consumption of polyunsaturated fats to lower your cardiac risk, calling into question all of the standard nutritional guidelines related to heart health.

Finding: 'Current evidence does not clearly support cardiovascular guidelines that encourage high consumption of polyunsaturated fatty acids and low consumption of total saturated fats'.

6.   2014, Tulane University School of Public Health and Tropical Medicine: Lydia A. Bazzano et al. 'Effects of Low-Carbohydrate and Low-Fat Diets, A Randomized Trial'.

Finding: 'The low-carbohydrate diet was more effective for weight loss and cardiovascular risk factor reduction than the low-fat diet. Restricting carbohydrate may be an option for persons seeking to lose weight and reduce cardiovascular risk factors'.

7.   2014: DiNicolantonio JJ. 'The cardiometabolic consequences of replacing saturated fats with carbohydrates or Ω-6 polyunsaturated fats: Do the dietary guidelines have it wrong?'

Finding: 'The benefits of a low-fat diet (particularly a diet replacing saturated fats with carbohydrates or Ω-6 polyunsaturated fatty acids) are severely challenged. Dietary guidelines should assess the totality of the evidence

Chapter 5 - Cholesterol, Saturated Fat, Sugar and Heart Disease

and strongly reconsider their recommendations for replacing saturated fats with carbohydrates or Ω-6 polyunsaturated fats'.

8.   2014, Schwingshackl L., Hoffmann G. 'Dietary fatty acids in the secondary prevention of coronary heart disease: a systematic review, meta-analysis and meta-regression'.

Finding: 'The present systematic review provides no evidence for the beneficial effects of reduced/modified fat diets in the secondary prevention of coronary heart disease. Recommending higher intakes of polyunsaturated fatty acids in replacement of saturated fatty acids was not associated with risk reduction'.

9.   2014, Dias CB., Garg R., Wood LG., Garg ML. 'Saturated fat consumption may not be the main cause of increased blood lipid levels'.

Finding: '.....evidence would lead therefore to the hypothesis that there is a beneficial effect on the combination of SFA and n-3PUFA in the diet with a concomitant reduction in the consumption of n-6PUFA' (n-3 PUFA = omega 3 fatty acids, n-6 = omega 6 fatty acids)

10.   2013, Malhotra A. 'Saturated fat is not the major issue'. An editorial in the British Medical Journal describing how the avoidance of saturated fat actually promotes poor health in a number of ways, compounding the health risks of following this completely outdated advice. Dr Aseem Malhotra, a heart specialist at Croydon University Hospital in London states: 'The mantra that saturated fat must be removed to reduce the risk of cardiovascular disease has dominated dietary advice and guidelines for almost four decades. Yet scientific evidence shows that this advice has, paradoxically, increased our cardiovascular risk... The aspect of dietary saturated fat that is believed to have the greatest influence on cardiovascular risk is elevated concentrations of low density lipoprotein (LDL) cholesterol. Yet the reduction

in LDL cholesterol from reducing saturated fat intake seems to be specific to large, buoyant (type A) LDL particles, when in fact it is the small, dense (type B) particles (responsive to carbohydrate intake) that are implicated in cardiovascular disease'.

Finding: 'Recent prospective cohort studies have not supported any significant association between saturated fat intake and cardiovascular risk. Instead, saturated fat has been found to be protective'.

11.   2013, Ramsden CE., Zamora D., Leelarthaepin B., et al. 'Use of dietary linoleic acid for secondary prevention of coronary heart disease and death: evaluation of recovered data from the Sydney Diet Heart Study and updated meta-analysis'.

Finding: 'In this cohort, substituting omega-6 linoleic acid for saturated fat did not provide the intended benefits, but increased all cause morality, cardiovascular death, and death from coronary heart disease... An updated meta-analysis incorporating these missing data showed no evidence of benefit, and suggested a possible increased risk of cardiovascular disease from replacing saturated fat with omega-6 linoleic acid... As expected, increasing n-6 LA from safflower oil in the SDHS significantly reduced total cholesterol; however, these reductions were not associated with mortality outcomes (results not shown). Moreover, the increased risk of death in the intervention group presented fairly rapidly and persisted throughout the trial. These observations, combined with recent progress in the field of fatty acid metabolism, point to a mechanism of cardiovascular disease pathogenesis independent of our traditional understanding of cholesterol lowering'.

12.   2012, Hoenselaar R. 'Saturated fat and cardiovascular disease: the discrepancy between the scientific literature and dietary advice'.

Chapter 5 - Cholesterol, Saturated Fat, Sugar and Heart Disease

Finding: 'Results and conclusions about saturated fat intake in relation to cardiovascular disease, from leading advisory committees, do not reflect the available scientific literature'.

13. 2011, Kuipers et al: 'Saturated fat, carbohydrates and cardiovascular disease'.

Finding: 'The dietary intake of saturated fatty acids is associated with a modest increase in serum total cholesterol, but not with cardiovascular disease. Replacing dietary saturated fat with carbohydrates, notably those with a high glycaemic index, is associated with an increase in cardiovascular disease risk in observational cohorts. We conclude that avoidance of saturated fatty acid accumulation by reducing the intake of carbs with high glycaemic index is more effective in the prevention of cardiovascular disease than reducing saturated fat intake per se'.

14. 2011, Hooper L., et al. 'Reduced or modified dietary fat for preventing cardiovascular disease.' Cochrane Review.

Finding: 'There is no significant evidence for concluding that dietary saturated fat is associated with an increased risk of coronary heart disease or cardiovascular disease'.

15. 2011, Frieden T. R. & Berwick D.M. 'The "Million Hearts" Initiative – Preventing heart attacks and strokes'.

Finding: 'The only dangerous fats to be avoided for the prevention of heart disease are the artificial trans-fatty-acids'.

16. 2011, Astrup et al .'The role of reducing intakes of saturated fat in the prevention of cardiovascular disease: where does the evidence stand in 2010?'

> *Finding:* 'Current dietary recommendations advise reducing the intake of saturated fatty acids (SFAs) to reduce coronary heart disease (CHD) risk, but recent findings question the role of SFAs'.
> 'Substituting polyunsaturated fatty acids (PUFAs) for SFAs is associated with lower CHD risk; substituting total carbohydrate for SFAs is associated with no or a moderately higher risk of CHD'.
> 'Industrially produced trans-fatty acids (TFAs) are consistently associated with a higher risk of CHD (on a gram-for-gram basis)'.
> 'The ratio of total cholesterol to HDL cholesterol is a powerful predictor of CHD and that this ratio is more predictive than is LDL'.

17. 2010, Siri-Tarino et al. 'Meta-analysis of prospective cohort studies evaluating the association of saturated fat with cardiovascular disease'.

> *Finding:* 'There is no significant evidence for concluding that dietary saturated fat is associated with an increased risk of coronary heart disease or cardiovascular disease or stroke'.

18. 2010, Siri-Tarino et al. 'Saturated fat, carbohydrate and cardiovascular disease.'

> *Finding:* 'High intake of refined carbohydrates has been associated with a high risk of CHD'.
> 'Dietary efforts to improve the increasing burden of cardiovascular disease ... should primarily emphasise the limitation of refined-carbohydrate intakes and the reduction in excess adiposity'.

19. 2009, Jakobsen MU., et al. 'Major Types of Dietary Fat and Risk of Coronary Heart Disease: A Pooled Analysis of 11 Cohort Studies', this was a meta-analysis of 11 studies in US & Europe totalling 344,696 subjects followed for 10 year'.

Chapter 5 - Cholesterol, Saturated Fat, Sugar and Heart Disease

Finding: 'Replacing saturated fat with carbohydrate increased the risk of coronary events but not coronary deaths'.

20. 2006, Howard BV., Van Horn L., Hsia J., et al. 'Low-fat dietary pattern and risk of cardiovascular disease: the Women's Health Initiative Randomized Controlled Dietary Modification Trial'. An 8-year study on 49,000 women with 20,000 in the study group eating a low fat diet.

Finding: 'The dietary intervention (a low-fat diet) did not reduce the risk of coronary events manifested by coronary heart disease deaths or nonfatal myocardial infarcts'.

As Nina Teicholz succinctly states in her brilliantly researched 2014 book, *The Big Fat Surprise*, 'The sum of the evidence against saturated fat over the past half-century amounts to this:

- *The early trials condemning saturated fat were unsound*
- *The epidemiological data showed no negative association*
- *Saturated fat's effect on LDL-cholesterol (when properly measured in subfractions) is neutral*
- *And a significant body of clinical trials over the past decade has demonstrated the absence of any negative effect of saturated fat on heart disease, obesity or diabetes*

In other words, every plank in the case against saturated fat has, upon rigorous examination, crumbled away'.

The 2015 Academy of Nutrition and Dietetics Comments on the Scientific Report of the 2015 Dietary Guidelines Advisory Committee states that 'While the body of research linking saturated fat intake to the modulation of LDL and other circulating lipoprotein concentrations is significant, this evidence is essentially irrelevant to the question of the relationship between diet and risk for cardiovascular disease'.

Sugar and Coronary Heart Disease: closer to the truth?

As far back as 1957, English physician and nutritional scientist, Dr John Yudkin, had published good quality research correlating sugar intake with an increased risk for coronary heart disease and related deaths. Even in Ancel Keys's Seven Countries Study, a significant correlation between the incidence of coronary heart disease and the percentage of calories from sucrose in the diets was noted. However, these researchers were so intent on associating saturated fat and cholesterol as the causes of heart disease, that these other inconvenient findings were simply overlooked or ignored.

Recent research findings show the risk of death from coronary heart disease increases in direct proportion to sugar intake. A 2014 study by Quanhe Yang et al., of the Division for Heart Disease and Stroke Prevention at the Centre for Disease Control and Prevention (CDC) suggests that individuals who consume high amounts of added sugar in their diet may be at increased risk of death from cardiovascular disease. Compared with people who consumed around 8% of daily calories from added sugar, the findings were the following:

- Those who consumed between 17-21% of daily calories from added sugar had a 38% higher risk of CVD mortality.
- Those who consumed more than 21% of daily calories from added sugar had double the risk of CVD mortality.
- The risk of CVD was almost tripled for those who consumed 25% of daily calories from added sugar.
- Regular consumption of sugar-sweetened drinks, defined as 7 or more servings every week, was linked to increased risk of CVD mortality.

Chapter 5 - Cholesterol, Saturated Fat, Sugar and Heart Disease

Research from the EPIC study (Khaw et al., 2004) shows the most accurate predictor of future heart disease to be the glycated haemoglobin HbA1c blood test (an index of average blood sugar over the past 90 days). HbA1c showed a significant and continuous relationship with cardiovascular disease and all-cause mortality in both men and women and therefore was proven to be much more predictive than cholesterol levels.

In support of a reduced carbohydrate intake, James DiNicolantonio and colleagues wrote in a recent 2015 review article 'To reduce the burden of CHD (*coronary heart disease*), guidelines should focus particularly on reducing intake of concentrated sugars, specifically the fructose-containing sugars like sucrose and high-fructose corn syrup in the form of ultra-processed foods and beverages'.

Summary of the main factors associated with increased Coronary Heart Disease risk

- Persistently elevated blood glucose and elevated HbA1c levels
- Elevated fasting insulin levels
- Metabolic syndrome (pre-diabetes)
- Type 2 Diabetes
- High blood pressure
- Arterial inflammation associated with
  - Smoking
  - Advancing age
  - High fructose intake
  - Elevated blood sugar (glucose) levels
  - Elevated insulin levels
  - High trans-fat and omega-6 rich vegetable oil intake
- Atherogenic dyslipidaemia including high LDL particle number
- Familial hypercholesterolaemia (FH)
- Significantly elevated cholesterol levels in men under 50 years of age

Table 10: Know Your Numbers That Count and What They Mean

Index	Good	Measure	Bad	Meaning
LDL	Large ++	Particle size & no.	Small dense ++	LDL Pattern B Increased heart disease risk
HDL	High > 1.2	mmol/L	Low < 1.0	Increased heart disease risk
Triglycerides	Low < 1.2	mmol/L	High > 1.5	Increased small dense LDL Increased heart disease risk
Total cholesterol : HDL ratio	Low < 4.5	ratio	High > 5.0	Increased heart disease risk
Triglycerides : HDL ratio	Low < 1.0	ratio	High > 3.5	Metabolic syndrome Increased heart disease risk
HbA1c	Low < 5.4	%	High > 5.5	Increased risk of diabetes Increased heart disease risk
Serum insulin	Low < 6.0	µIU/mL	High > 10	Insulin resistance Increased heart disease risk

Chapter 5 - Cholesterol, Saturated Fat, Sugar and Heart Disease

Key Points: Cholesterol and Heart Disease

1. **Cholesterol is essential to human life. Without cholesterol in your body you would have no functioning cells, no bone structure, no muscles, no hormones, no sexual function, no reproductive system, no digestion, no brain function, no memory, no nerve endings, no movement, no life processes!**
2. **Dietary cholesterol intake makes no significant difference to circulating cholesterol levels and is not a risk factor for heart disease.**
3. **Elevated total blood cholesterol levels are associated with coronary heart disease but are not the proven cause of the disease.**
4. **Low HDL, small LDL particle size, increased LDL particle number and elevated triglycerides are associated with, and more predictive of, increased coronary disease risk.**
5. **Elevated cholesterol does not appear to be a significant heart disease risk factor in women of any age or in men aged over 50 years.**
6. **Statins do not significantly prevent heart attacks in people who do not already have established coronary heart disease.**

Key Points: Fats and Heart Disease
1. Dietary saturated fat makes little difference to circulating triglyceride levels.
2. Saturated fat is not associated with increased risks of heart disease.
3. Trans-fats, margarines and vegetable oils increase heart disease risk.

Key Points: Sugar and Heart Disease
1. Arterial inflammation is a major factor in coronary heart disease.
2. Sugar, refined carbs and insulin are significant role players in coronary heart disease because of the adverse, combined effects of elevated blood sugar, insulin and atherogenic lipid profiles on arterial health.

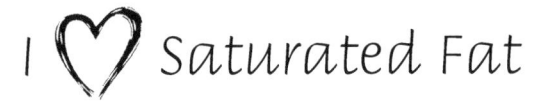

I ♥ Saturated Fat

Chapter 5 - Cholesterol, Saturated Fat, Sugar and Heart Disease

The Low-Carb Companion

SECTION TWO:

THE DIET

Chapter 6
LOW-CARB, HIGH-FAT NUTRITIONAL GUIDELINES

'In treating a patient, let your first thought be to strengthen his natural vitality'.
Rhazes, Persian Physician

....

Low-Carb Nutrition by other names:
- Low-carb diet (LCD)
- Low-carb, high-fat (moderate protein) diet (LCHFD)
- Very low-carbohydrate ketogenic diet (VLCKD)
- Commercialised and popularised versions – *the Atkins Diet, the Paleo Diet, the Dukan Diet, the Banting Diet or to 'Bant', the Noakes Diet*

Low-Carb Programs – there are three broad categories according to the level of carb restriction:
- A reduced carbohydrate diet: 130g - 200g of carbs per day
- A low-carbohydrate, high-fat diet (LCHFD): 30g - 130g of carbs per day
- A very low-carbohydrate ketogenic diet (VLCKD): < 30g of carbs per day

Individual carbohydrate tolerances vary widely, but it is safe to assume that the worse your disease of lifestyle, the less carbs your body will tolerate. Low-carb programs for general weight loss will restrict carbs simply based on cutting out the principal starches and sugar. If you have type 2 diabetes, metabolic syndrome (pre-diabetes) or childhood epilepsy, then a more controlled restriction to less than 30g of carbs per day (a ketogenic diet) is necessary for good results.

Who may benefit from a low-carb nutrition program?

Research and clinical evidence supports the use of LCHFD or VLCKD in the following conditions:

- Acne
- ADHD
- Age related macular degeneration
- Alzheimer's dementia
- Asthma
- Autism
- Cancer (colon, breast, prostate)
- Childhood epilepsy
- Coeliac disease
- Coronary heart disease
- Depression
- Fibromyalgia
- Gallbladder disease
- Gastro-oesophageal reflux (GORD, GERD)
- Gestational diabetes
- Gout
- Hypertension
- Irritable bowel syndrome
- Metabolic syndrome
- Migraines
- Non-alcoholic fatty liver disease (NAFLD)
- Obesity
- Parkinson's disease
- Polycystic ovary syndrome (PCOS)
- Rheumatoid arthritis
- Schizophrenia
- Sleep apnoea
- Type 2 Diabetes

> *'White flour is better suited to glue for primary school art projects than for nutrition'.*
>
> — *New Atkins New You*

What to eat: EAT REAL FOOD! √√
- Food in its natural form as much as possible
- As organic as possible (grass-fed beef, free-range chickens & eggs)
- Full fat dairy
- Food cooked and dressed in natural fats
- Unlimited fresh vegetables
- Cooked vegetables (especially those grown above ground)
- Healthy nuts and seeds
- Occasional fruit, mostly berries, citrus or apples

Eat the *'SUPERFOODS'* often: √√
- Butter
- Eggs (free range is best)
- Liver (especially chicken livers)
- Kidneys
- Fatty fish (salmon, mackerel)
- Lard
- Bacon (ideally nitrate/nitrite free)
- Coconut oil
- Avocados

What *NOT* to eat: XX
- Processed / baked grain-based foods including bread, cereals, rice, maize, pasta, refined oats
- Processed meats

- Sweets, milk chocolate, carbonated drinks, fruit juices
- Low-fat dairy / low-fat anything
- Vegetable (seed) oils, margarine
- Starchy root vegetables (grown underground)
- Dried fruit
- Soya (unfermented)
- Synthetic sweeteners
- Sugary alcoholic drinks and beer

No grain... No pain!

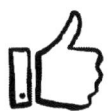

Table 11:
THE LOW-CARB COMPANION: THE 'YES' LIST

MEATS (grass-fed or organic is best)	VEGETABLES	VEGETABLES
 • Bacon (charcuterie, non-nitrated) • Beef, lamb, pork, venison • Biltong (beef jerky) • Broths • Chicken, duck, turkey • Cured meats with minimal sugar (pancetta, Parma ham) • Organ meats (liver, kidneys) • Sausages (containing meat & spices only, salami, chorizo) **FISH & SEAFOOD** • Calamari • Fish (the oilier the better) • Shellfish • Tuna in brine (not sunflower oil)	• Artichoke hearts • Asparagus • Aubergines (Eggplant) • Broccoli • Brussel sprouts • Cabbage • Cauliflower • Celery • Courgettes • Kale • Leeks • Marrows • Patty pans • Peppers • Pumpkin • Radishes • Rape / Kovu • Spinach • Spring onions	• Avocado • Cucumber • Green beans • Lettuce • Mange tout • Mushrooms • Olives • Onions • Rocket • Sauerkraut • Sugar snaps • Tomatoes **FRUIT** • Apples • Berries • Citrus • Coconut • Pears

Chapter 6 - The Low-Carb, High-Fat Nutritional Guidelines

EGGS	**NUTS** *(raw & unsalted)*	**SEEDS**
Free range best	• Almonds	• Chia
	• Brazils	• Flaxseeds
NUT & SEED FLOURS	• Hazelnuts	• Psyllium husk
	• Macadamias	• Pumpkin
• Almond flour	• Marula nuts	• Sesame
• Coconut flour, flakes, desiccated	• Mongongo nuts	• Sunflower
• Flax flour (Linseed)	• Peanuts	
• Hazelnut flour	• Pecans	**HERBS & SPICES**
• Pumpkin flour	• Pine nuts	
	• Pistachios	• Herbs, spices
	• Walnuts	• Salt ½ tsp/day
		• Vinegar
FATS & OILS	**DAIRY (FULL CREAM)***	
		SWEETENERS
• Avocado oil	• Butter	
• Beef / lamb tallow	• Buttermilk	• Erythritol
• Bone broths	• Cottage cheese	• Stevia
• Coconut oil, coconut cream / milk	• Cream	• Xylitol
• Duck fat	• Cream cheese	
• Ghee	• Crème fraiche	**BEVERAGES**
• Lard	• Fermented milk (amasi/lacto)	• Cocoa
• Macadamia oil	• Milk	• Coconut water
• Marula oil	• Soft & hard cheeses	• Coffee
• Mayonnaise (home-made)	• Yoghurt (Greek)	• Sparkling water
• Nut butters – almond, macadamia, organic peanut, pecan	*(for weight loss, restrict dairy intake initially, except for butter)*	• Teas
• Olive oil		• Water

Table 12:
THE LOW-CARB COMPANION: THE 'NO' LIST

GRAINS & CEREALS	VEGETABLES	FRUIT
• 'Gluten-free' - cornflour, tapioca, ricestarch, potato starch • All wholegrains • Barley • Bran • Bread, crackers • Breakfast cereals, muesli • Buckwheat • Couscous • Gravy thickeners, stock cubes • Maize (corn) • Millet • Oats • Pasta, noodles • Popcorn • Quinoa • Rice • Rye • Semolina • Sorghum • Wheat & all grain flours	• Baked beans • Beans • Carrots (cooked) • Chickpeas • Lentils • Parsnip • Peas (tinned) • Potatoes • Veggie juices **FOOD ADDITIVES*** • Food dyes esp. E102,E104,E110, E122,E124,E129 • MSG (E621) • Textured vegetable protein • Yeast extract *Food additives specified by E nos. on food labels	• Bananas (ripe) • Dried fruit • Fruit juices • Pineapples • Tinned fruit **JUNK FOOD** • Biscuits • Cakes • Chutney • Corn curls • Crisps, chips • Doughnuts • Energy bars • Fried fast foods • Jam • Jellies • Milk chocolate • Pizza (flour based) • Sweet desserts • Sweets, candy • Tomato ketchup

Chapter 6 - The Low-Carb, High-Fat Nutritional Guidelines

SOYA	*NUTS & DRIED FRUIT*	*MEATS*
• All unfermented soya products • Edamame beans • Soy milk • Soya sausages, soya mince • Tofu	• Flavoured / sugared nuts • Raisins, dates, sultanas, glazed cherries	• Battered fish • Cured meats • Luncheon meats • Processed meats • Vienna sausages
FATS & OILS	*DAIRY*	**SWEETENERS**
• Canola oil • Commercial salad oils & sauces • Corn oil • Cottonseed oil • Flaxseed oil • Grapeseed oil • Hempseed oil • Hydrogenated oils • Margarine • Peanut oil • Rapeseed oil • Safflower oil • Soybean oil • Sugar-added peanut butter • Sunflower oil • Tinned fish in vegetable oil	• Cheese spreads • Chocolate milk • Condensed milk • Fruit yoghurt • Ice-cream • Low-fat anything **BEVERAGES** • All carbonated drinks • Beer, Cider • Energy drinks • Fruit juices • Horlicks, Milo • Liqueurs & cocktails • Sweet wines	• Acusulfame K • Agave syrup • Aspartame • Dextrin • Dextrose • Fructose • Glucose • HFCS • Honey • Malt • Maltodextrin • Saccharin • Splenda • Sucralose • Sucrose • Syrup, Maple syrup

Table 13:
THE LOW-CARB COMPANION: THE 'SOMETIMES' LIST

Can be eaten occasionally and in small quantity. To be avoided if trying to lose significant weight.

DAIRY	VEGETABLES	FRUIT
• Milk (full cream) ½ cup	• Beetroot • Butternut • Carrots (raw) • Peas (raw) • Sweet potato	• Cherries • Clementines • Figs • Gooseberries • Grapes • Guavas • Kiwi • Litchis • Mangos • Nectarines • Pawpaw • Peaches • Pears • Plums • Pomegranate • Prickly pear • Quince • Watermelon

SWEETS	NUTS	BEVERAGES
	(with higher carb content)	
• Dark chocolate (>80% cocoa)	• Cashews	• Brandy
• Honey (1 tsp, only in cooking)	• Chestnuts	• Champagne
		• Dry wine
		• Rum
		• Sparkling wine
		• Tequila
		• Vodka
SOY		• Whiskey
• Organic soy sauce (in cooking)		

Table 14: THE LOW-CARB COMPANION '25 GRAMS OF CARB' LIST for a Very Low-Carb Ketogenic Diet (VLCKD)

Carbs restricted to 25g daily. For obesity, type 2 diabetics and childhood epilepsy.

DAIRY	VEGETABLES	FRUIT
• Fresh milk 2C • Yoghurt, full cream ⅔C **NUTS** • Almonds 230g • Cashews 150g • Macadamias 270g • Peanuts 200g • Pecans 270g **NUT BUTTERS** • Almond 8 Tbsp • Cashew 5 Tbsp • Macadamia 12 Tbsp • Peanut 7 Tbsp • Pecan 12 Tbsp	• Artichokes 2 • Avocadoes 3 • Butternut 1½C • Sweet potato ½ C Below: 5C raw/2½C cooked • Bean sprouts • Beans (green) • Beets • Broccoli • Brussels sprouts • Cabbage • Carrots • Cauliflower • Celery • Cucumber • Eggplant • Greens • Lettuce • Mushrooms • Okra • Onions • Pea pods	• Apples 1½ • Banana (small) 1 • Blackberries 3½C • Blueberries 1½C • Cherries 1½C • Clementines 3 • Figs (small) 3 • Gooseberries 1½ C • Grapefruit ¾ • Grapes green 1C • Guavas 2 • Kiwi fruit 2 • Litchis 18 • Mangos sliced 1C • Naartjies 4 • Nectarines 2 • Oranges 2

Chapter 6 - The Low-Carb, High-Fat Nutritional Guidelines

SWEETENER	VEGETABLES	FRUIT
• Honey (1 tsp, only in cooking)	• Peppers • Radishes • Rutabaga • Spinach • Tomatoes • Zucchini	• Papaya 1½C • Pawpaw 1 • Peaches 1½ • Pears 1 • Plums 4 • Pomegranate ½ • Prickly pears 4 • Quince 2 • Raspberries 2C • Strawberries 2C • Sweet melon 1½ • Watermelon 2C
KEY *C = Cup per day* *Tbsp =Tablespoon per day* *tsp = teaspoon per day* *g = grams per day*	------>	*AMOUNTS INDICATE approx. 25g OF NET CARBS**

* *For example, on a on a very low-carb ketogenic program with a restriction of 25g of carbs per day, a total of 2 oranges would be the total carbs allowed for one day.*

Table 15: Macronutrient Content of Real vs Processed Foods*

REAL FOOD 100g	CARB g	FAT g	PROTEIN g	PROCESSED FOOD 100g	CARB g	FAT g	PROTEIN g
Chicken (skinless)	0	1.5	23	Pork Pie	24.6	30.6	8.8
Beef	0	2.8	22	Sausage & Onion Lattice	20.3	27.7	8.7
Milk	5	3.4	3	Ice cream	22.9	10.1	3
Liver (chicken)	0	4.8	17	Chocolate Éclair	31.2	28.1	6.7
Eggs	1	10	13	Biscuits	62.7	23.4	6.7
Salmon (pink)	0	3.5	20	Crisps	50	34	3.9
Avocado	9	15	2	Savoury Cheese Snack	49.8	30.8	11.1
Cheese (Cheddar)	0.1	33	25	Choc Chip Chewy Bars	65	18.4	7
Cream	3	37	2	Chocolate	56.3	32.5	6.6
Butter	0	75	trace	Shredded Wheat cereal	80	2	11
Olive oil	0	100	0	Carrot Cake	79	10	5
Coconut oil	0	100	0	Strawberry Jam	64	0	0
Lard	0	100	0	Chocolate Milk	10	3	3

*Note the low-carb content of the unprocessed nutritious real foods vs. the high-carb content of the multi-ingredient processed foods.

Table adapted from *The Obesity Epidemic* by Zoe Harcombe

Chapter 6 - The Low-Carb, High-Fat Nutritional Guidelines

Table 16: The Macronutrient Composition of Nuts & Nut Butters

MACRONUTRIENTS IN NUTS BY CALORIE RATIO and FIBRE CONTENT

NUT	Fat % by calories	Protein % by calories	Carb % by calories	Fibre % by weight
Almond	73%	13%	14%	11%
Macadamia	88%	4%	8%	9%
Pecan	87%	5%	8%	9%
Brazil	85%	8%	7%	5%
Walnut	81%	8%	11%	5%
Peanut*	73%	16%	11%	8%
Cashew	67%	12%	20%	3%

peanuts (groundnuts) are legumes, not true nuts

MACRONUTRIENT COMPOSITION OF NUT BUTTERS
Quantity = 2 tablespoons

NUT BUTTER	Calories	Fat (g)	Protein (g)	Carb (g)	Fibre (g)
Almond	190	16	7	6	4
Macadamia	230	24	2	4	3
Pecan	213	20	3	4	2.5
Hazelnut	180	17	4	5	3
Peanut	190	16	8	7	3
Cashew	190	15	5	10	1.5

Key Points: Low-Carb Nutrition
1. Eat real foods.
2. Eat the 'superfoods' often.
3. Avoid processed foods as they often contain high amounts of sugar and refined carbs.

Chapter 6 - The Low-Carb, High-Fat Nutritional Guidelines

Chapter 7
LOW-CARB NUTRITION – GETTING STARTED

'Do the difficult things while they are easy and do the great things while they are small. A journey of a thousand miles must begin with a single step'.
Lao Tzu

....

Lifestyle change is about embarking on a new way of life. For some of you, it might be quite radical, for some a gentle transition. For families, it can be a challenge to separate your new eating habits from those of the family, but it's not as hard as you think. More often than not, the family eventually joins you on the journey. Below are five basic steps to get you started and to keep you going on a low-carb, high fat, moderate protein nutrition program. Begin a real food, healthy-fat nutrition journey that will become a lifestyle.

1. Clear out the pantry

Out with the 'old' and in with the 'new'! Clearing out the pantry and kitchen cupboards of all the things you should not eat is a must. This way, you reduce the chances of error, temptation, giving in to cravings or just eating the wrong things. Start by clearing out the following:
- All wheat and grain-based foods, including wholegrain and whole wheat varieties of bread, noodles, pastas, pastries, baked foods and cereals

- All other processed carbs, sugar and starches such as rice, corn products, maize meal, popcorn, potatoes, chips, crackers, biscuits, pastries, muffins, pizza bases, cakes, doughnuts, sweets, energy bars, ice-cream, sweetened low fat yoghurts, jellies, jams, marmalades, chocolate spreads, peanut butter, tomato sauce, processed cheese spreads, gravy powders, stock cubes, dried fruit, fruit juices, soft drinks, energy drinks, honey, sugar (brown or white), syrups, agave
- All 'gluten-free', 'low-fat' and 'fat-free' foodstuffs
- Margarine and vegetable oils
- Processed meats
- Soy products (non fermented) like tofu and soy milk

2. Restock the pantry

Your shopping list will include the following (the more organic and pasture-fed, the better):

- Healthy natural fats and oils (olive oil, coconut oil)
- Nuts and seeds, coconut chips
- Fruits and vegetables
- Meats, offal and fish
- Eggs
- Full-fat dairy
- Coconut cream & coconut milk
- Nut & coconut flours
- Nut butters
- Herbs, spices & condiments
- Sweeteners like Xylitol or Stevia
- Tea, coffee & cocoa
- Dark chocolate & red wine!

3.   Establish your baseline health profile

See your doctor, dietician or contact a Low-Carb Nutrition Program near you to have your baseline biometric (body) measures and blood tests done (see page 32). Biometric measures can be repeated monthly and blood tests can be repeated every 3-6 months. There is nothing more rewarding and motivating than steady and positive measured improvements in your health profiles. These measures are also very useful to your health and nutrition advisor to monitor your progress (or lack of) and to give you further constructive evidence-based data-driven advice.

4.   Follow Dr Jeans's Beginner 'Low-Carb Rules'

These rules are guidelines that will apply differently to each individual. For example, what constitutes too much dairy for you may be different to the next person. If you are on a 'self-help' program then follow the guidelines in the food lists on pages 124 - 133. More specific information can be obtained from your nutrition advisor.

1. Eat primarily real (whole) foods. Where required, cook them from scratch.
2. Eat fat at every meal. Natural fats are your friend.
3. Eat non-starchy vegetables and add fat to them (olive oil / butter).
4. Eat when you are hungry, stop when you are full, fast in-between.
5. Eat eggs often. Every day if you like!
6. Eat food cooked in healthy, heat-stable fats.^
7. Add a small pinch of salt to main meals.

Chapter 7 - Low-Carb Nutrition - Getting Started

8. Avoid processed foods (if not, avoid added carbs by reading food labels†).
9. Avoid snacking in between your 2 or 3 main meals.
10. Avoid sugar or grains as these will likely stop fat burning for 3-5 days.
11. Avoid overeating beyond feeling full.
12. Avoid excess protein (the palm-sized portion rule applies, this is not a high protein diet).
13. Avoid too many fruits* and nuts. Do not eat them in large quantities or daily.
14. Avoid too much fresh dairy* (see food lists for guidance).
15. Avoid alcohol binges.*

^ *Healthy, heat-stable cooking fats are avocado oil, ghee, refined coconut oil, beef tallow, duck fat, extra light olive oil, lard, butter see Table 5 on page 62.*

† *Food labels - the many names for sugar added to processed food*

* *For obese people and people with type 2 diabetes, a total restriction of fruit & alcohol and very limited fresh dairy is recommended for the first 4-6 weeks*

'Sugar by any other name is still sugar'!

Table 17: The Many Names For Sugar Added To Processed Food

Sucrose	Dextrose	Fructose	HFCS
Buttered syrup	Cane sugar	Cane juice	High fructose corn syrup
Maple syrup	Grape sugar	Fruit juice	Refiner's syrup
Lactose	Diastase	Icing sugar	Date sugar
Confectioner's sugar	Maltase	Honey	Demerara sugar
Dehydrated cane juice	Beet sugar	Golden sugar	Raw sugar
Galactose	Sugar syrup	Cane crystals	Crystalline fructose
Dextran	Glucose	Maltose	Maltodextrin
Corn syrup	Caramel	Treacle	Agave nectar
Diastatic malt	Sorbitol	Sorghum syrup	Carob syrup
Barley malt	Castor sugar	Mannitol	Fruit juice concentrate
Malt	Yellow sugar	Molasses	Glucose solids
Corn sweetener	Granulated sugar	Turbinado sugar	Invert sugar
Evaporated cane juice	Corn syrup solids	Malt syrup	Ethyl maltol

Any food label showing a sugar content exceeding 5g per 100g (or per 100ml) should be avoided.

Chapter 7 - Low-Carb Nutrition - Getting Started

5. Follow the Easy Low-Carb 'Substitution' Options

Find and follow easy low-carb options to substitute for common high-carb foodstuffs, such as those listed below. More options can be found in Part Two, *The Food Companion*.

Table 18: Easy Low-Carb Substitution Options

Low-Carb, Healthy-Fat Option	To Replace
Almonds, pecans, macadamia nuts, peanuts	*Cashews, choc peanuts & dried fruit*
Avocado oil, Coconut oil, Olive oil, Lard for frying	*Vegetable cooking oils*
Berries, apples, pears, citrus fruits - fresh	*Tinned fruit, fruit juices, bananas, grapes*
Bone broths, low-carb soups	*Canned soups*
Butter	*Margarine*
Cauliflower mash	*Mashed potato*
Cauliflower rice	*Rice*
Cocoa with full cream milk	*Chocolate milk (sweetened)*
Coconut battered fish	*Crumbed / flour battered fish*
Coconut flour wraps, pancakes	*Wheat flour wraps, pancakes*
Courgette pasta / noodles	*Pasta*
Cream	*Sweetened cream, condensed milk*
Cream, coconut cream, low-carb ice cream,	*Ice cream*
Dark (80%+) chocolate	*Milk chocolate*

Low-Carb, Healthy-Fat Option	To Replace
Dried goji berries	Dried fruit
Dried meat (biltong, jerky), nuts, coconut pieces	Crisps, junk snacks
Fatty cuts of meat, mince or liver	Burgers, cured & processed meats
Full cream milk	Low fat / no fat / skimmed milk
Full cream yoghurt	Low fat (sweetened) yoghurt
Hard cheeses – cheddar, feta, halloumi	Processed cheese, cheese spreads
Homemade low-carb mayonnaise, Olive oil	Commercial mayonnaise & salad oils
Hot cocoa with cream	Hot chocolate (sweetened)
Low-carb (egg and cheese / cauliflower) pizza bases	Wheat flour or gluten free flour pizza bases
Low-carb breads & seed crackers	Bread & crackers
Low-carb confectionaries & desserts	High-carb sugared confectionary & desserts
Low-carb smoothies	Milkshakes
Nut butters – macadamia, pecan, almond	Jam, chocolate spreads, honey
Nut, seed & coconut granola/muesli	Cereals
Sparkling water, still water, tea, coffee	Soft drinks (colas), fruit juices, energy drinks
Sweet potato chips baked in olive oil	Potato chips fried in vegetable oil
Xylitol, Stevia	Sugar, Fructose, Synthetic sweeteners

Chapter 7 - Low-Carb Nutrition - Getting Started

Low-Carb On A Budget

Many of the common foods associated with a low-carb, high-fat program are deemed expensive, but it is quite simple to manage a cost effective low-carb program with the following options:

- Bone broths
- Beef fat, tallow, suet for cooking
- Cheaper cuts of fatty meat like shin and brisket
- Pork products (pork fat, pork belly)
- Home reared poultry (chicken, turkey)
- Eggs
- Organ meats (offal) such as liver, kidney or heart
- Any fish
- Fresh milk
- Fermented milk products (lacto, amasi) & homemade live culture yoghurt
- Home grown vegetables – sweet potatoes, cauliflower, cabbage, tomatoes, onions, rape, etc.
- Avocadoes and wild fruits
- Nuts - groundnuts (peanuts), Marula nuts, Mongongo nuts
- Marula nut oil
- Peanut butter (organic, unsweetened)
- Coconuts – raw, whole or coconut flakes
- Unrefined starches – sorghum, millet, maize, oats (where your low-carb program permits)

In relation to low-carb food costs, bear in mind that lower quantities of food are eaten with less frequency because of the lack of hunger. The long-term savings on health costs need to be considered as well. The costs of obesity, diabetes and heart disease are significant.

Not Losing Weight? – The '12 Step' Checklist to Find The Problem

An inability to achieve early weight loss (or hitting a weight-loss plateau) can be very frustrating! Work through the 12-step checklist below either on your own or with your nutrition advisor. 'Stubborn weight loss' is often a result of one or more of the following issues:

1. **Carb intake still too high** - You may still be exceeding your individual carb tolerance and therefore need to cut back further on the amount of carbs you are eating; this may include moving downwards from a low-carb to a very low-carb intake.
2. **Inadequate fat intake** - Often, women remain reluctant to increase their fat intake because of old habits and mistaken beliefs, and men are reluctant for fear of cholesterol and heart disease, but once you cut down total carb intake, your healthy natural fat intake must increase to restore 'metabolic energy balance' to the body. If you do not increase the fat intake, you will not see healthy weight loss as your body holds onto its stored fuel in 'starvation' mode.
3. **Excessive food portions** - Habitual large food portions need to be cut down; appetite suppression happens naturally in most people with a higher fat and moderate protein intake after the first two weeks or so. Cutting meals to two per day also helps. If it does not help, then progress to intermittent fasting (water only) for 24 hours every couple of days at a time to reduce insulin levels and mobilise fat stores.
4. **Frequent snacks** - Avoid snacking, especially lots of nuts, as this leads to excessive calorie intake. Remember to eat when hungry and not in between.
5. **Excessive dairy** - For some, especially if you are obese or have type 2 diabetes, restricted fresh dairy milk and cream cheese intake is needed to reduce the potential weak sugar effects of lactose (milk sugar).

6. **Excessive protein intake -** Ingestion of large amounts of protein may cause insulin spikes and the conversion of amino acids to glucose (via the process of gluconeogenesis) with weight gain effects. Limit protein to a moderate intake (palm-sized portions).
7. **High fruit intake -** Fruits contain a variety of sugars including glucose and fructose; certain fruits are more sugary than others. If weight loss is not achieved, then restrict fruit intake.
8. **Alcohol intake too high -** Avoid alcohol, especially beer, sweet or fortified wine, liqueurs and cocktails, which are high in carbs.
9. **Slow fat adaptation -** For some severely carb-intolerant people, the best way to initiate or promote metabolic change is to start by fasting (no food, only water) for 24 hours.
10. **You may be overweight but not carb-resistant -** If you have no insulin resistance issues and have 'pear shaped' subcutaneous weight distribution in the buttocks and the thighs, rather than central 'visceral' belly fat, then you may have the type of body that does not always respond to dietary manipulation. Fortunately, this type of fat is not associated with the adverse health effects of central 'belly' fat.
11. **An underactive thyroid gland -** Your doctor can test this.
12. **Medications -** Certain medical drugs encourage weight gain and discourage weight loss; the most common ones are beta-blockers, diuretics, corticosteroids (e.g. prednisolone), anti-depressants (e.g. SSRIs such as Prozac), hormone therapy (oestrogen, HRT, oral contraceptives) and insulin.

Key points: How to get started on a low-carb program
1. Clear out the pantry.
2. Restock with the 'good' things.
3. Establish your baseline health profiles.
4. Stick to the basic beginner rules.
5. Follow easy low-carb options to replace high carb foods.
6. Follow the 'low-carb on a budget guidelines' if cost is an issue.
7. Look to the '12 Steps' if weight loss is stubborn or hits a plateau.

Chapter 7 - Low-Carb Nutrition - Getting Started

The Low-Carb Companion

SECTION THREE:

SPECIAL POPULATIONS

Chapter 8
LOW-CARB FOR BABIES, CHILDREN, TEENS & PREGNANT MUMS

'I prefer the company of peasants because they have not been educated sufficiently to reason incorrectly'.
Michel de Montaigne

....

Low-carb, higher healthy-fat nutrition is perfectly healthy for younger age groups and pregnant women and provides them with the essential macronutrients plus the vitamins and minerals they require for healthy growth and development.

> Babies and children should not be exposed to a diet high in sugary processed foods that may leave them addicted, allergic, behaviourally compromised, prone to weight gain and unhealthy for life.

BABIES – The first year
Under 6 months of age

- 'BREAST IS BEST' for babies whose mother's breast milk supply is adequate. Breast milk can be the sole provider of nutrition for up to six months, and then used in conjunction with foods until two years of age.

- The energy (or calories) in breast milk comprises 54% (mostly saturated) fat, 38% carb and 8% protein.
- Commercial baby formulas are not an ideal substitute for breast-feeding.
- Be aware that commercial baby formula milk is often 'carb-heavy' and is heavily sugared.
- For example, two popular commercial baby formulas list their constituents as:
  - Baby Formula A: 43% corn syrup solids + 10.3% sucrose (+ water)
  - Baby Formula B: 50% corn syrup + 14.2% soy protein + 10.4% high oleic safflower oil + 9.7% sucrose + 8.2% soy oil + 7.5% coconut oil
  - => Effectively, these two baby formulas expose the child to a diet of 60% sugar!
- Soy-based formulas should be avoided until after six months of age.
- Alternatives to cow's-milk formulas are extensively hydrolysed cow's-milk formula or a whey-based formula.

6 – 9 months: Breast-feeding and weaning

- Weaning babies onto healthy fats and healthy carbs is important. Start with pureed or mashed vegetables (broccoli, baby marrow, butternut, pumpkin, green beans, squash, carrots), avocados, beef, lamb, chicken, fish and chicken liver. Extra fat can be added in the form of butter, olive oil, coconut oil or ghee.
- Bone broth is a very nutritious liquefying food to add to baby puree.
- Introduce flax cereal and creamy porridge.
- Introduce mashed whole eggs or egg yolk. (Previous evidence suggested egg whites should be limited until the babies are older, but more recent research does not support this).
- Water is the healthiest drink for babies and is certainly a healthier alternative to most baby formulas that comprise water, flour and sugar.

- Fruit purees other than apple should probably be delayed until 9 or 10 months old to avoid early exposure to fructose, but this is not a hard and fast rule; mixing fruit puree with pureed vegetable combinations is tasty and nutritious.

10 – 12 months: Introduce more solid foods and continue breast-feeding

- Full cream dairy – milk, cream, yoghurt, hard cheeses
- 'Finger foods' - diced chicken pieces, stewed meat pieces, steamed/baked vegetable and fruit (apple, strawberries) cubes, raw carrots, low-carb bread cubes, avocado pieces, low- carb bread
- Whole eggs
- Fruit, pureed or grated (apple, pear, nectarine), cooked or raw, mixed with cream
- Fish, unsalted nut butter (not if allergic to nuts)

FOODS TO AVOID IN THE 1ST YEAR: salt, fried food, honey, spinach, beetroot, leafy celery, soft cheeses (like Brie and Camembert), liver pâté, sugar, sugared high-carb baby food, sweeteners, possibly egg whites.

FOODS THAT CAN CAUSE ALLERGIES: citrus fruits, shellfish, legumes (peanuts), strawberries and gluten grains (including cereals). Traditional teaching has been to introduce these potentially allergenic foods only after one year of age, and one at a time to determine sensitivity. Recent research, however, suggests that earlier introduction between 4 – 8 months under controlled conditions may significantly reduce the risk of food allergies (G Du Toit et al., D Da Silva et al.).

TODDLERS: 1 – 3 years old

- Protein and fat are essential nutrients in this key stage of physical growth and on-going brain development.
- **Over 60% of the brain is comprised of fat.**
- Omega-3 fatty acids that come from fatty fish, crushed nuts or nut butters and pasture-fed beef are essential for the developing brain, both structurally and functionally.
- Animal protein is an important component of the toddler's diet and provides key amino acids.
- Eggs, avocados, berries and dairy products are all 'superfoods' for this age group.
- Toddlers need a variety of brightly coloured vegetables.
- Adding butter and salt to food is a great way to enhance flavour.
- Small infrequent amounts of unrefined non-gluten grains such as quinoa, millet, buckwheat, oats, or brown rice may be incorporated into toddler nutrition.
- Most importantly, avoid exposing your child to junk (processed) food, sugar or gluten grains (wheat, rye, barley, baked foods).

SCHOOL AGE CHILDREN

For children going to school, choose healthy snacks and treats for their lunch boxes comprising low-carb, real food alternatives instead of processed junk food.

Healthy lunch box ideas:
- Almonds, coconut & seed clusters
- Apple slices with nut butter

- Avocado, feta & tomato salad
- Bacon and cheddar cheese mix
- Basted chicken wings
- Biltong (jerky) and nuts
- Cheese cubes rolled in ham
- Chicken cubes & avocado
- Cream cheese balls
- Dried boerewors / sausage
- Full cream yoghurt & fruit
- Low-carb pizza
- Low-carb bread and nut butter
- Low-carb brownies
- Low-carb muffins like coconut and berry muffins
- Low-carb wraps with healthy tasty fillings
- Mini beef cubes & cherry tomatoes
- Mini meatballs
- Mini quiches
- Nuts, seeds and coconut mix
- Seed crackers with homemade cream cheese

TEENAGERS

The teenage years are characterised by increased growth-driven appetites (especially in boys between the ages of 14 -18 years, who require 20 - 40% more calories than girls!), increased self-awareness and body consciousness, a search for independence, intense peer pressure, and an acute susceptibility to media marketing, including that of the fast food industry.

> Teens in Europe and the USA ingest up to 34 teaspoons of sugar per day from soft drinks and junk food!

Chapter 8 - Low-Carb Nutrition and the Family

A recent UK study on weight perception among 5000 teenage boys and girls found that 47% of overweight boys, and 32% of overweight girls, perceived themselves to be 'about the right weight'. The study authors noted that 'this lack of awareness of excess weight among overweight and obese adolescents could be a cause for concern' (SE Jackson et al.).

Parents can best serve their teenagers by:

- Acting as role models regarding healthy food choices and lifestyles.
- Teaching them that troublesome skin conditions, like acne, are aggravated by sugar and junk food but improve with low-sugar, healthy-fat choices (RN Smith et al., K Stevenson et al.).
- Showing teenagers in search of protein supplements for 'mirror muscles' that better food options like 'egg milk' and homemade, low-carb chocolate milk are easy to make. (NOTE: Many commercial protein supplements also contain high amounts of carb and can lead to significant weight gain if taken excessively).
- Talking to them gently about sensitive subjects like being overweight and helping them to understand the concept of *what* they eat matters more than how much they eat.
- Positively, but not authoritatively, providing tips and advice about good food and choices.
  - Cheese & ham instead of *bread and jam*
  - Cheese chips instead of *potato crisps*
  - Dark chocolate rather than *sweets / candy*
  - Homemade hot cocoa with cream rather than *commercial hot chocolate*
  - Low-carb ice-cream in place of *commercially made ice-cream*
  - Low-carb pancakes with cream instead of *flour based pancakes and jam*
  - Low-carb wraps instead of *hamburgers*

- ➢ Mixed nuts instead of *chocolate peanuts*
- ➢ Nuts, even peanuts instead of *chips*
- ➢ Sparkling water in place of *colas, fruit juices and energy drinks*
- ➢ Sweet potato buttered chips instead of *vegetable oiled French fries*

PREGNANCY

Wholesome real food based on low-carb, healthy-fat nutrition is perfectly nutritious for the pregnant mum and her in-utero baby, and provides all the required macronutrients and micronutrients for maternal health and baby's growth and development.

- Avoiding processed foods becomes even more important during pregnancy.
- The risks of high blood pressure, eclampsia and gestational diabetes are reduced with low-carb nutrition.
- Overweight women who eat a high-refined carb diet during pregnancy tend to deliver overweight babies who become overweight adults with increased risks of metabolic syndrome, coronary heart disease and diabetes.
- The baby in-utero who is exposed to high maternal blood sugars and insulin levels is likely to be born with a high risk of future insulin resistance.

Guidelines for low-carb nutrition in pregnancy include:
- Increased intake of eggs, bone marrow and healthy animal fats. Fat is important for the baby's brain development.

Chapter 8 - Low-Carb Nutrition and the Family

- Fatty fish rich in omega-3 fatty acids like salmon, mackerel, herring, sardines and anchovies (omega-3s may also help to reduce post-partum depression) are important.
- Liver in small, infrequent amounts (<30g) is an excellent source of fat and retinol (Vitamin A). ***see cautionary note**
- Meat, fish, chicken, eggs, organ meats and game are all excellent sources of high-quality protein and haeme iron.
- On a low-carb program in pregnancy your carb intake should be more than 50 grams daily, i.e. lower-carb but not very low-carb (ketogenic) levels; there is, as yet, inadequate research on nutritional ketosis in pregnancy for it to be medically recommended. An adequate carb intake can easily be obtained by increasing your starchy vegetable, fruit and dairy intake. Occasional non-gluten grains are also OK but not necessary.
- High fibre vegetables of all colours should be included in the daily diet.
- Fruits should be limited to two per day. If you are struggling with weight issues, avoid eating too much of the very sweet fruits like grapes and pineapples.
- Sauerkraut (cabbage) and fermented foods create healthy maternal gut bacteria (the 'gut biome') that prime the baby's digestive flora during natural birth.
- During the first 6-12 weeks of pregnancy when morning nausea may be a problem, eating fatty food later in the day is usually better than at breakfast.

*Caution regarding liver: *There is some evidence that suggests that eating liver or liver products (paté or liver sausage) during pregnancy should be very minimal or not at all, because of the potential risks of excessive retinol ingestion (retinol is the pure form of Vitamin A found in relatively high concentrations in liver). High doses of retinol pose potential risks to the developing foetus.*

> **Key Points: Low-Carb for Babies, Kids, Teens and Pregnant Mums**
> 1. Low-carb nutrition is healthy for babies, young children and teens.
> 2. A balanced lower-carb, high-fat moderate protein program during pregnancy is healthy but carb intake should exceed 50g daily.
> 3. Pregnant women should not eat too much liver.

Chapter 8 - Low-Carb Nutrition and the Family

Chapter 9
LOW-CARB NUTRITION AND DIABETES

'Let food be thy medicine and let thy medicine be food'.
Hippocrates

Type 2 Diabetes Mellitus - *fast facts:*

- 'Diabetes' means 'passing water like a siphon' and was named by the ancient Greek physician Aretaeus. 'Mellitus' means 'tasting like honey' and was added by the English doctor, Dr Thomas Willis in 1674.
- There are three types of diabetes - type 1, type 2 and gestational (in pregnancy).
- Although they share the same name, type 1 and type 2 diabetes have different disease origins and profiles.
- Type 1 diabetes is caused by a failure of the pancreas to produce insulin as a consequence of viral or autoimmune destruction of the pancreatic beta cells. It is characterised by very low or absent levels of insulin with associated elevated blood sugar.
- Type 2 diabetes
  - is a disease of progressive insulin resistance (IR) with elevated levels of insulin and blood sugar.
  - is the most common form of diabetes constituting 90 - 95% of all diabetes cases; it is categorised as a 'disease of lifestyle'.

- has a genetic trend as over 50 genes that increase risk have been identified to date.
- is strongly associated with obesity; 80% of type 2 diabetics are obese.

> Diabetes, along with obesity, is the fastest growing disease in the world (the term coined is 'DIABESITY') and diabetes cases worldwide are projected to more than double in the next decade.

- In the USA:
  - The dramatic rise in obesity and diabetes occurred within 5 years of the introduction of the low-fat, high-carb US Dietary Guidelines for Americans in 1977.
  - The total cost of treating a diabetic over the age of 50 yrs. is estimated to be $150,000 - $250,000 in direct and indirect health costs.
- Among American children, parallel with soaring childhood obesity rates, the prevalence of type 2 diabetes has increased dramatically.
  - It is estimated that 1 in 3 boys and girls born after 2000 will develop diabetes.
- For every diabetic, it is estimated that there are 3-4 pre-diabetics 'waiting in the wings'.
- Consuming one to two sugar sweetened drinks per day increases the risk of developing diabetes by up to 26% (Romaguera et al., Malik et al., Hu et al.).
- Habitual consumption of sugar-sweetened beverages is associated with a greater incidence of type 2 diabetes, independent of body weight in a recent Cambridge review study (Imamura et al.).
- Statin therapy increases the risk of developing diabetes (up to 48% increased risk in a 2012 study on 160,000 post-menopausal women by Culver AL. et al.).
- Two out of three diabetics die from cardiovascular disease.

- In **TYPE 2 DIABETES**
  - The **DISEASE is SEVERE INSULIN RESISTANCE** caused by chronic **ELEVATED INSULIN.**
  - The **SYMPTOM is ELEVATED BLOOD SUGAR** caused by a high refined carb intake and increased liver glucose secretion in the presence of insulin resistance.

- Type 2 diabetics have high levels of insulin (in contrast to type 1 diabetics who suffer insulin deficiency) and only in the late stages of severe disease do insulin levels fall as the pancreatic beta cells suffer increasing damage and dysfunction.
- High blood sugar, elevated insulin and belly fat in diabetes wreak havoc on the body through insulin toxicity, glucotoxicity, lipotoxicity and inflammation.
- Insulin is both ATHEROGENIC (directly causes arterial disease) and OBESOGENIC (belly fattening), whether elevated in the body naturally or through insulin treatment.
- The development of diabetes is preceded by fat accumulation in both the liver (NAFLD) and pancreas, a result of, and indeed a further cause of, increasing insulin resistance.
- According to diabetes expert, Dr Roy Taylor, 'Type 2 diabetes can be understood as a potentially reversible metabolic state precipitated by the single cause of chronic excess intra-organ fat'.
- Blood tests of liver function such as a rising Gamma-glutamyl transferase (GGT*) level, even within the 'normal' range, can be an early indication of fatty liver disease and thereby predictive of insulin resistance, metabolic syndrome and eventual type 2 diabetes (Grundy; Steinvil et al.). *See page 33 for your optimal GGT test results.
- Recent evidence shows that obese type 2 diabetics have significantly more fat accumulation in the liver and pancreas compared to obese non-diabetics. This evidence also shows that weight loss can result in a significant reduction in this intra-organ fat accumulation, and

- is accompanied by a normalisation of liver insulin sensitivity and pancreatic beta cell function (Fung; Steven et al.).
- Liver fat accumulation and insulin resistance predict worse atherogenic dyslipidaemia (Bril et al.).
- Heart disease in diabetics today is no less frequent than it was prior to 1921, the year insulin was discovered and subsequently used to treat type 1 and severe type 2 diabetes.
- When the fat content of a diabetic's diet is reduced and the carb content increased (as happened in the 1970s with the 'fear of fat and heart disease') the incidence of arterial disease increases 5 fold (Albrink MJ, as described by Gary Taubes in *The Diet Delusion*).
- Diabetic drugs that reduce blood sugar levels but increase insulin DO NOT TREAT THE DISEASE, WHICH IS INSULIN RESISTANCE!

- **Diabetes is a 'DIETARY DISEASE' and diet is therefore the 'CURE'!**

Diabetes results in:
- Accelerated ageing
- Atherogenic dyslipidaemia (small dense LDL (high LDL-P), low HDL, high triglycerides)
- Coronary heart disease (risk increased 2-5x)
- Circulatory disease and limb amputations
- Hypertension
- Kidney disease
- Increased cancer risk (notably breast & colon cancer)
- Nerve damage (diabetic neuropathy)
- Increased risk of Alzheimer's (2x risk)
- Infections & foot ulcers
- Blindness
- Premature death (usually from heart disease)

Figure 17: Insulin, Insulin Resistance and the Development of Type 2 Diabetes

EXCESSIVE INSULIN CAUSES DIABETES

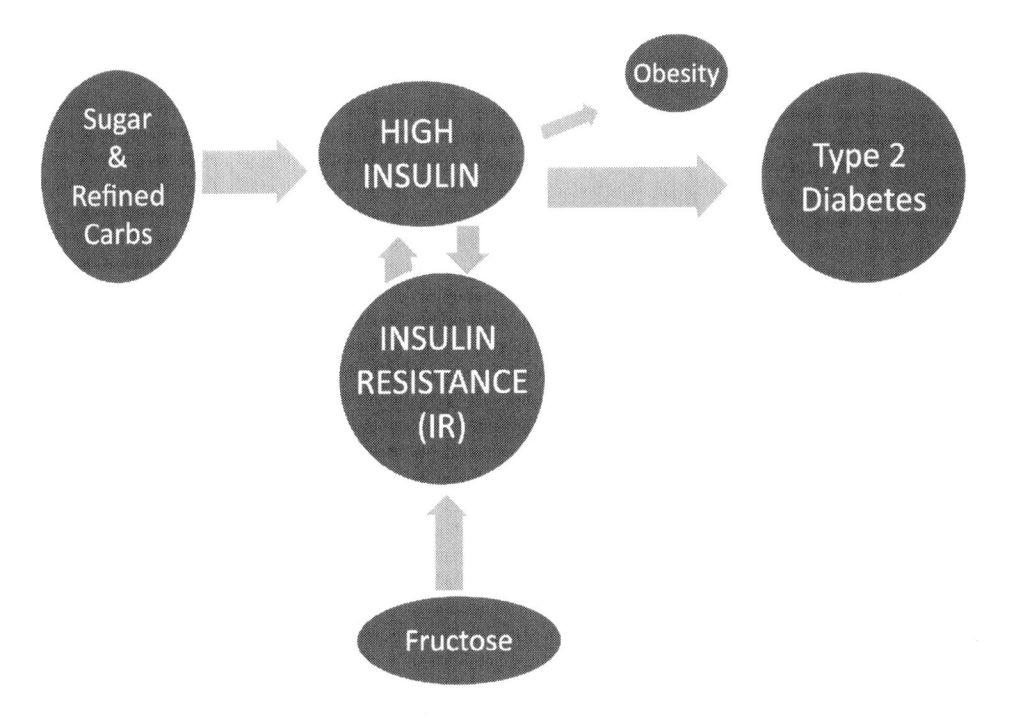

Over 80% of people with type 2 diabetes suffer a thrombotic death (heart attack, stroke or peripheral vascular complication)! This may be explained by the following effects of sugar and insulin on blood clotting:
- Excessive fructose results in hyperuricemia (high uric acid levels), which is associated with reduced blood vessel endothelial nitric oxide causing vasoconstriction, endothelial dysfunction and insulin resistance.
- Hyperglycemia allows IGF-1 to stimulate smooth muscle proliferation in blood vessel walls, a hallmark of atherosclerosis.
- Blood coagulability (clotting) is increased by hyperglycemia.
- Hyperinsulinaemia is associated with reduced fibrinolysis and increased risk of thrombosis (Crofts, et al.).

Summary of risk factors for developing diabetes

- Family history of type 2 diabetes
- Obesity (belly fat) – if your BMI is over 30 kg/m² your diabetes risk increases ten times
- Age (70% of diabetics are over 50 yrs. old)
- Metabolic Syndrome (pre-diabetes)
- Gestational diabetes (80% will go on to develop permanent diabetes)
- Being born of an obese mother or a mother who developed gestational diabetes
- High-carb diet with lots of sugar / high fructose corn syrup & refined carbs*
- High intake of sugared carbonated drinks
- Being inactive
- Taking statins

*A recent, extremely large, epidemiological study reported that diabetes risk is directly correlated, in an apparently causative manner, solely to sugar intake, regardless of weight or sedentary lifestyle (Basu S. et al.).

Take-home message: Prevention is better than cure.

If you have a family history of diabetes, do yourself a favour and endeavour to PREVENT its onset by living a healthy lifestyle.

- Do not eat significant amounts of sugar, refined carbs or processed foods
- Eat real food (low-carb, healthy-fat) nutrition
- Maintain a healthy weight
- Exercise regularly
- Be cautious about taking statins (unless you have Familial Hypercholesterolaemia or established coronary artery disease)

Using very low-carb nutrition as a treatment strategy for type 2 diabetes

Medical nutrition goals in diabetes are to attain & maintain optimal metabolic outcomes measured as:
1. Reduced insulin levels and increased insulin sensitivity
2. Reduced fat accumulation in the liver and pancreas
3. Blood sugar in normal range (or as close to normal as safely possible)
4. Weight reduction, especially belly fat
5. Heart-friendly lipid profiles
6. Normal blood pressure
7. Normal metabolic state
8. Normal healthy life, free of complications

Chapter 9 - Low-Carb Nutrition and Diabetes

The 'traditional' nutritional approaches to type 2 diabetes have been based on diets that reduce fat intake and correspondingly increase carb intake. The success of this approach has been limited, not surprisingly, since diabetes is a disease of severe carb intolerance! Ironically, we treat lactose intolerance with restricted lactose intake; likewise, we treat gluten intolerance with restricted wheat intake. However, we have been allowing diabetics to consume up to 150g of carbs daily because of an out-dated and unjustified fear that fat causes heart disease, and also because of a limiting belief that the brain can only utilise glucose for energy. As the diabetic state worsens over time, the traditional therapeutic approach is more likely to progress to the use of oral drug treatments to control blood sugars and eventually insulin therapy in the more severe cases. Yet all the evidence points clearly to the fact that weight gain and diabetic cardiovascular complication rates worsen with insulin therapy.

The mounting research-based evidence shows that **very low-carb, higher-fat nutrition** in diabetics produces the following positive results (Schofield, et al.) :

- Reduced insulin fluctuations
- Improved blood sugar control
- Reduced or eliminated diabetes medications
- Effective weight loss
- Improved risk markers for cardiovascular disease
- Reduced blood pressure and medications
- Initial beneficial effects of carb restriction, like lower blood sugars and reduced blood pressure, occur before significant weight loss

Very low-carb, higher-fat nutrition in action: At the Duke University Lifestyle Medicine Clinic, Dr Eric Westman and his colleagues use a very low-carb ketogenic diet (VLCKD), without calorie restrictions, to treat diabetics.

Their results show that insulin treatment requirements drop by up to 50% in the first 24 hours of carb restriction (less than 20g carb/day) and that by 6 months, 95% of patients are able to reduce or eliminate their glucose-lowering medications (Westman et al., Feinman et al.).

The American Diabetes Association (ADA) acknowledged the use of low-carb diets in diabetes management in their 2008 Guidelines stating:

- Modest weight loss has been shown to improve insulin resistance in overweight and obese insulin-resistant individuals.
- Weight loss is recommended for all overweight individuals who have, or are at risk for, diabetes.
- Low-carb diets may be effective for weight loss in the short term (up to one year).
- Patients on low-carb diets should have their lipid (cholesterol) profiles, kidney function and protein intake (for those with kidney damage) monitored regularly.
- To avoid hypoglycaemia, patients who follow a low-carb diet and who take blood sugar lowering medications, need to have them monitored and adjusted as needed.

The practical points about low-carb nutrition for a type 2 diabetic.

1. You will need to utilise a very low-carb ketogenic dietary program (VLCKD) with carbs restricted to < 25g/day to induce nutritional ketosis.
2. You will need to stick rigidly to the YES food list on page 126 and be guided by the 25g carbs/day list (page 132).
3. If you are a 'diet controlled' diabetic, you can introduce the VLCKD, although it is highly recommended that you seek the advice and guidance of an experienced dietician who is familiar with low-carb programs.

4. If you take oral glucose-lowering medication like metformin or glibenclamide, then you should definitely consult your doctor before you begin a program.
5. If you are using insulin, then it is mandatory from the outset that you engage your doctor to monitor your progress; there is a real danger of hypoglycaemia in the early stages of a VLCKD as insulin requirements can drop dramatically in the first days of restricted carbs.

Nutritional KETOSIS

- Nutritional ketosis is a perfectly normal physiological metabolic state that occurs during prolonged fasting or when carbohydrates are restricted below 50g/day (on a very low-carb, high-fat ketogenic diet program).

- When carb stores become depleted after 3-4 days, the liver produces higher than normal levels of ketone bodies (beta-hydroxybutyric acid, acetoacetate and acetone) from fat in a process called ketogenesis.
- Ketone bodies provide an efficient and 'clean' fuel source for the brain, heart and tissues; they are able to produce more energy than glucose because of the metabolic effects of ketosis.
- During nutritional ketosis, normal fasting blood sugar levels are maintained by two mechanisms. The first one is the production of glucose from amino acids (protein) in a process called gluconeogenesis. The second mechanism is the utilisation of glycerol that is liberated in the breakdown of triglycerides.
- In nutritional ketosis, blood ketone levels will normally range from 0.5-3mmol/l; they do not exceed 8mmol/l and blood pH remains in normal limits.
- Physiologically normal nutritional ketosis must be differentiated from the pathologically abnormal condition of DIABETIC KETOACIDOSIS, a

dangerous state that occurs in type 1 diabetes and is characterised by very high blood ketone levels exceeding 10mmol/l, often progressing to over 20mmol/l, associated with acidic blood pH. Ketoacidosis does not occur in non-diabetics.

The weight loss effects of a VLCKD seem to be caused by the following factors:

1. Reduction in appetite due to
    - A higher satiety effect of proteins
    - The effects of appetite-control hormones
    - A possible direct appetite suppressant effect of ketone bodies
2. Reduction in fat production and storage (lipogenesis) and increased release of fat from fat stores (lipolysis)
3. A greater metabolic efficiency in utilising fats for energy
4. Increased metabolic costs of gluconeogenesis and the 'thermic effect' of proteins (greater energy cost to digest proteins)

Chapter 9 - Low-Carb Nutrition and Diabetes

Key Points: Low-Carb & Type 2 Diabetes

1. The onset of type 2 diabetes can be prevented in high-risk individuals who follow a low-carb, high-fat nutritional lifestyle.
2. Type 2 diabetes is a potentially curable disease once we recognise that insulin resistance is the cause and that elevated blood sugar is a symptom.
3. Diabetic drugs that reduce blood sugar levels but raise insulin levels, DO NOT TREAT THE DISEASE, WHICH IS INSULIN RESISTANCE!
4. Diet is the 'CURE'! Reducing carbs reduces insulin which abolishes insulin resistance = the end of type 2 diabetes.
5. Type 2 diabetes should more accurately be renamed Type 2 *insulin-resistant* diabetes and Type 1 diabetes renamed Type 1 *auto-immune* diabetes.

LOW-CARB NUTRITION – A ROLE IN TYPE 1 DIABETES?

'To avoid sickness, eat less; to prolong life, worry less'.
Chu Hui Weng

....

Type 1 diabetic patients have conventionally been instructed to follow a low-fat, high-carbohydrate diet for the following reasons:

1. Most type 1 diabetic patients eventually develop heart disease and die of complications related to heart disease.
2. The conventional 'healthy heart' diet has, to date, been a low-fat diet, which meant a high-carbohydrate diet. This high-carb diet meant that more insulin would be needed to control blood sugar levels.

We now appreciate that there are two main problems with this reasoning:

1. Dietary cholesterol and saturated fat have minimal impact on serum cholesterol or the risk of coronary heart disease. There was never any conclusive and compelling evidence to support the low-fat diet (Harcombe et al.).
2. There is strong evidence that high doses of insulin are harmful to the body.

Persistent high levels of insulin over many years lead to insulin resistance and 'Insulin Toxicity' (Fung).

Chapter 9 - Low-Carb Nutrition and Diabetes

There are far fewer published studies on low-carb diets for the management of type 1 diabetes. However, clinical studies have shown the metabolic benefits of carbohydrate-restricted diets, including the ketogenic diet (Nielsen et al., Toth et al.). A 2012 clinical audit by Nielsen et al. concluded that there is **no evidence for the following:**

- The use of the widely recommended high-carbohydrate, low-fat diet in type 1 diabetes.
- The belief that dietary animal fat causes cardiovascular disease.
- The belief that protein intake causes kidney disease; in fact, hyperglycaemia results in a 3½ times higher incidence of kidney dysfunction.

The audit also stated that there is strong evidence for the following:
- The aggressive development of damage in all organs in poorly regulated type 1 diabetics.
- That a low-carbohydrate diet lowers the need for insulin, and reduces the number of hypoglycaemic episodes (low blood sugar attacks).
- That a low-carbohydrate diet is sustainable in the long-term.

Toth et al. presented a case of a 19-year-old male with newly diagnosed type 1 diabetes (T1DM) who was put on a standard insulin treatment regime and then, after twenty days, was put on a low-carb 'paleolithic ketogenic' diet. With strict adherence to the diet, the patient was able to discontinue insulin treatments, had normal glucose levels and exhibited biochemical evidence of restored pancreatic insulin production. By 6½ months, no symptoms, signs or side effects had emerged. The conclusion was 'that the paleolithic ketogenic diet was effective and safe in the management of this case of newly diagnosed T1DM...that the paleolithic ketogenic diet may halt or reverse autoimmune processes destructing pancreatic beta cell function in T1DM'.

Research shows that type 1 diabetics who require high insulin dosages to manage their high-carbohydrate, low-fat intake, eventually develop similar problems to type 2 diabetics such as weight gain (belly fat), hypertension and coronary heart disease, all of which are features of insulin resistance.

> As diabetic specialist, Dr Jason Fung, postulates, 'In type 1 diabetes the persistent exposure to high levels of insulin eventually leads to type 2 diabetes'!

A 2014 study by Larry Distiller titled 'Why do some patients with type 1 diabetes live so long?' identified the following features of long-surviving patients with type 1 diabetes:

- Reasonable (not necessarily ideal) glycaemic control
- High HDL-cholesterol levels
- No evidence of metabolic syndrome (insulin resistance)
- Low daily insulin requirements ('insulin sensitive')
- Normal body weight
- Non-smokers
- Lower blood pressures
- No evidence of kidney disease (nephropathy) after 15-20 years with diabetes
- Family history of longevity

The key points that can be deduced from the above are that:

1. Elevated blood sugars and 'glucotoxicity' are factors, but not the major factors, in type 1 diabetes disease complications.
2. Low daily insulin requirements are significantly correlated to survival, indicating that insulin sensitivity is maintained by lower insulin dosages.
3. The presence of insulin resistance (metabolic syndrome features) negatively affects survival, which means that 'insulin toxicity' is a major factor that influences disease progression and associated complications.

Take-home messages for people with type 1 diabetes

- Reasonable, but not tightly controlled, levels of blood sugars are important.
- Insulin therapy will always be required but the less insulin required, the better.
- A low-carbohydrate (ketogenic) nutrition program will minimise insulin requirements.

The Food Insulin Index

A potentially useful tool for diabetics may be found in the concept of a 'Food Insulin Index' or Insulin Score, which is a measure of the insulin demand of different foodstuffs (Holt et al., Bell, Kendall). In these studies, the postprandial (after eating) insulin responses to measured portions of several common foods were compared to those of white bread and glucose.

Interesting findings in Holt's research are the following:
- The consumption of fat or protein with carbs increased more insulin secretion compared to the insulinogenic (insulin stimulating) effects of these nutrients alone.
- Within food groups with similar nutrient compositions (carb/fat/protein)
    - there was a wide range of insulin responses.
    - bread and potatoes were amongst the most insulinogenic foods.
    - highly refined bakery products and snack foods induced substantially more insulin secretion than other foods.

- Equal carb servings of food do not necessarily stimulate insulin to the same extent; this challenges the scientific basis of carb exchange tables, since these assume that portions of different foods containing 10-15g of carb will have equal physiological effects and will require equal amounts of exogenous insulin in order to be metabolised.
- Post-eating insulin response is not necessarily proportional to the blood glucose response (GI).
- The glycaemic (blood glucose) response is a significant predictor of insulin response but together with the macronutrient (protein/fat/carb/sugar/starch/water) content of food only accounts for 33% of the variation in insulin responses to food. In other words, in whole foods with multiple constituents there are other factors that influence insulin response.
- Western diets high in refined carb are likely to be more insulinogenic than more traditional diets higher in unrefined foods.

Bell's research found the food insulin index to have the following practical applications:

1. Calculating insulin dose using the food insulin index data provided better blood sugar control for type 1 diabetics than normal carbohydrate counting.

2. Type 2 diabetics improved their blood sugar control by choosing foods that caused a lower insulin secretion, regardless of calories or carbohydrates.

Kendall's writings detail specific foods and their insulinogenic effect. From these, it can be concluded that:

Chapter 9 - Low-Carb Nutrition and Diabetes

- The carbohydrate content of a food alone does not accurately predict insulin response.
- The food insulin index data indicates that dietary fat is the one macronutrient that does not require a significant amount of insulin.
- Net carbohydrates plus approximately half protein correlates well with observed insulin demand.
- **Knowing the insulinogenic effect can be used to help select low insulin foods and more accurately calculate insulin doses for diabetics.**
- The importance of dietary fibre should not be underestimated, especially when trying to reduce insulin demand. Fibrous non-starchy vegetables provide vitamins and minerals that cannot be obtained from other foods (unless you're consuming a significant amount of organ meats), as well as feeding the gut bacteria, which is also important to help improve insulin sensitivity and the body's ability to digest fats.
- The more carbohydrates and/or protein ingested, the more insulin is required.
- In the carbohydrate vs. insulin relationship, the outliers are the high protein foods that trigger a higher insulin response than can be explained by considering carbohydrates alone.
- Choosing higher protein foods will generally reduce insulin.
- For most people, transitioning to a reduced carbohydrate whole foods diet will give them most of the results they are after. For type 1 diabetics, however, or people trying to design a therapeutic ketogenic diet, consideration of protein may be important to further refine the process to achieve the desired outcomes.
- For someone struggling to lose weight on a low-carb diet, considering the insulinogenic effect of protein might be what is needed to reduce insulin, normalise blood sugars and reach their goals.

Kendall proposes two practical applications of the food insulin index:
1. Individual foods can be ranked and prioritised based on their proportion of 'insulinogenic calories'. Foods with the lowest proportion of insulinogenic calories will have the least impact on blood glucose and have the lowest insulin demand. Some common food examples are shown in Table 19. A list of the percentage of insulinogenic calories of nearly 8000 foods on the USDA Foods List is available as a link on Kendall's Optimising Nutrition website.
2. Diabetics and people looking to reduce the insulin demand of their diet can determine the total 'insulin load' (as opposed to carbohydrate counting) using the following formula:

Insulin load = [carbs (g) – fibre (g)] + [0.56 x protein (g)]

The total insulin load can be reduced to achieve target blood glucose levels by:
- Decreasing carbohydrates
- Increasing fibre
- Moderating protein
- Increasing fat

The key points are to focus on eating foods that lower insulin requirements. This means taking into account the carbohydrate, protein and fibre content of specific foods. The lower the carb and higher the fibre content, the lower the insulin demand. Some lean protein foods may increase insulin requirements. This provides a more comprehensive method of measuring insulin requirements than simply measuring carb intake.

Chapter 9 - Low-Carb Nutrition and Diabetes

Key Points: Low-Carb and Type 1 Diabetes
1. Most type 1 diabetic complications are linked to the levels of insulin required for treatment; type 1 diabetes may progress to the development of progressive insulin resistance.
2. Foods that reduce insulin requirements also produce better outcomes.
3. A low-carb ketogenic diet improves type 1 diabetes and reduces insulin requirements.
4. Some protein foods may be insulinogenic.
5. The Food Insulin Index, % insulinogenic calories and calculating insulin load may be better measures of insulin requirements than carb counting.

Table 19: Insulin Responses of Common Foods
Data sources: Bell K; Holt S et al.

VERY SMALL INSULIN RESPONSE	LOW INSULIN RESPONSE	MODERATE INSULIN RESPONSE
Avocado	Peanut Butter	Beef steak (lean)
Bacon	Eggs	Carrot juice
Butter	Full cream milk	Cheddar cheese
Gin	Tuna	Muesli
Olive Oil	Cream cheese (full fat)	White fish
Walnuts	Peanuts	Apples
Wine	Chicken	All bran cereal
	Prawns	Raisins
	Porridge	Muffin
		Pasta (white/brown)
		Beer
		Milk chocolate
		Snickers bar

Chapter 9 - Low-Carb Nutrition and Diabetes

HIGH INSULIN RESPONSE	VERY HIGH INSULIN RESPONSE	VERY HIGH INSULIN RESPONSE
Low fat cottage cheese	Skim milk	Bread (white/brown)
Oranges	Vanilla ice-cream	White rice
Chocolate milk	Low fat ice-cream	Cornflakes
Cheese pizza	Low fat strawberry yoghurt	Shredded wheat
Lentils	Mars bar	Water crackers
Rice (brown/white)	Jam (raspberry)	Tinned peas
Popcorn	Bananas	Baked beans
Potato chips	Grapes	Potato
Croissant	Melon	Fat free pretzels
French fries	Iced tea	Jelly beans
Doughnut	Fruit juice	Cake
Coca cola	Pancake & Waffle Mix	Choc chip cookies

Table 20: % Insulinogenic Calories in Common Foods
Source: www.optimisingnutrition.wordpress.com

FOOD	% INSULINOGENIC CALORIES	FOOD	% INSULINOGENIC CALORIES
Fats & Oils		**Dairy**	
Olive oil	0%	Heavy whipping cream	3.5%
Butter	0%	Sour cream	8%
Coconut oil	0%	Full fat Greek yoghurt	25%
Lard	0%	Full cream milk	40%
Sugary foods		Skim milk, 1% fat	63%
Rice Crispies cereal	97%	Chocolate milk, low fat	65%
Jellies	98%	Vanilla ice-cream	75%
Jams and preserves	98%	Low fat yoghurt	76%
Sugar	100%	Fruit, low fat yoghurt	83%
Cranberry juice	100%	**Vegetables**	
Honey	100%	Broccoli	29%
Maple syrup	100%	Lettuce	36%
Cheeses		Mushroom	42%
Cream cheese	8%	Cauliflower	49%
Cheddar	15%	Carrots	62%
Gouda	18%	Onions	78%
Feta	18%	**Nuts & Seeds**	
Mozzarella	19%	Macadamia nuts	5%
Swiss	21%	Coconut meat	6%
Cream cheese, low fat	25%	Coconut cream	7%

Chapter 9 - Low-Carb Nutrition and Diabetes

FOOD	% INSULINOGENIC CALORIES	FOOD	% INSULINOGENIC CALORIES
Swiss, low fat	43%	Flaxseed	8%
Cottage cheese, low fat	55%	Peanuts	13%
Cream cheese, fat free	63%	Chia seeds	13%
Meats		Pumpkin seeds	14%
Pork, ham	11%	Almonds	14%
Duck	12%	Sesame seeds	14%
Liver pate	12%	Sunflower seeds	15%
Salami	12%	Cashew butter	22%
Pork sausage	13%	**Egg**	
Chorizo	13%	Whole egg	21%
Beef, rib eye	15%	**Fish & Seafood**	
Bacon	15%	Mackerel	13%
Fruits		Herring	19%
Olives	3%	Salmon	24%
Avocados	6%	Sardine	26%
Raspberries	42%	Trout	31%
Blackberries	47%	Tuna	32%
Gooseberries	51%	Squid	41%
Rhubarb, raw	55%	Sea bass	42%
Pears	63%	Crab	46%
Strawberries	67%	Tilapia (bream)	47%
Oranges	73%	Shrimp	49%
Apples	75%	Whitefish	50%
Bananas	84%	Haddock	50%
Watermelon	100%	Oyster	51%

Chapter 10
LOW-CARB NUTRITION AND CANCER

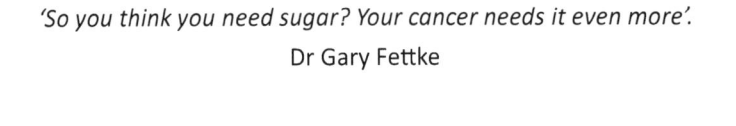

'So you think you need sugar? Your cancer needs it even more'.
Dr Gary Fettke

....

Cancer rates are rising worldwide. It is estimated that there will be a 70% increase in cancers over the next 20 years, especially in developing nations. There is already a 3% increase in cancer occurrence in children per annum. One in two men, and one in three women, will develop cancer.

As we move towards a greater understanding of the metabolic basis of cancer growth and development, cancer is being considered more of a metabolic disease. Modern cancer research is moving away from the area of genetics and DNA mutations that were once thought to be the bedrock of cancer genesis. The research is focusing more on understanding the metabolism of cancer with its implications for treatment.

We certainly need to be doing something different since statistics show that the current death rate from cancer is still the same as it was in 1950, and as a departure from current 'targeted' anti-cancer drug therapies, metabolic therapies have the potential to treat many, if not all, types of cancer by exploiting the dysfunctional metabolism that is common to every cancer cell (Christofferson).

Chapter 10 - Low-Carb Nutrition and Cancer

Some interesting facts about cancer:
- A recent paper in the journal, *Nature*, provides '... evidence that intrinsic risk factors contribute only modestly (less than 10-30% of lifetime risk) to cancer development' (Wu et al.). This suggests that up to nine out of ten cancers are caused by unhealthy lifestyles rather than bad genes.
- Diseases of lifestyle like obesity and type 2 diabetes are associated with an increased incidence of cancers, notably of the breast, colon, ovary, uterus and prostate.
- Coeliac disease (a condition of severe wheat intolerance) is associated with a significant increased risk of bowel cancers.
- Body weight and cancer risk:
  - Waist circumference is a powerful predictor of cancer, especially breast (2-4x increased risk) and colon cancer.
  - The World Health Organisation (WHO) says that after tobacco, being overweight or obese are the most important known, avoidable causes of cancer. In other words, OBESITY is the second highest risk factor for cancer after smoking.
  - Cancer Research UK data suggests that 274 in every 1000 obese women are expected to develop a weight-related cancer (bowel, breast, kidney) in their lifetime compared with 194 in every 1000 healthy weight women; this amounts to a 41% increased risk in obese women.
  - Obese women have a 30% higher risk of postmenopausal breast cancer than women with a healthy weight.
- Overweight women with breast cancer
  - have higher recurrence rates.
  - have five times increased death rates.
  - respond poorly to chemotherapy.
  - suffer more side effects from radiotherapy.
- A high trans-fat intake doubles the risk of breast cancer.
- Women with elevated blood sugars and breast cancer do not respond well to cancer treatment.

- Both hyperglycaemia (elevated blood sugar) and hyperinsulinaemia (elevated blood insulin) are predictors of cancer occurrence and cancer-related mortality.
- Fasting insulin levels predict outcome in women with early breast cancer.
- Elevated blood triglycerides are associated with an increased prevalence of breast cancer.

Cancer as a metabolic disease:

- Normal cells in the body do not take up essential nutrients such as glucose and glutamine without the appropriate growth signals, but cancer cells acquire mutations that allow them to take up nutrients autonomously.
- In a recent review, Pavlova & Thompson postulate that this altered metabolism may lie at the very heart of cancer by allowing cancer cells to maintain both viability and the capacity to build new cancer cells independent of the body's controlling mechanisms.
- **Cancer cells proliferate faster in a high-sugar environment.**
- There is increasing evidence linking cancer growth with insulin and IGF-1 (Insulin-like Growth Factor).
- The role of sugar in cancer cell metabolism was identified in the 1920s by German scientist Otto Warburg, who won the Nobel Prize in 1931 for his work showing that cancer cells use primitive and inefficient cellular glycolysis (a process of biological fermentation of glucose) for energy (ATP) production. This is known as the 'Warburg Effect'.
- Cancer cells do not use normal mitochondrial processes for ATP production.
- By doing so, cancer cells avoid the normal processes of programmed or

controlled cell death (apoptosis), which any other irreparably damaged or abnormal cell would undergo.
- As stated by oncologist Dr Robert Nagourney in his book, *Outliving Cancer*, 'Cancer cells don't grow too much, they die too little'.
- The 'Warburg Effect' allows cancer cells to divert glucose away from energy production to cell growth, facilitating the production of phospholipids required for cell structure.
- The glycolysis energy pathway also allows rapidly growing cancer cells to 'flourish' in an anaerobic environment where their rate of growth exceeds the available blood oxygen supply.
- Therefore, cancer cells need more and more sugar and can 'burn' up to 200 times more sugar than normal cells.
- In effect, cancer cells 'corrupt' cellular metabolism by having increased receptors for insulin and IGF-1 on their cell membranes, which enables them to command the sugar supply.
- There is increasing recognition of the association of diet and cancer; the chief culprits are sugar, particularly fructose, refined carbohydrates and polyunsaturated (omega-6 rich) vegetable oils that create a highly inflammatory environment in the body and result in significant amounts of DNA-damaging free radicals.
- Cancer cells invade surrounding cells and use free radicals to cause cell death. They, in turn, cause the release of the building materials required for their further growth.
- The 'voracious appetite' of cancerous cells for sugar is seen on a PET scan, frequently used in cancer diagnosis and monitoring, which demonstrates the uptake of radiolabelled glucose into tumours; virtually all cancers have the same PET scan appearance.
- 95% of cancer cells need glucose to survive; they cannot metabolise fat or ketone bodies.
- Existing cancer treatments have largely ignored the area of glucose metabolism. There is growing evidence to show that future cancer treatments will target how to starve cancer cells of their supply of

glucose and the stimulatory effects of insulin and IGF-1, including the use of low-carb nutritional ketosis as a therapeutic strategy.
- Nutritional ketosis has also been shown to be protective of normal cells during chemotherapy and radiotherapy treatment.
- The modern high-carb, seed-oil rich diet is inflammatory and chronic inflammation is the underlying link to cancer; inflammation is considered 'fertiliser' for cancer.
- Low-carb, healthy-fat ketogenic nutrition is not yet the cure for cancer, but it should be considered as part of a broad-based cancer management strategy alongside conventional chemotherapy and radiotherapy options.

- 'Diet changes the *nurture* rather than *nature* of cancer'.
  Dr Robert Nagourney *Outliving Cancer*

- Researchers have found that reducing carbohydrate intake could reduce the risk of breast cancer recurrence among women whose tumour tissue is positive for the IGF-1 receptor. They found an association between increased breast cancer recurrences in women with a primary breast cancer tumour that was positive for the IGF-1 receptor, which is consistent with other studies. They also found that a decreased carbohydrate intake was associated with decreased breast cancer recurrence for these women (Edmond JA et al.).

*Do you want the carbs...
or the cancer?*

Chapter 10 - Low-Carb Nutrition and Cancer

> **Key Points: Low-carb and Cancer**
> 1. Sugar, insulin, IGF-1 and inflammation facilitate the growth and spread of cancer cells.
> 2. By reducing the amount of sugar, refined carbohydrates and seed oils in the diet, the emergence of cancer can potentially be suppressed or delayed, or the proliferation of already existing tumour cells can be slowed down, stopped and reversed.

Chapter 11
LOW-CARB NUTRITION AND THE ATHLETE

'It's what we know already that often prevents us from learning'.
Claude Bernard

The use of low-carb/ketogenic diets for exercise, training and sports performance is the subject of increasing volumes of published research. It is the topic of numerous anecdotal reports by athletes in many disciplines who have been using a LCHFD successfully for years, even at the top level of sporting performance. The evidence supporting low-carb, high-fat regimens in various sports is growing. This evidence is not yet overwhelming, but it is certainly enough to challenge the traditional facts, dogmas and doctrines regarding optimal sports nutrition for athletes. Ketogenic diets may offer significant benefits to athletes in training and sports performance.

The evidence sometimes produces disparate results; this is often a result of studies that are conducted over periods of time that are too short. Studies that are done in less than 2 weeks may not allow sufficient time for true physiological fat adaptation to be measured in terms of training or performance benefits. Other studies have been limited by suboptimal intakes of protein and minerals (Phinney 2004).

In this chapter we will look at the potential roles of low-carb nutrition in the areas of:
1. Macronutrients as fuels for exercise
2. Endurance training and performance
3. Sport and weight control
4. Strength and power
5. Muscle mass

1. Macronutrients as fuels for exercise

Carbohydrate

The consensus view on carbohydrate and exercise, supported by numerous scientific studies in the past 80 years, suggests that carbs must constitute a major component of one's daily energy intake if optimum physical performance is to be maintained. This view is reinforced by the concept of muscle glycogen as the limiting fuel for high intensity exercise. This traditional view further holds that humans are physically impaired if given a low-carbohydrate diet since fat has limited utility as a fuel for vigorous exercise. For the past 50 years we have therefore been advised that glucose is the most important muscle fuel for exercise, especially at intense exercise levels and as a result, the belief that a high-carb diet is best for active individuals and athletes has prevailed. The body absorbs glucose from carbohydrates and stores it in the liver and muscles as glycogen. Circulating blood glucose, liver glycogen and muscle glycogen provide glucose for anaerobic and aerobic energy production to fuel muscle energy (ATP) requirements for exercise.

Traditional high-carb diets in athletes have several potential drawbacks such as:

1. There is a susceptibility to 'hitting the wall' in prolonged exercise; this term describes the fatigue that results from liver and muscle glycogen depletion and insufficient glucose for the muscles and brain. The body can only store about 2000kcal of carb as fuel (enough for 2-3 hours of exercise), despite having in excess of 50,000kcal of fat stores (enough for 4-7 days of continuous exercise). University of Connecticut researcher Jeff Volek calls 'hitting the wall' an 'inexcusable metabolic failure'! Since the athlete has not truly run out of fuel, this represents a failure of inter-organ fuel partitioning.
2. A reliance on regular carb/sugar refuelling during prolonged exercise often results in gastrointestinal upset.
3. Refuelling with carbs does not reliably prevent 'hitting the wall', as muscle glycogen depletion still occurs during intense levels of exercise.
4. There is no proven improvement in performance, even with 'carb-loading' nutritional strategies. We just burn the extra carbs faster!
5. An athlete can experience increased body weight from carb-loading strategies since each stored gram of carb is stored as glycogen with three grams of water. This can reduce an athlete's power-to-weight ratio.
6. There is a reduced physiological oxidation of fat since a high-carb intake blocks the utilisation of our more efficient and longer-lasting fat stores for exercise; burning fat is the best way to spare stored muscle glycogen and thereby prevents 'hitting the wall'.
7. Overweight athletes remain overweight despite high training volumes; the fact is, they are likely to be insulin-resistant and will fatten on carbs.
8. There is an increased risk of adverse health outcomes like diabetes, heart disease and dental problems.

Note: Exercise is not all about the CARBS!

Chapter 11 - Low-Carb Nutrition and The Athlete

Low-carb nutrition for sports training and performance is supported by strong scientific evidence and there are plenty of anecdotal reports from athletes who have successfully used a LCHFD. When carbs are restricted as an energy source, even at ketogenic levels of < 20g of carb daily, the main requirement is for the diet to have sufficient alternative sources of energy in order to adequately fuel exercise and positively influence performance. This occurs with an adequate fat intake and 'fat adaptation'.

Fat

Our fat stores are considerably larger (20 - 40 times larger in calorie terms) than our carbohydrate reserves. Fat is a very efficient fuel that supplies 9 kcal of energy per gram, which is more than double that of carbs. Utilisation of fat-derived ketone bodies creates more energy than glucose because of greater mitochondrial ATP energy production from ketone bodies by up to 31% (Veech, 2004).

A low-carb, high-fat program promotes fat adaptation and physiologically increases the capacity of the body to utilise fat for fuel to provide energy for exercise.

FAT ADAPTATION on a low-carbohydrate / ketogenic diet:
- There is a wide individual variance in time and degree with respect to fat adaptation.
    - Upon starting a low-carb, higher-fat program, an athlete takes about 7 days to show early fat adaptation, and up to 2 weeks to resume effective training, after experiencing a period of fatigue and weariness during this early fat adaptation phase.
    - It can take 2 - 4 weeks to exercise at previous endurance performance levels or to resume hard training.

> It can take 2 - 6 months for full fat adaptation to occur on a level commensurate with high performance in ultra-distance sport.
- A fat adapted athlete will satisfy their fuel energy needs from fat (fatty acid) oxidation, blood lactate, ketone bodies and gluconeogenesis.
- During exercise, fat derived ketone bodies provide efficient 'clean' fuel to the brain (supplying up to half of its energy needs) and to the heart as well.
- Fat adaptation results in markedly reduced rates of muscle glycogen utilisation, effectively sparing muscle glycogen stores.
- Protein (and thereby muscle mass) sparing is achieved because of the reduced requirement for gluconeogenesis.

Protein

Protein is not used as a fuel to energise exercise, but it is primarily important for athletes to maintain or build muscle (lean body) mass. However, dietary protein and possibly lean muscle is utilised in the early stages (first 7-14 days) of low-carb, higher-fat adaptation to provide glucose to the brain via gluconeogenesis (the conversion of protein to glucose in the liver). Later on, the increased use of fat and ketone bodies for energy substantially reduces the need for protein conversion.

How much protein is required?
- Optimal protein requirements in athletes are between 1.2 - 1.7 grams per kg body weight per day, and in some sports up to 2.5 grams per kg body weight. This amount ensures the availability of sufficient dietary protein for body protein replacement and for gluconeogenesis. A mid-range intake of 1.5 grams per kg body weight translates to 90-120g of protein per day.
- An insufficient intake of protein may impair performance. A 1990 study by Davis and Phinney showed that subjects consuming 1.1 grams of protein per kg of body weight experienced a significant reduction in

VO2max (aerobic endurance capacity) during a 3-month period on a very low-carb diet, compared with subjects given 1.5 grams per kg body weight who maintained their VO2max.
- An excessively high-protein intake of more than 25% of daily energy expenditure may actually act to suppress ketone body production from fat (possibly a result of insulin stimulation by the excessive protein).

The importance of mineral intake:

It has been demonstrated that protein metabolism in exercise with muscle mass preservation also hinges upon an adequate intake of both sodium (3-5g/day) and potassium (2-3g/day). These two minerals can be ingested from food or supplements. In a study by Phinney in 2004, he reported that with 'these supplements maintaining daily intakes for sodium at 3-5 g/day and total potassium at 2-3 g/day, our adult subjects were able to effectively maintain their circulatory reserve (i.e. allowing vasodilatation during submaximal exercise) and effective nitrogen balance with functional tissue preservation'.

The common misconception that a low-carb diet is unsafe because it is a 'high-protein, high-saturated fat' diet is false. The key feature of a correctly structured low-carb, or ketogenic dietary program, is an energy-sufficient diet with a relatively low-carbohydrate intake; this is completely compatible with normal protein consumption and a balanced nutritional intake of macronutrients and essential micronutrients.

2. Endurance Training and Performance

Fuel change:
- Once an athlete is fat adapted, muscle glycogen is used at a quarter of the rate during exercise compared to the rate glycogen is used in an

athlete on a high-carb diet. This lower rate of use amounts to effective muscle glycogen sparing.
- Significantly high rates of fat oxidation can be achieved, which would be sufficient to allow an athlete to cover their fuel requirements during an Ironman Triathlon event without the need for extra fuel consumption during the race. In contrast, a carb-fed athlete would require approximately 100g/hour of ingested carbs to maintain exercise performance at a similar level.
- Studies on low-carb runners show that they can use fat for fuel at high exercise intensities up to 80% of VO2max.

Other advantages:
- Less oxidative muscle damage occurs causing less DOMS (delayed onset muscle soreness).
- Faster recovery from prolonged exercise is achieved.
- Less central fatigue occurs as a result of
  - Muscle glycogen sparing
  - Ketone bodies and lactate that provide a reliable brain fuel supply
  - Increased brain serotonin levels from branched chain amino acids
- There is a reduced likelihood of gut distress as there is a reduced need for (carb) fuel ingestion during prolonged exercise.
- A reduced ventilatory drive occurs as fat oxidation increases, which makes the perception of effort seem easier.
- Better altitude tolerance is reported.
- A LCHFD is associated with improved health biomarker levels of HbA1c, HDL-cholesterol, triglycerides, fasting insulin and increased insulin sensitivity.
- Weight loss may increase an athlete's power-to-weight ratio, which can be increased further if the athlete's program includes appropriate resistance training.

Chapter 11 - Low-Carb Nutrition and The Athlete

Fine Tuning a LCHFD for sport:
- Athletes on a LCHFD require added sodium (salt) in their food to compensate for increased sodium losses and dilution effects of increased plasma volume in exercise.
- A 'Train-Low-Race-High' strategy may benefit shorter-distance, higher-intensity athletes. This involves a low-carb, higher-fat diet during training, and then an increased carb intake immediately before and/or during an event. The term 'sugar trickle' has been coined to describe the intake of small volumes of sports carb drinks during an event to improve performance during high intensity bursts of exercise.
- Research into 'Train-Low-Race-High' strategies suggests that carefully scheduled periods of training under conditions of low-carbohydrate availability may be beneficial for inducing skeletal muscle adaptations and improving subsequent performance. Some evidence suggests that the carbs taken may be affecting the brain rather than acting as metabolic fuel in the fat adapted athlete (Baar & McGee, 2008), (Burke LM et al., 2011).
- In a fat adapted athlete, taking carbs during races does not appear to affect fat adaptation or health.

In the Vermont Study (2004) conducted on cyclists by low-carb researcher, Dr Steve Phinney, findings show that 'despite four weeks of eating no visible carbs, in the four week test of the bike racers, their VO2max was unimpaired, and their endurance to exhaustion was pretty much the same as it had been initially, on the high-carb diet. But there was a change, and that involved what their cells used for fuel. At the start, when they were eating mostly carbs, the muscle cells of those bicycle racers were burning 50:50 carbs to fats. After four weeks, they're doing the same amount of work but almost 95% of the energy is coming from fat. This is quintessential evidence for keto(fat) adaptation. Meanwhile, in the muscle glycogen, they drop the total amount of glycogen in the muscles, compared to when they started. But doing exercise, they use far less of the glycogen for fuel'.

A recent study by Zajac et al., using a ketogenic diet in trained off-road cyclists showed:
- '... favourable changes in body mass and body composition, as well as in the lipid and lipoprotein profiles'.
- '... a significant increase in the relative values of maximal oxygen uptake (VO2max) and oxygen uptake at lactate threshold (VO2 LT) after the ketogenic diet, which can be explained by reductions in body mass and fat mass and/or the greater oxygen uptake necessary to obtain the same energy yield as on a mixed diet, due to increased fat oxidation or by enhanced sympathetic activation'.

In a 2014 review article 'Low-carbohydrate diets for athletes: what evidence?' by Noakes, Volek and Phinney, they comment on '...the key difference in the low and high carbohydrate dietary approach for endurance athletes. Once they deplete their endogenous carbohydrate reserves, athletes chronically adapted to high carbohydrate diets likely become entirely dependent on exogenous carbohydrate for their performance. In contrast, athletes adapted to a low-carbohydrate diet carry all the energy they need in their abundant fat reserves. And because they live and train with chronically low blood insulin concentrations, they have instantaneous access to those fat reserves at all times'.

3. Sport and Weight Control

Weight loss in certain athletes is desirable for different reasons:
- Weight loss improves an athlete's power-to-weight ratio in endurance sports and sprint and power activities.
- An athlete has to compete in a specific weight category like combat sports such as judo, karate, taekwondo, boxing and wrestling.
- In bodybuilding, an athlete needs to achieve an aesthetically pleasing, lean, low body fat appearance.

Unfortunately, many common methods that athletes use to reduce weight rapidly, like drastic energy reduction or rapid dehydration using saunas or diuretic drugs and other medications, may also have significant and detrimental side effects on sports performance and health. These methods are usually employed very close to competition time and with potentially negative consequences such as:
- energy (glycogen) depletion and weakness
- performance reduction
- electrolyte disturbances and water imbalance
- lean body mass (muscle) loss
- doping violations through the use of prohibited medications

Use of a low-carb diet for weight loss in athletes:
A LCHFD is an effective weight loss tool, but to be used effectively in weight-category sports, it cannot be used for rapid weight loss. It should be considered as a medium to long-term nutritional strategy for gradual body weight reduction and maintenance. Athletes should schedule a low-carb diet for weight loss at least 2 weeks before competition.

In the first few days on a LCHFD, initial weight loss is a result of muscle glycogen and stored water loss; initial fat loss starts after about 7 days and increases over time. Available data (Paoli, 2015) suggests that weight loss between 1.2 to 1.6 kg is possible in lean subjects, who weigh between 70 to 73 kg of body weight, during 3 to 4 weeks on a VLCHFKD without performance loss.

In a recent 2015 review article by Antonio Paoli et al., entitled 'The Ketogenic Diet and Sport: A Possible Marriage?', the authors state, 'We can propose some interesting fields of action of KD (ketogenic diets) in sports. It is a type of diet that appears to have several advantages over other types of extreme energy-restricted "crash" diets; the latter, even if used for just a few days, can create situations of undernutrition for essential nutrients (vitamins, minerals, essential fatty acids, and amino acids) as well as depriving the body of other macronutrients that help control oxidative stress and inflammatory processes. An energy-sufficient KD with an adequate amount of protein (minimum 1.3 - 1.5 g per kg of body weight) is not an "extreme" diet apart from the very low-carbohydrate levels (<20 g carbohydrates per day) and, as such, it does not lead to metabolic imbalances that can have irreversible effects if nutrient-deficient weight loss diets are repeated on a regular basis'.

4. Strength and Power

Limited studies are available on low-carb and strength or power development and performance. As mentioned already, low-carb nutrition may positively affect power by reducing body (fat) weight and increasing an athlete's power-weight ratio. One study on gymnasts demonstrated that compared with a standard ad libitum diet, a 30-day ketogenic diet did not negatively affect explosive and strength performance in a group of high-level gymnasts (Paoli A. et al., 2012).

Strength and power athletes may require higher protein intakes on a low-carb program. Intakes in the region of 2.5 grams of protein per kg body weight will meet body protein requirements and will preserve muscle mass.

It is interesting to note that Dr Nic Gill, the strength and conditioning coach for the 2015 Rugby World Champions, the New Zealand All Blacks, has found success with the LCHFD. He is an Ironman Triathlete who has significantly reduced the sugar and processed food intake of these elite rugby players. In an October 2015 interview for whatthefatbook.com he said, 'The movie "The Sugar Film" has influenced the players quite a lot I think. Most of the guys now understand that we need to get the sugar out. We've come a long way. I would say we are in a low-sugar environment. That's a big change. We now have nuts on the sideline after training, not lollies. I wouldn't say we've made it all the way to high fat, but we have healthy fat on hand when we need it. We (the team) go through 6-7 tins of coconut oil a week. We travel with peanut butter and nut butters for the guys to use in smoothies and wherever else it can fit in'. He went on to comment, 'I'd say most professional sports teams are now at least low-sugar, lower to low-carb. That's not always high fat, but it's healthy fats. Nutrition for sport is really changing fast'.

5. Muscle Mass

Currently there is very little evidence associating a low-carb, high-fat diet with significantly increased muscle mass development. Short-term low-carb studies on men by Volek et al., Rauch et al. and Silva et al. did show increased free testosterone in test subjects and increases in lean muscle mass. An individual's 'observed' muscular appearance may also improve as a cosmetic effect of reduced subcutaneous body fat, i.e. looking 'ripped'.

> **Key Points: Low-carb for Athletes**
> 1. A low-carb, high-fat nutrition program may be beneficial for athletes especially in endurance sport and is a healthier weight loss tool in weight category sports.
> 2. Athletes can take longer to achieve full fat adaption on a low-carb program (as measured by performance) than inactive individuals.
> 3. Fat adaptation leads to muscle glycogen sparing and lean body (muscle) mass sparing.

The Low-Carb Companion

Chapter 12 - Questions and Answers

SECTION FOUR:

QUESTIONS AND ANSWERS

Chapter 12
THE 'TOP 40' MOST FREQUENTLY ASKED LOW-CARB QUESTIONS

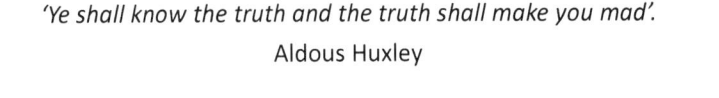

'Ye shall know the truth and the truth shall make you mad'.
Aldous Huxley

....

This section deals with the commonly asked questions regarding low-carb, high-fat nutrition. These answers are as accurate as the current level of knowledge permits. It is important to understand that the world of nutrition is constantly evolving, and as our knowledge expands and transforms, these answers may change as well.

Q.1. What are the main sources of carbs to eliminate from my diet?
A. Eliminating all sugar, sugar sweetened drinks, fruit juices, bread, cereals, pasta, rice, potatoes and refined maize meal, the so called 'sugar & white starches', will make 80% of the difference to cutting carbs in your diet.

Q.2. How much fat can I eat?
A. As long as you eat natural, healthy fats (e.g. animal, fish, dairy, olive oil, coconut) and remain within the boundaries of eating only to fullness and only when hungry, you can eat as much as you want. The natural appetite suppressant effects, combined with the 'superfuel' energy content of fats, make it unlikely that you will overeat fat. Fat intake does not provoke insulin secretion and is not likely to lead to weight gain unless it is combined with a high-refined carb intake.

Q.3. How much protein can I eat?
A. On a low-carb, higher-fat, moderate protein diet program for healthy

weight loss the recommended maximum protein portion is up to a palm-size width and thickness per meal. In athletes, protein requirements are determined by specific needs (see page 192).

Q.4. How many calories can I eat if I'm trying to lose weight?
A. Firstly, focusing only on calorie intake as a factor in effective and sustainable weight loss ignores the critical component of the metabolic effects of the food. Unlike fat and protein, carbs stimulate the sugar-insulin-fat storage cycle. Secondly, the available evidence shows clearly that low-calorie and low-fat diets fail miserably to produce sustainable weight loss. If you are carb-resistant and eat a high-sugar and refined-carb diet, you are likely to gain a lot more weight than if you eat the same amount of calories from protein and healthy fat. The current evidence suggests that people on a low-carb, healthy-fat nutrition program generally eat up to 25% less calories than those on a high-carb diet, which implies that they enjoy healthy weight loss as a result of the dual benefits of reduced sugar-insulin-fat storage metabolism and reduced total daily caloric intake. Simply put, don't worry about the calories; concern yourself with what you eat.

Q.5. How much exercise will help me lose weight?
A. The answer to this question hinges on what you eat, not how much energy you burn. Studies on exercise for weight loss in people on a high-carb, low-fat diet show disappointing results with long-term net weight loss of only 1.5-3kg. This is because exercise makes you hungry! This has two potential pitfalls; firstly, you are likely to overeat, and secondly, by satiating your hunger with carbs, you maintain a 'fattening' stimulus in the body: the sugar-insulin-fat cycle. Moderately intense exercise may boost calorie intake by up to 383 kcal/day (Whybrow S. et al.). Exercise is not a useful weight loss intervention for carb-resistant people who eat carbs. Physical activity is, however, a very important fitness and health tool in the prevention and therapy of conditions like heart disease, diabetes, osteoporosis, colon cancer, lower back pain and depression. Regular, safe and effective exercise is highly recommended.

Q.6. Is constipation a problem on a low-carb program?
A. Some people do find their bowel habits tend towards intermittent constipation. The main causes of this and their related solutions are the following:
- Inadequate water intake – drink enough water or tea daily to maintain hydration.
- Excessive protein intake – limit protein to palm-size portions per meal.
- Salt depletion – add a pinch of salt to meals.
- Changes in fibre intake – it can be helpful to add psyllium husk (soluble fibre) to yoghurt, smoothies, nut mixes, gravies and other low-carb recipes. Eat fibrous vegetables.
- Eating too much food – remember to eat only when you're hungry, stop when full and to fast in between.

Q.7. How long will it take for my body to adapt to a higher-fat way of eating?
A. Fat adaptation varies widely from person to person. On average, inactive people take about 2-3 weeks to feel 'change'. Active people (athletes) take 3-6 weeks for early fat adaptation and up to 3-6 months for complete fat adaptation compatible with high levels of sports performance.

Q.8. How do I know when my body has 'fat adapted'?
A. You will feel energised. You will notice an absence of hunger and a sharp reduction in cravings, and you will see the start of progressive weight loss if you are overweight, and an improvement in exercise performance if you are an active individual.

Q.9. I understand that the human brain needs glucose for energy and cannot burn fat, so how will my brain manage on a low-carb program?
A. It is a gross oversimplification and a factually incorrect statement that the brain can only use glucose for fuel. On a high-carb diet, the brain will

utilise 100-150g of glucose per day. The brain can also effectively use ketone bodies that are naturally produced from fat when on a very low-carb ketogenic diet (VLCKD). On a very low-carb program, the brain will be fuelled by glucose (20g/day) produced from two sources. The first source is amino acids (protein), which produce glucose in a process called gluconeogenesis. The second source is glycerol, the biochemical 'backbone' of broken down triglycerides. The balance (up to 75%) of its energy requirements will be met by ketone bodies. Ketones can make the brain 25% more efficient from a fuel perspective.

Q.10. What is the effect of 'cheating' once in a while on carbs while on a low-carb program?

A. If, as a carb-resistant (intolerant) person, you eat sugar and carbs in amounts over your individual 'carb threshold', then it is likely that your fat burning metabolism will be 'shut down' for 3-5 days at a time. 'Cheating' once a week may halt the fat burning process for up to a week, and you will not lose weight.

Q.11. I'm not losing weight but I have cut back on my sugar and refined carb intake for 4 weeks. What's the problem?

A. An inability to achieve early weight loss (or hitting a plateau) is often because of one or more of the following: (see page 146 for more details)

- Carb intake still too high
- Inadequate fat intake
- Excessive food portions
- Frequent snacks
- Excessive dairy
- Excessive protein intake
- High fruit intake
- Alcohol intake too high
- Slow fat adaptation
- You may be overweight but not carb intolerant
- An underactive thyroid gland
- Medications that affect weight loss

Q.12. How much alcohol and what type is OK to drink on a low-carb program?

A. *If you are very overweight and/or diabetic, then all alcohol should be eliminated for the first 4 - 6 weeks of the program. If you are enjoying weight loss, or are at a stable weight, then adhere to the following guidelines:*

- *Do not exceed medically safe guidelines of alcohol intake per week (21 units/week for men and 18 units/week for women, where beer and wine are, on average, 2 units and spirits are 1 unit per standard tot).*
- *Spirits like whiskey, gin, vodka, rum, brandy, cognac, tequila have no carbs. Consume these occasionally and within safe limits.*
- *Mixers need to be restricted to non-sweetened beverages, like sparkling water, as opposed to sweetened soft drinks.*
- *Avoid beer, which is generally high in carbs; German traditional brews and some 'lite' beers are lower in carbs and may be a better choice.*
- *Wines are acceptable as they are generally low in carbs, especially dry varieties of red and white wine, including sparkling wine; red wines have other potential health benefits since they contain antioxidants and resveratrol.*
- *Avoid fortified wines, ciders, liqueurs and cocktails, which are concentrated sugar sources.*
- *Elevated blood triglycerides may point to excessive alcohol intake.*

Q.13. Do I need to see my doctor or dietician before starting a low-carb program?

A. *If you are overweight, but otherwise healthy and not on any medication, then you can start quite safely on your own, following the basic guidelines in this and other similar books. If you are obese, type 2 diabetic, hypertensive or have any kidney disorder, then it is advisable to seek the advice of a knowledgeable medical professional in the field of low-carb nutrition in order to monitor your condition and medication requirements. Medication needs may change quite significantly. Insulin dosages in type 2 diabetes and blood pressure medication will more than likely be reduced in most people on a low-carb program.*

Chapter 12 - Questions and Answers

Q.14. Is low-carb, higher-fat nutrition suitable for babies and children?
A. Yes, it is! Babies start with high-fat, lower-carb nutrition in the form of human breast milk, which by energy is 54% fat (mostly saturated fat), 38% carbs and 8% protein. They should continue to be weaned onto whole foods rich in healthy natural animal fats, protein and vegetables. Real foods are the most nourishing for children. Babies and children should not be exposed to sugary processed foods which may leave them addicted, allergic, behaviourally compromised, prone to weight gain and unhealthy for life. (see page 152)

Q.15. What will happen to my blood cholesterol with a higher fat intake?
A. Firstly, according to the bulk of modern research, neither dietary cholesterol nor saturated fat intakes are significant risk factors for coronary heart disease. Secondly, dietary cholesterol does not make a significant difference to blood cholesterol levels. The measured effects of a low-carb, high-fat nutrition program on blood cholesterol levels can be divided into the following three subgroups:
1. Most people experience no increase in their total blood cholesterol and see positive improvements in their other heart disease risk markers.
2. Some people experience a transient increase (20-30%) in blood cholesterol that declines to normal levels after about 4-6 weeks.
3. A small number of people see an 'outlier' response of significant (>50%) elevation in total cholesterol levels (and LDL*), but at the same time they see improvements in other biomarkers like increased HDL and larger LDL particle size. The ratio of total cholesterol: HDL is important to consider in risk analysis, as is LDL particle size. These 'outlier' cases are still being investigated.

*Note that elevated LDL cholesterol levels may also reflect, in part, the mathematical way in which LDL is calculated from **the Friedewald equation (LDL = Total cholesterol − HDL − Triglycerides/5)** because if triglyceride levels fall, as they usually do on a low-carb program, then the LDL estimate will rise. (read the section on cholesterol and heart disease on page 94)

Q.16. Can I eat honey, which is reputed to be so healthy?
A. Despite the 'healthy' reputation of honey, it comprises over 50% fructose, which for a carb-intolerant, overweight person is not likely to contribute to healthy weight loss. Cut it out, as with other sweeteners. Small quantities (1 tsp.) used in cooking are permitted.

Q.17. I had my gallbladder surgically removed. How will I cope with a high-fat intake?
A. Initially, see how you fare. Introduce increased fats slowly, and if you struggle, then consider using a commercial digestive enzyme blend with lipase. Most livers respond with increased bile production to an increased fat intake, even without a gallbladder, to store the bile. Some people may experience intermittent nausea if too much fat is consumed initially. Interestingly, there is good evidence to suggest that gallbladder disease is initially provoked by a dysfunction associated with low-fat, high-carb eating patterns.

Q.18. What's the truth about low-carb diets and bad breath?
A. It is true that a very low-carb ketogenic program can produce a temporary 'acetone breath' (sweet smell like nail varnish remover) from early ketone formation, but this often settles over time. Persistent bad breath (halitosis) may have other causes including excessive protein intake, lactose intolerance, poor dental hygiene and dental disease.

Q.19. What are healthy fats and oils for cooking?
A. Fats and oils that have the following 3 properties are the best for cooking:
1. High smoking points that maintain their 'chemical stability' at higher cooking temperatures
2. A 'healthy' ratio of omega-3 to omega-6 fatty acids (not too many omega-6s)
3. Natural antioxidants and vitamins

Chapter 12 - Questions and Answers

These include avocado oil, ghee (clarified butter), animal fats (tallow, duck fat) and refined coconut oil. Olive oil is stable at moderate to high cooking heat, depending on which type of olive oil. Butter and lard are suitable at moderate heat. The unrefined seed (vegetable) oils are the least healthy, the least heat stable, and are also high in omega-6 fatty acids.

Q.20. Vegetable oils are said to be 'toxic'. In what way are they toxic?
A. Vegetable (seed) oils have unhealthy effects on the body in four main ways:
1. In their unrefined forms, they are unstable oils when heated and smoke at relatively low temperatures, which produces toxic fumes and chemicals like aldehydes and AGEs, especially when used for deep-frying. Repeated use for deep-frying dramatically increases the toxicity.
2. They are high in omega-6 fatty acids, which are inflammatory in the body in excess.
3. Their polyunsaturated fats displace saturated fats from cell membranes, making cells more susceptible to oxidation damage.
4. High intakes of omega-6 rich polyunsaturated vegetable oils are associated with increased risks of cardiovascular disease, diabetes, cancer and arthritis.

Q.21. Are all grains bad for health and weight?
A. Good question! The general answer is YES, especially if you are a carb-resistant person challenged by overweight issues, pre-diabetes, diabetes, hypertension or heart disease. If the grains are in any way refined or processed into foodstuffs, they are bad. If, however, you are of normal weight and in general good health, but wish to adopt a low-carb program for health reasons, then small quantities (a tablespoon) of lower GI unrefined starches like sweet potatoes or brown or wild rice, eaten infrequently are unlikely to 'upset the applecart'. Bear in mind that such meals must still contain sufficient healthy fat and protein to limit the effects of ingested carbs on

blood sugar and insulin. Wheat, in all its forms and products including 'wholewheat', is considered unhealthy because of significant blood glucose-elevating properties. Remember that two slices of wholewheat or brown bread will elevate blood glucose more than six teaspoons of sugar will.

Q.22. What's the deal with artificial sweeteners as a substitute for sugar?
A. *Healthier, low-calorie sweeteners that have the least effect on blood sugar are Xylitol, Erythritol and Stevia. These can be used in beverages (tea/coffee/cocoa) or in recipes. Be aware that Xylitol, in excess, can have a laxative effect! All other artificial sweeteners (including aspartame, saccharin, cyclamate and sucralose) are best avoided from the standpoint of health risks (cancer, metabolic syndrome, diabetes) plus their potential to stimulate an insulin response, create carb cravings and stimulate appetite. Recent research has linked artificial sweeteners to glucose intolerance through effects on intestinal bacteria (the gut biome), disturbing the composition and functions of your gut's microorganisms.*
*Note that Xylitol is highly toxic to dogs.

Q.23. How much sugar is too much?
A. *While there is no exact and finite answer to this important question, we can confidently conclude that sugar intake needs to be controlled to maintain good health. What we do know, however, is that diabetes is rare in populations that consume less than 18g of sugar per day (<5 teaspoons per day or <5kg of sugar per year). On this basis, it makes sense to broadly advise that sugar intake be limited to less than 15g (3 heaped teaspoons) per day. Note that a can of cola has upwards of 32g (=10 teaspoons) of sugar and the problem is that so many processed foods have added sugar. When you increase your sugar intake from 8 teaspoons per day to 20 teaspoons your risk of dying from coronary heart disease increases by 38%, and the risk doubles at over 20 teaspoons and triples when over 25 teaspoons.*

Chapter 12 - Questions and Answers

Q.24. How does a low-income family make a low-carb, high-fat diet affordable and sustainable?
A. The answer to this important question comes in three parts. Firstly, it is not true that a healthy, sustainable low-carb program hinges on relatively expensive foods like olive oil, salmon and coconut cream. It is equally effective with bone broths, beef fat, cheaper cuts of fatty meat like shin and brisket, pork fat, home-reared poultry, eggs, organ meats (offal) such as liver or kidney, any fish, fermented milk products, home grown vegetables, avocados, groundnuts (peanuts), other indigenous nuts (in Africa) like Mongongo nuts and Marula nuts, wild fruits and raw coconuts. Secondly, the lack of hunger associated with low-carb, healthy-fat nutrition also reduces the quantity of food required to remain fed and healthy. Thirdly, we need to consider the long-term health costs of a diet high in sugar and refined carbs that can result in obesity, diabetes and heart disease, which can be financially crippling to low-income families.

Q.25. Is an increased protein intake bad for my kidneys?
A. If you are healthy with normal functioning kidneys, then the moderate protein intake recommended as part of a low-carb program will not harm your kidneys. In people with kidney disease or diabetics with kidney dysfunction, a medical professional will need to monitor dietary protein and kidney function. Recent research in diabetics has not shown that a moderate protein intake adversely affects kidney function.

Q.26. Can a vegetarian manage a low-carb, higher-fat program?
A. Absolutely. There are, of course, different types of vegetarianism, ranging from pure vegans to others who eat some animal products like eggs and dairy. There are plenty of vegetable sources of healthy fats such as olive oil, avocados, coconuts and nuts. The more extreme the vegetarianism, the more challenging it can be to assemble enough protein to provide essential amino acids, as it takes at least two different vegetable sources of protein

daily to provide the spectrum required. Many vegetable protein sources like quinoa are also high in carbs (60%), which is an issue when trying to follow a LCHFD. A heavy reliance on non-fermented soya products may also present health challenges.

Q.27. Is ketosis an unhealthy metabolic state?
A. There is 'nutritional ketosis', which is a perfectly healthy metabolic state achieved through very low-carb programs. There is also 'ketoacidosis', which is a dangerous condition that occurs when type 1 diabetes is out of control. These are two very different conditions. (see page 162 for more details)

Q.28. How do I manage a low-carb program whilst the rest of the family eat 'normally'?
A. It is not as difficult as you may think. At the simplest level, if the family main meal consists of meat, vegetables and starch (e.g. rice or potatoes) then you can eat the meat and vegetables and omit the starch. Add some extra butter or olive oil to the vegetables and you are perfectly 'on program'! Often, with exposure to and experimentation with the full range of recipes and meals available as low-carb options, the rest of the family jump on board the low-carb program, making it much easier to manage. This generally happens when they see just how much healthier, lighter and happier you are whilst eating less carbs and more healthy fat.

Q.29. No grain-based cereals, no bread, no sugar added food. What am I going to feed the kids?
A. Hopefully, you will feed the children healthy, wholesome, real foods as the mainstay of their nutrition program. Explore the whole new 'universe' of low-carb food as there are low-carb options for breads, rolls, pizzas, pancakes, wraps, muffins, cakes, cookies, ice cream, smoothies and even treats like marshmallows. Most children can also have unrefined carbs in small amounts like sweet potatoes, brown or wild rice, oats and the full spectrum of fruit and vegetables without significant problems. (see page 152 for more on low-carb nutrition options for children)

Chapter 12 - Questions and Answers

Q.30. I read that soya products are not recommended on a low-carb program because of health concerns. What are the issues with soy?
A. Soy (soya) eaten in the traditional fermented form (like miso, natto and tempeh), is not considered a health issue. However, most soy is ingested in non-fermented forms like tofu, bean curd and soy milk, or as food additives in many processed foods as textured or hydrolysed vegetable protein and lecithin. Soy is a poor quality 'vegetable' protein, and 98% of the world's soy is GMO (genetically modified) primarily to make it herbicide resistant. The potential health problems associated with a high intake of non-fermented soy are:
- Nutritional deficiencies – phytates in soy have 'anti-nutrient' effects causing poor absorption of protein, vitamins (B12), zinc, calcium, magnesium, and iron
- Suppression of thyroid function
- Isoflavone induced oestrogen-like metabolic effects associated with infertility in men and breast cancer in women
- Mental effects – ADD/ADHD, depression and anxiety
- Allergies
- Kidney stones
- Immune system dysfunction
- Fat storage
- Increased cancer risk (www.westonprice.org)

Q.31. Do I need to take supplements on a low-carb program?
A. As Henry E. Siegerist once said, 'Nicotinic acid cures pellagra, but a beefsteak prevents it'. Different schools of thought exist on the requirement for supplements. To some extent, the advice depends on who you are, what you eat and what level of carb restriction you follow. In our 'Weight Lite' very low-carb weight management program that eliminates fruit and limits fresh dairy products in the beginning to promote early weight loss, we recommend a limited supplement program consisting of a basic multivitamin and mineral supplement (without iron), Vitamin C and Fish oil Omega-3s. Additionally, in obese individuals, we recommend supplementary Vitamin D. There is no hard

scientific evidence to show that people develop vitamin deficiencies, even on very low-carb programs or that supplements are absolutely necessary. Seek advice specific to you from your low-carb nutrition advisor.

Q.32. I have been advised to add extra salt to my low-carb meals. Will this affect my blood pressure?

A. At an individual level, people vary in their blood pressure response to salt. Higher salt intakes in some individuals may be associated with blood pressure elevations of up to 6mmHg. Long-term low-salt diets are associated with small reductions in blood pressure of 1-3mmHg. A person who eats a high-refined carb diet is likely to eventually develop high blood pressure as a consequence of insulin-induced salt retention by the kidneys, fructose and uric acid effects on arteries and sympathetic nervous system effects. When a person with high blood pressure adheres to a low-carb program, their blood pressure will often reduce by up to 20mmHg; most of this improvement occurs before significant weight loss. Sugar and carb restriction result in the excretion of salt from the body by the kidneys; in reaction to this excretion, salt depletion can occur over time and cause fatigue. On a low-carb program it is therefore advisable to add a small pinch of salt to your main meals. If, however, you have high blood pressure and are on medical treatment, it is recommended that you consult a medical professional to monitor your blood pressure and medication whilst on a low-carb program.

Q.33. Eating at restaurants can be challenging on a low-carb program. What advice can you give me?

A. With the increasing number of people who follow low-carb programs, there are increasing numbers of restaurants that offer low-carb or 'Banting' options on their menus. If you do not have these options, avoid the following: basting sauces, marinades and meat sauces, gravies, glazed meats, sugared or caramelised vegetables, potatoes, mayonnaise, sweetened or seed oil-based salad dressings, crumbed or battered food or fried food (restaurants generally use vegetable oil for frying) and margarine. Many restaurateurs

Chapter 12 - Questions and Answers

will happily oblige if you ask for butter and olive oil at the table or for cooking your food. Ask for your food not to be basted, battered or crumbed. Keep a look out for low-carb only restaurants.

Q.34. Can people gain weight on a low-carb, high-fat (LCHF) program?
A. *Examples of weight gain on a LCHF diet are recorded, but are most unusual. It is possible for individuals to have abnormal metabolisms, but it is more likely that weight gain occurs because they are overeating (large portions, frequent meals and snacking, ignoring lack of hunger signals) or eating excessive protein, which is converted to sugar, and/or eating excessive carbs from sources like nuts or processed foods, sauces, marinades and low-fat products.*

Q.35. Does a low-carb, high-fat program influence a woman's fertility?
A. *Positive effects on female fertility are possible with an increased fat intake and improved hormonal balance. Low-carb nutrition is used as a treatment strategy for Polycystic Ovary Syndrome (PCOS), a cause of infertility in women.*

Q.36. Why is fructose considered a 'toxic' sugar?
A. *Fructose is considered 'toxic' for the following reasons:*
- *We consume too much of it as a result of the excessive addition of sucrose and high fructose corn syrup to processed foods and carbonated drinks.*
- *As we cannot metabolise it for energy, 80% of fructose is converted to fat in the liver and is secreted in VLDL. This raises blood triglyceride levels and increases fat storage.*
- *High fructose intake is associated with a tenfold increase in advanced glycation end products (AGEs), which cause oxidative damage to many tissues including arteries.*
- *High fructose intake is associated with insulin resistance in the liver, obesity, diabetes and heart disease.*

- The effects of fructose are worsened when combined with glucose intake (in sucrose and HFCS) as glucose stimulates insulin secretion.

Q.37. How do I bake without wheat flour?
A. Easy. Grain-based flours are not the only flours available. Explore the low-carb world of flour-based baking using nut flours (almond, coconut) and seed flours (sunflower, pumpkin).

Q.38. Is coconut flour a refined carb?
A. No, it is a low-carb foodstuff. 28g (2 Tbsp) of coconut flour consists of 4g fat and 6g of net carb (actually 17g total carb of which 11g is fibre & 2g is sugar = 6g net carb); it has a low glycaemic load (GL) value of 3 (GL= total carbs which impact on blood sugar), compared to that of a baguette 48, potato 15 and rice 50!

Q.39. I'm looking at the 'mainstays' of my diet. What can I eat instead of bread, rice, potatoes, pasta, cereal and crackers?
A. You can eat low-carb bread, 'cauli-rice' and 'cauli-mash' (made from cauliflower), courgette 'pasta or noodles', nut and seed granola and seed crackers. All are low-carb options! Lower GI unrefined starches like sweet potatoes, brown or wild rice in small infrequent quantities are also acceptable.

Q.40. Is 'sugar addiction' a real addiction?
A. Frightfully so! Many experts in the field who treat patients with morbid obesity are convinced that carb/sugar addiction is the bigger problem, and that the cure of their weight issues is not possible unless the addiction is effectively addressed. It is estimated that sugar may be 4 - 8 times more addictive than cocaine. Brain scans show that sugar brightly lights up the same parts of the brain as cocaine does in a cocaine addict. In neuroscience research done on rats, sugar fulfils the following four behavioural criteria

that classify a substance as addictive: bingeing, withdrawal, craving and cross-sensitisation. (See page 31 for the Sugar and Carb Addiction Screening Questionnaire)

Chapter 13
IN SEARCH OF GREATER LOW-CARB KNOWLEDGE

'The facts of the present won't sit still for a portrait. They are constantly vibrating, full of clutter and confusion'.
William Macneile Dixon

....

To further advance your knowledge and to develop an increased insight into the evolving arena of nutritional science and medical care, I highly recommend that you keep reading! The following informative sources are pertinent and relevant whether you are a patient, a doctor, a relative, a dietician, an athlete or a health-conscious person.

Low-Carb Science

- **The Big Fat Surprise** by Nina Teicholz
- **The Diet Delusion** by Gary Taubes, also published as **Good Calories, Bad Calories**
- **The Obesity Code** by Jason Fung
- **Why We Get Fat and What To Do About It** by Gary Taubes
- **Challenging Beliefs** by Tim Noakes with Michael Vlismas
- **The Real Meal Revolution** by T. Noakes, S. Creed, J. Proudfoot and D. Grier
- **New Atkins New You** by Drs Westman, Phinney and Volek

Chapter 13 - In Search of Greater Low-Carb Knowledge

- **The Art and Science of Low-carbohydrate Living** by Drs Volek and Phinney
- **The Obesity Epidemic** by Zoe Harcombe
- **Grain Brain** by Dr David Perlmutter with Kristin Loberg
- **Wheat Belly** by William Davis
- **Always Hungry** by David Ludwig
- **What the Fat?** by Prof Grant Schofield, Dr Caryn Zinn, Craig Roger
- Review Articles:
  - **Low-carbohydrate nutrition and metabolism** by Eric Westman et al., *American Journal of Clinical Nutrition* 2007
  - **Low-carbohydrate diet review: shifting the paradigm** by Adele Hite et al., *Nutrition in Clinical Practice*, June 2011
  - **The science of obesity: what do we really know about what makes us fat?** An essay by Gary Taubes, *British Medical Journal BMJ*, April 2013
  - **A new look at carbohydrate-restricted diets: separating fact from fiction** by Jeff Volek, and Stephen Phinney, *Nutrition Today,* March / April 2013
  - **Beyond weight loss: a review of the therapeutic uses of very-low-carbohydrate (ketogenic) diets** by A. Paoli et al., *European Journal of Clinical Nutrition* June 2013
  - **How calorie-focused thinking about obesity and related diseases may mislead and harm public health. An alternative** by Sean Lucan and James DiNicolantonio, *Public Health Nutrition*, March 2015
  - **Hyperinsulinemia: A unifying theory of chronic disease?** by Catherine A.P Crofts et al., Diabesity, October 2015.
- *www.authoritynutrition.com*
- *www.eatingacademy.com*
- *www.dietdoctor.com*
- *www.westonprice.org*

Sugar in Food and Sugar Addiction

- **Salt Sugar Fat: How the food giants hooked us** by Michael Moss
- **Fat Chance: Beating the Odds Against Sugar, Processed Food, Obesity and Disease** by Robert Lustig
- **Sugar Free** by K. Thomson, K. Hammerton and T. Campbell
- **That Sugar Film** (2014 movie)
- The documentaries **Cereal Killers** (2013) and **Cereal Killers 2** (2015)

Low-Carb and Diabetes

- Review Articles:
  - **Very low-carbohydrate diets in the management of diabetes revisited** by Grant Schofield et al., *NZMJ*, April 2016.
  - **Dietary carbohydrate restriction as the first approach in diabetes management: critical review and evidence base** by Richard D. Feinman et al., *Nutrition*, January 2015
  - **Type 2 Diabetes, Etiology and Reversibility** by Roy Taylor, *Diabetes Care*, April 2013
  - **Dietary carbohydrate restriction in type 2 diabetes mellitus and metabolic syndrome: time for a critical appraisal** by Anthony Accurso et al., *Nutrition & Metabolism*, April 2008
- *www.intensivedietarymanagement.com*

Low-Carb, Fat, Cholesterol and Coronary Heart Disease

- **The Great Cholesterol Con** by Dr Malcolm Kendrick
- **Ignore the Awkward: How the Cholesterol Myths are Kept Alive** by Uffe Ravnskov
- **Cholesterol Clarity** by Jimmy Moore and Eric Westman
- Review Articles:
  - **Diverging global trends in heart disease and type 2 diabetes: the role of carbohydrates and saturated fats** by Dariush Mozaffarian, *Lancet Diabetes Endocrinol*, June 2015
  - **The 2015 US Dietary Guidelines lifting the ban on total dietary fat** by Dariush Mozaffarian and David Ludwig, *JAMA*, June 2015
  - **Insulin resistance and coronary heart disease in nondiabetic individuals** by Gerald Reaven, *Arteriosclerosis, Thrombosis, and Vascular Biology*, August 2012
  - **Dietary carbohydrate restriction induces a unique metabolic state positively affecting atherogenic dyslipidaemia, fatty acid partitioning and metabolic syndrome** by Jeff Volek et al., *Progress in Lipid Research*, September 2008
  - **The Evidence for Saturated Fat and for Sugar Related to Coronary Hear Disease** by JJ DiNicolantino, et al. *Prog Cardiovasc Dis*, November 2015
  - **Dietary and Policy Priorities for Cardiovascular Disease, Diabetes, and Obesity. A Comprehensive Review** by Dariush Mozaffarian. Circulation, January 2016.
- *www.eatingacademy.com*

Low-Carb and Cancer

- **Anticancer A New Way of Life** by Dr David Servan-Schreiber
- **Outliving Cancer** by Robert A. Nagourney
- **Nature's Cancer-Fighting Foods** by Verne Varona
- **Tripping over the Truth: The Metabolic Theory of Cancer** by Travis Christofferson
- Review Articles
  - **The Emerging Hallmarks of Cancer Metabolism** by Natalya N. Pavlova and Craig B. Thompson, *Cell Metabolism*, 12 January 2016
  - **Is there a role for carbohydrate restriction in the treatment and prevention of cancer?** by Rainer J Klement & Ulrike Kämmerer, *Nutrition & Metabolism*, October 2011

Low-Carb and Athletes

- **The Art and Science of Low-carbohydrate Performance** by Drs Volek and Phinney
- **What the Fat?** Sports Performance by Prof Grant Schofield, Dr Caryn Zinn, Craig Roger
- Review Article: **Low-carbohydrate diets for athletes: what evidence?** by Timothy Noakes, Jeff Volek and Stephen Phinney, *British Journal of Sports Medicine BJSM*, October 2014
- Review Article: **The ketogenic diet and sport: a possible marriage?** by Antonio Paoli, Antonino Bianco and Keith Grimaldi, *Exercise & Sport Sciences Reviews*, July 2015.

Chapter 13 - In Search of Greater Low-Carb Knowledge

Low-Carb Recipes and Cooking

- **Low-carb is Lekker** by Ine Reynierse
- **Low-carb Living for Families** by Monique le Roux Forslund
- **Raising Superheroes** by T. Noakes, J. Proudfoot, B. Surtees
- **The Real Meal Revolution** by T. Noakes, S. Creed, J. Proudfoot and D. Grier
- **200 Low-Carb, High Fat Recipes** by Dana Carpender
- *www.carbsmart.com*
- *www.ditchthecarbs.com*
- *www.realmealrevolution.com*

Chapter 14
GLOSSARY OF TERMS AND ABBREVIATIONS

ACC: American College of Cardiology

ADD/ADHD: Attention Deficit (Hyperactivity) Disorder. A condition more commonly diagnosed in children, which is characterised by a poor concentration span, learning difficulties and overly active behaviour patterns; this disorder has strong links to a high dietary intake of sugar, refined carbs, junk food, food additives and food colourings.

Adiponectin: A protein hormone that is produced and secreted by fat cells. Adiponectin regulates the metabolism of lipids and glucose. It influences the body's response to insulin, it reduces insulin resistance and it also has anti-inflammatory effects on blood vessel walls. Elevated levels of adiponectin are associated with a reduced risk of coronary heart disease, hypertension and diabetes. Low levels are found in obese people.

Adipose tissue: Collections of fat cells (adipocytes) in the body that store fat in the form of triglycerides.

Advanced Glycation End products (AGEs): Abnormal complexes of sugars joined by cross-linkages to proteins, which result in tissue damage and dysfunction; they are created in high blood sugar states and by heating vegetable oils. These complexes are thought to be the cause of much of the bodily damage seen in the complications of diabetes and in ageing itself.

Examples of AGE damage: in the kidneys (kidney failure), eyes (cataracts), brain (dementia), nerves (polyneuropathy), arteries (coronary artery disease) and LDL cholesterol oxidation. Fructose is a potent generator of AGEs.

AHA: American Heart Association

Alpha-linolenic acid (ALA): Alpha-linolenic acid is a polyunsaturated essential omega-3 fatty acid.

Alzheimer's dementia: A slow insidious brain disease that usually affects older people and causes progressive memory loss, personality change and mental dysfunction. Associated with type 2 diabetes, coronary heart disease, high blood pressure and head injury. The Alzheimer's brain has increased deposition of beta amyloid plaque and neurofibrillary tangles. Brain levels of advanced glycation end products (AGEs) in Alzheimer's are threefold higher than normal. It was first described by, and later named after, German psychiatrist and pathologist, Alois Alzheimer, in 1906.

Amino acids: The building blocks of proteins.

Antioxidant: A molecule that is capable of inhibiting the oxidation of other molecules.

Apolipoprotein B: Apo B, a protein that serves as the structural foundation for LDL, IDL and VLDL lipoproteins. Apo B can be measured in specialised laboratory testing to determine LDL particle number.

Apoptosis: Programmed cell death which occurs normally in damaged cells.

Atherogenic: Something that causes atherosclerotic plaque in arteries.

Atherogenic dyslipidaemia: A combination of predominantly small dense LDL particles + low HDL + elevated triglycerides; associated with an increased risk of coronary artery disease and found in people with metabolic syndrome, diabetes and more often associated with a diet high in sugar and refined carbohydrates.

Atherosclerosis: The degenerative narrowing of arteries by plaque deposits which form in the artery wall.

ATP: Adenosine Tri-Phosphate, a high-energy organic compound that provides energy for muscle work and metabolic processes in the body. It is mostly produced from glucose and fat in cellular energy metabolism.

Banting (or to 'Bant'): Term used to denote the practice of following a low-carbohydrate, high-fat diet predominantly for weight loss; named after William Banting, a 19th Century English undertaker who in his 1863 Letter on Corpulence, publicly documented his remarkably successful weight loss on a carbohydrate-restricted diet prescribed for him by the surgeon William Harvey.

Beta-blocker: A class of drugs which act to restrict the heart rate and to reduce blood pressure; these are commonly used to treat hypertension and heart disease; commonly used examples are propranolol, atenolol and bisoprolol.

Beta cells: Specialised cells of the pancreas that produce the hormones insulin and glucagon.

Biometrics: Refers to measurements or metrics related to human characteristics such as height or weight.

Blood pressure: A combined measure of the heart-pump pressure into arteries (systolic pressure) and of the recoil pressure of the arteries (diastolic pressure); measured in mmHg (mm of mercury); normal adult blood pressure <120/80mmHg.

Body Mass Index (BMI): A measure of body size relating weight to height; calculated as weight divided by height squared [weight (kg)/height (m²)]. A 'healthy' BMI is less than 24kg/m², an overweight BMI is >25 kg/m², an obese BMI is >30 kg/m².

Calorie: A measure (in nutrition) of the energy content of nutrients and food, units - kilogram calorie or 'kilocalorie' (kcal) or calorie (Cal); defined in physics as the amount of energy required to raise the temperature of one kilogram of water by one degree Celsius.

Carbohydrate: A macronutrient comprising starches, sugars and fibre.

Carbohydrate intolerance: A genetically influenced level of intolerance to carbohydrates, predisposing to progressive insulin resistance over time. The onset of carbohydrate intolerance may be triggered by diet, age, stress, menopause and pregnancy.

Cell membrane receptors: Sites located on the outer cell wall which act as attachments for signalling molecules that influence cell function.

Cholesterol: A lipid substance essential to life that is found in certain foods, but mainly manufactured in the body by the liver and cells.

Chylomicrons: Large lipoproteins that transport dietary fat and cholesterol from the intestines to the lymphatic ducts and then into the bloodstream.

Coeliac disease: A disorder of severe intolerance to wheat gluten causing abdominal cramping, diarrhoea, weight loss, failure to thrive in children, plus a host of other system abnormalities; associated with a higher risk of gastrointestinal cancer.

Coronary arteries: The system of arteries that supply blood to the heart muscle (myocardium).

Coronary heart disease (CHD) / Coronary artery disease (CAD): A complex process of atherosclerotic plaque formation and potential obstruction in the heart's coronary arterial blood supply; increases the risk of a heart attack.

Corticosteroids: A class of drugs related to bodily cortisol used in a variety of conditions for their anti-inflammatory properties; examples are hydrocortisone and prednisolone.

DGAC: Dietary Guidelines Advisory Committee.

Diabetes mellitus: An endocrine disease of insulin deficiency (type 1 diabetes) or insulin resistance (type 2 diabetes). Also occurs in pregnancy (gestational diabetes).

Diuretic: A class of drugs that act mainly by increasing urine output from the kidneys; used commonly to treat hypertension and heart failure; examples are hydrochlorothiazide and furosemide.

Endocrine: Means hormone-secreting. The endocrine system is made up of eight hormone-secreting glands: pineal, pituitary, thyroid, thymus, adrenals, pancreas, ovaries (female) and testes (male).

Endothelium: The inner lining of an artery wall consisting of a single layer of endothelial cells.

Enzyme: A protein/protein-based molecule that speeds up (catalyses) a chemical reaction.

Epidemiological study: An observational study that identifies the incidence of a disease or other condition across different populations or groups. These studies can demonstrate associations but not causation.

Familial Hypercholesterolaemia (FH): A hereditary condition of high-circulating cholesterol levels caused by a deficiency in LDL uptake receptors on cell membranes; associated with an increased risk of early onset coronary heart disease in some individuals, especially those with homozygous inheritance of the defect (i.e. from both parents).

Fat: A macronutrient comprising chains of fatty acids of various lengths; may be monounsaturated, polyunsaturated or saturated; essential to life and cellular structure, stored in the body as triglycerides and supplies fuel for energy as free fatty acids or ketone bodies.

Fibre: Indigestible carbohydrate found naturally as intact fibre in foods or as isolated fibre added to processed food.

Fibrinolysis: The normal process in the body of breaking down blood clots that occur naturally, which prevents those clots from growing larger and causing problems.

Food Insulin Index: A measure of the post-eating insulin response of an ingested food.

Free radicals: Highly reactive oxygen molecules that potentially cause cellular damage.

Friedewald equation: A mathematical formula named after William Friedewald, who developed it; used in the laboratory determination of cholesterol to calculate LDL levels that are not measured directly.

Fructose: A simple sugar that occurs naturally in fruit, honey and cane or beet sugar (sucrose). It is the main constituent sugar in high fructose corn syrup (HFCS).

Gallbladder: A bag-like structure located beneath the liver used by the body to store bile that is secreted into the intestine for fat digestion.

Genes: Regions on DNA (deoxyribonucleic acid), the fundamental building block of life, which code for a specific protein; genes control the development and regulatory functions of living cells.

Gestational: During pregnancy.

Glibenclamide: A sulphonylurea drug used in the treatment of type 2 diabetes; acts by stimulating the pancreas to secrete insulin.

Glucagon: Hormone secreted by the beta cells of the pancreas that acts to elevate blood sugar when levels are low.

Gluconeogenesis: The conversion of amino acids (protein) to glucose in the liver.

Glucose: A simple sugar; the measured sugar in human blood represented as blood sugar or blood glucose.

Glucotoxicity: Toxic effects of elevated blood glucose.

Gluten: Proteins (gliadin and glutenins) found in wheat, barley, rye and triticale.

Glycaemic Index (GI): An index that ranks carbohydrate-containing food depending on the rate at which the body digests it to form glucose; glucose is assigned a GI of 100.

Chapter 14 - Glossary of Terms and Abbreviations

Glycaemic Load (GL): A measure that incorporates the amount of carbohydrate in a portion of food together with how quickly it raises blood glucose levels. Glycaemic load helps to work out how different sized portions of different foods compare with each other in terms of their blood glucose raising effect. GL = GI x grams of carbohydrate /100.

Glycation: The toxic effects of elevated blood sugars binding to body proteins and disrupting or damaging cellular function in the process; examples of glycation damage are eye cataracts, arterial inflammation and skin wrinkles.

Glycerol: A sugar alcohol derived from carbohydrate metabolism; used by the body to form triglycerides by adding three fatty acids to one glycerol molecule.

Glycogen: The storage form of glucose in liver and muscles.

Glycolysis: The breakdown of sugars in a series of enzyme activated steps for cellular energy production that takes place in the cell cytoplasm.

Grains: Wheat, corn (maize), oats, barley, rye, amaranth and quinoa are all common examples of agriculturally grown grains used for flour and food production; wholegrains refer to a reduced level of milling, refining or processing of grains. All grains are high in carbohydrate; the more refined the grain, the higher the 'carb' availability or GI.

Gynecomastia: Breast tissue development in males.

HbA1c: Glycated (or glycosylated) haemoglobin; an example of glycation-induced damage to protein (in this case haemoglobin, the pigment found in red blood cells); its measurement as a percentage of total haemoglobin is used as a tool to plot average blood glucose levels over a previous 90-day period; used to monitor diabetic blood glucose control and to screen for pre-diabetes /diabetes.

High Density Lipoprotein (HDL): The transport lipoprotein that returns cholesterol from body tissues back to the liver; a process called reverse cholesterol transport. HDL also acts as an antioxidant.

High Fructose Corn Syrup (HFCS): Manufactured from corn as a cheaper alternative to sugar since the 1970s. The most widely used varieties are HFCS 55 (mostly used in carbonated drinks), approximately 55% fructose + 42% glucose, and HFCS 42 (used in beverages, processed foods, cereals, and baked goods), approximately 42% fructose + 53% glucose.

Hydrogenated Oil (or partially hydrogenated oils): Industrially processed polyunsaturated oils that are solid at room temperature; they are created by chemically bombarding polyunsaturated fats with hydrogen, a process that produces trans-fatty acids. Margarine is an example.

Hyperglycaemia: Elevated blood sugar (glucose).

Hyperinsulinaemia: Elevated levels of insulin in the bloodstream, usually a result of excessive pancreatic secretion.

Hypertension: A condition of persistent high blood pressure.

Hyperuricaemia: Elevated levels of uric acid in the bloodstream.

Hypoglycaemia: Low blood sugar (glucose).

Inflammation: A complex reaction that occurs in response to tissue injury or infection; resolution of an acute inflammatory response is crucial for normal healing; failure to resolve an inflammatory response results in chronic inflammation.

Immune system: Cells, tissues and organs that normally act to protect the body against disease and in response to cellular damage.

Intermediate Density Lipoprotein (IDL): A lipoprotein transporting triglycerides and cholesterol, derived from VLDL; normal composition approximately 31% triglycerides, 29% cholesterol, 22% phospholipids & 18% protein.

Insulin: Hormone secreted by the beta cells of the pancreas in response to a rise in blood glucose from digested foods. Insulin is the principal regulator of glucose, amino acid and fat metabolism; it has glycogenic, lipogenic, anabolic, atherogenic and obesogenic properties. Insulin has different effects on different parts of the body but acts principally on muscles, liver, fat cells and the brain.

Insulinogenic: The capacity of a nutrient or food to stimulate an insulin response.

Insulin-like Growth Factor (IGF-1): Insulin-like substances secreted by cells and tissues that play a key role in facilitating the supply of energy from foods to cells for growth; thought to be derived from circulating Growth Hormone; IGF-1 is a role player in cancer cell growth.

Insulin Resistance (IR): A state in which greater than normal amounts of insulin are required to elicit a normal glucose uptake response from cells, tissues and organ systems in the body and characterised by increasingly impaired cellular glucose uptake over time. IR is caused by persistently elevated levels of insulin and usually affects the liver and muscles more than the fat stores; it may initially be a cellular defence mechanism to protect cells from excessive glucose uptake in the presence of hyperglycaemia. IR is the primary metabolic defect leading to central obesity, metabolic syndrome and type 2 diabetes.

Isoflavones: Powerful plant substances found in soy (soya) that are chemically similar to the female hormone oestrogen.

Keto-adaptation: The adaptation of the cells of the body to increased use of fat-derived ketones for energy production.

Ketoacidosis: A dangerous metabolic state of very high ketone production and accumulation in the bloodstream that occurs in uncontrolled type 1 diabetes.

Ketogenic: Causing increased ketone production from fats.

Ketones (ketone bodies): Substances produced from fat in the liver during metabolic states of increased fat utilisation, e.g. fasting or carbohydrate restriction. Ketone bodies provide an effective source of energy fuel to cells especially the brain and heart.

LCD: Low-Carb Diet, but also used in some texts as an acronym for Low-Calorie Diet.

LCHFD: Low-Carb, High-Fat Diet.

Lactate: A chemical by-product of glycolytic energy production in active skeletal muscle; used as a metabolic fuel by muscles and the heart; can be used by the liver to produce blood glucose.

Lactose: A relatively weak sugar found in milk and dairy products; a disaccharide of glucose and galactose. Highest levels are found in fresh dairy, reduced levels are found in fermented dairy products. Lactose intolerance affects some individuals.

Lard: Rendered pig fat; a stable cooking fat that contains 47% monounsaturated, 41% saturated and 12% polyunsaturated fats.

Low Density Lipoprotein (LDL): Lipoproteins that carry 70% of the blood cholesterol to the body's cells, including the brain; normal composition is approximately 45% cholesterol, 8% triglycerides, 22% phospholipids and 25% protein. LDLs occur in a range of sizes from small, dense particles to larger particles; most LDL is derived from IDL that is derived from VLDL.

Leptin: A hormone released from fat stores which, in a normal functioning system, signals the brain to suppress appetite when well fed; in obese individuals, leptin is involved in inflammatory responses and leptin resistance when released from visceral (belly) fat.

Linoleic acid (LA): A polyunsaturated essential omega-6 fatty acid.

Lipid: An insoluble (i.e. does not dissolve in water or plasma) compound in the body such as fat (triglycerides) and cholesterol.

Lipidaemia: A high level of lipids (cholesterol or fat) in the bloodstream.

Lipo: Prefix meaning fat.

Lipogenesis: The creation and storage of fat in the body; 'de novo' lipogenesis refers to the conversion of sugars (especially fructose) to fat (triglycerides) in the human liver.

Lipolysis: The breakdown and release of fat from fat stores in the body; at a biochemical level, the conversion of stored triglycerides to fatty acids for release from fat stores.

Lipoprotein: A protein designed to transport cholesterol and triglycerides (lipids) in the bloodstream; there are different types of lipoproteins of different sizes, ranging from chylomicrons, VLDL, IDL, LDL to HDL.

Lipotoxicity: A process of fat-induced cell damage that occurs in the pancreatic beta cells in advanced type 2 diabetes.

Liver enzymes: Protein-based molecules in the human liver that speed up chemical reactions.

Macronutrient: The collective term for carbohydrate, fat and protein, the three major nutrients obtained from food.

Metabolic Syndrome: Dietary induced metabolic dysfunction associated with fatty liver infiltration (NAFLD) that predisposes to type 2 diabetes and coronary heart disease. The occurrence of three out of five conditions [high blood pressure, central (belly) obesity, high blood sugar, high blood insulin or atherogenic dyslipidaemia (small dense LDL + low HDL + elevated triglycerides)] meets the criteria for diagnosis. Also called pre-diabetes or Syndrome X, as first described by Dr Gerald Reaven in 1996.

Metabolism: Complex bodily processes that convert food into energy or building blocks for tissues under the control of a range of hormones.

Metformin: A biguanide drug commonly used in the treatment of type 2 diabetes; acts to reduce blood sugar by increasing insulin sensitivity and peripheral glucose uptake by tissues.

Mitochondria: An organelle structure inside cells responsible for supplying the bulk of cellular energy via oxidative ATP production; mitochondria are also involved in other tasks such as signalling, cellular differentiation, cell death, cell growth and maintaining the control of the cell cycle.

Monounsaturated fats: Fatty acids containing a single double bond in their chemical structure; commonly found in foodstuffs like olive oil, nuts and avocados.

Non-Alcoholic Fatty Liver Disease (NAFLD): A condition of the liver associated with insulin resistance and obesity; has a high prevalence in people who have metabolic syndrome or diabetes. The liver tissues become invaded by fatty infiltrations that result in simple fatty liver (steatosis) or steatohepatitis; the latter may progress to liver fibrosis and cirrhosis. NAFLD may be the direct cause of insulin resistance in the liver.

Nutritional ketosis: A physiological state of low to moderate levels of ketones (ketone bodies) in the bloodstream that provide fuel to the brain, heart and tissues and occurs with fasting, starvation and carbohydrate restriction.

Obesity: A state of being severely overweight; defined as having a BMI that exceeds 30 kg/m².

Oestrogen: The primary female sex hormone produced in the ovaries, chiefly responsible for female reproductive physiology and also involved in body fat distribution. Some oestrogen is also produced in smaller amounts by other tissues such as the liver, adrenal glands, breasts and fat cells.

Omega-3 Fatty Acids: Essential polyunsaturated fatty acids required from food that are principally obtained from fatty fish and fish oils; also found in much smaller bioavailable amounts in flaxseed and chia seeds. The three types of omega-3 fatty acids involved in human physiology are alpha-linoleic acid (ALA) (found in plant oils), eicosapentaenoic acid (EPA) and docosahexaenoic acid (DHA) (both found in fish oils); optimal levels are associated with health benefits including anti-inflammatory effects and reduced heart disease risk.

Omega-6 Fatty Acids: Essential polyunsaturated fatty acids such as linoleic acid (LA) required from food; principally obtained from seed (vegetable) oils, animal products and eggs from corn-fed or soya-fed livestock and poultry; excessively high intakes are associated with inflammation, heart disease and cancer.

Oxidation: A chemical process of cell or molecular damage by highly reactive oxygen molecules.

Paleo (paleolithic) diet: Also known as the 'caveman diet'; a low-carb, high-fat nutrition program based on a postulate of what type of food our ancient ancestors might have eaten; the diet emphasises meat, nuts and berries but excludes dairy foods.

Pancreas: An abdominal organ that functions as both exocrine (secreting digestive enzymes like amylase, protease and lipase into the gut) and endocrine (secreting hormones like insulin and glucagon).

PET scan: Positron Emission Tomography Scan; a nuclear medicine imaging technique that shows radiolabelled glucose uptake into cancerous tumours; used for cancer detection and treatment monitoring.

Polyneuropathy: A syndrome of nerve damage and dysfunction that occurs in diseases like diabetes.

Polyunsaturated fats: Fatty acids with more than one double bond in their chemical structure; tend to be liquid at cooler temperatures.

Processed food: Foodstuffs that are no longer in their natural form, but are refined by milling and/or mixed with other ingredients or additives in industrial food production.

Prolactin: A hormone produced in the pituitary gland, named for its role in lactation (milk production). It also affects the reproductive system, influences behaviour and regulates the immune system.

Protein: A macronutrient consisting of different arrangements of chains of amino acids; proteins are essential to life as the building blocks of body tissues and for multiple functions in bodily processes.

Quinoa: Pronounced 'kinwa' or 'kinuwa', a grain crop grown primarily for its edible seeds; a pseudo-cereal rather than a true cereal, as it is not a member of the true grass family; it is related to and resembles amaranth, also a pseudo-cereal. Quinoa is relatively high in protein when compared to other grains but whether or not it constitutes a 'complete protein' is currently debated.

Real food: Food in its natural form that has not been processed.

Refined carbohydrates: Carbohydrate-based foods produced by refining the base grain, for instance polished rice and milled wheat or maize. Refining leads to a loss of fibre, protein and micronutrients.

Retinol: An animal form of Vitamin A that is produced in the body from the hydrolysis of retinyl esters found in animal food sources like liver and eggs.

Resveratrol: A compound found in red wine and red grapes with antioxidant and heart protective effects.

Resistin: Also known as adipose tissue-specific secretory factor (ADSF), an adipose (fat)-derived peptide hormone that, in humans, is associated with belly fat obesity, inflammation, insulin resistance and type 2 diabetes.

Rhabdomyolysis: A condition in which skeletal muscle cells rupture as a consequence of traumatic crush injury, electrocution, drugs, toxins, excessive muscle exercise or disease. The release of muscle enzymes can result in kidney failure. It is a documented side effect of statin drugs.

Salt: In the dietary context, refers to table salt (sodium chloride) or sea salt used as a condiment for food.

Saturated fats: Fatty acids containing no double bonds in their chemical structure; found commonly in animal products (meat, dairy, eggs) as well as coconut and palm oil.

Selective Serotonin Re-uptake Inhibitors (SSRIs): A class of drugs used as antidepressants; a common example is fluoxetine (Prozac).

Starch: Carbohydrate that consists of chains of sugars; biochemically, a polysaccharide composed of glucose units that occurs widely in plant tissues in the form of storage granules, consisting of amylose and amylopectin.

Statins: Drugs known as HMG-CoA reductase inhibitors that act to reduce cholesterol levels in the body by blocking cholesterol production in the liver and cells.

Steatosis: A condition of 'fatty liver' produced by infiltration of liver tissue with fat; it is associated with insulin resistance, obesity, diabetes and metabolic syndrome and created by increased de novo triglyceride production by the liver.

Stroke: A bleed (haemorrhage) or blockage (embolus, clot) in a brain artery causing neurological deficit.

Subcutaneous Fat: Storage and distribution of body fat (triglycerides) beneath the skin.

Sucrose: A disaccharide sugar that contains equal portions of glucose and fructose; commonly known as table sugar; used to sweeten food and beverages.

Sympathetic Nervous System: Part of the body's autonomic nervous system that regulates 'unconscious' actions, especially 'fight and flight' responses mediated by both neuronal and hormonal mechanisms.

Tallow: Fat made from suet; the raw hard fat from cattle or sheep. Beef tallow is also called dripping.

Chapter 14 - Glossary of Terms and Abbreviations

Thermic Effect (of foods): The caloric cost of digesting and processing different macronutrients in your diet; protein has the highest thermic effect and fats have the lowest. When comparing calories burned through processing, protein accounts for 20-35%, carbohydrates 5-15% and fats 0-5%.

Thyroid gland: An endocrine gland located in the anterior neck that produces thyroid hormones responsible for multiple metabolic functions in the body.

Trans-fat: Fatty acids with a double bond in a 'trans' configuration that creates a zig-zag molecular shape and results in an unsaturated fat that is solid at room temperature; manufactured in processed foods and associated with increased risks of heart disease.

Triglyceride: The storage form of fat manufactured in the liver and in fat cells; biochemically, a triglyceride consists of three fatty acid molecules attached to a 'backbone' of glycerol.

Tumour Necrosis Factor (TNF): A cell-signalling protein (cytokine) involved in systemic inflammation and immune cell regulation.

USDA: United States Department of Agriculture.

Ventilatory drive: The central brain control of the respiratory cycle.

Visceral fat: Body fat stored around and between organs usually in the abdominal cavity ('belly' fat) and also around the heart; markedly increased in obesity; associated with inflammation, insulin resistance and heart disease.

VLCKD: Very Low-Carbohydrate Ketogenic Diet.

Very Low Density Lipoprotein (VLDL): A lipoprotein secreted by the liver to transport triglycerides manufactured in the liver (usually from carbohydrate). VLDLs leave the liver with a composition of approximately 50% triglyceride, 22% cholesterol, 18% phospholipid & 10% protein. VLDL progressively 'give up' triglycerides to become IDL and then LDL.

VO2max: The maximum amount of oxygen utilised by exercising muscles; a measure of maximum aerobic capacity (aerobic fitness).

Chapter 14 - Glossary of Terms and Abbreviations

The Low-Carb Companion

PART 2:

THE FOOD COMPANION

LOW-CARB COMPANION RECIPE BOOK

Table of Contents | Page

1. Broths & Soups — 253
2. Eggs — 271
3. Fish — 287
4. Poultry — 299
5. Beef — 319
6. Lamb — 337
7. Pork — 345
8. Sides, Salads & Vegetables — 353
9. Salad Dressings, Sauces, Marinades & Rubs — 371
10. Bread — 393
11. Pizza, Quiches & Pasta — 401
12. Pancakes & Muffins — 413
13. Cupcakes, Cakes & Cookies — 421
14. Desserts — 433
15. Smoothies & Shakes — 441
16. Snacks & Miscellaneous — 447
17. Conversion Tables — 461

The Low-Carb Companion

SECTION 1:

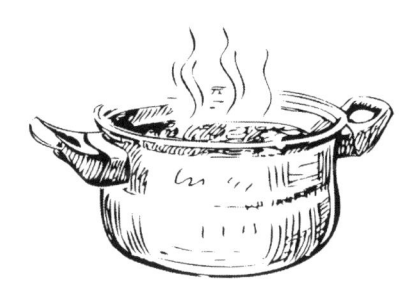

BROTHS & SOUPS

A hearty broth is one of the most nutritious things you can eat.

Broths & Soups

Broths | Page
Basic Bone Broth	255
Chicken Broth	256
Tom Yum Prawn Broth	257
Vegetable Broth	258

Soups | Page
Butternut or Pumpkin Soup	259
Avocado Pear Soup	260
Broccoli & Coconut Soup	260
Carrot & Leek Soup With Coriander	261
Cream of Spinach Soup	262
Mussel Soup	262
Tomato & Prawn Soup	263
Creamy Cauliflower Soup with Bacon Bits	264
Creamy Chicken Soup with Seasonal Vegetables	265
Cream of Tomato Soup	266
Italian Meatball Soup	267
Minestrone Soup	268
Fish, Tomato & Chorizo Soup	269

Section 1 - Broths & Soups

Broths

Basic Bone Broth *Serves 4*

INGREDIENTS
- 500g bones of any kind
- 1 carrot
- ½ onion
- 1 stick celery
- 1 bay leaf
- 5 peppercorns
- 1 head garlic

METHOD: If the bones are not already roasted, roast them in the oven until they are lightly browned. Place everything into a medium-sized pot and cover with water; place on the lowest heat and let it simmer for up to 12 hours. When you taste the broth, it should taste strongly of the animal meat used. Avoid boiling the broth to maintain its clarity. Once the broth has taken on the flavour, strain it through a sieve and freeze or use it right away.

Tip: Add lemon and white wine to flavour fish broth; add rosemary to flavour beef broth, and add thyme to flavour chicken broth.

Chicken Broth

Serves 4

INGREDIENTS
- *1 x 1.8kg chicken*
- *2 small onions*
- *2 centre celery sticks with leaves*
- *2 garlic cloves*
- *2 Tbsp. salt*
- *4 litres water*
- *5 parsley sprigs*
- *5 thyme sprigs*
- *2 bay leaves*
- *10 black peppercorns*

METHOD: Combine chicken, onions, celery, garlic, salt, water, seasonings and peppercorns in a large pot over medium heat. Bring to the boil. Reduce heat to low and simmer, covered, for 2 hours. Stir to break up large pieces of chicken. Add enough water to return to original level and simmer 2-4 hours longer. Restore water level again; bring to the boil and remove from heat. After stock has cooled slightly, strain and discard all solids, including chicken. Chill in the fridge until the fat congeals. Skim off fat and discard. Transfer broth to small containers; refrigerate for up to 3 days or freeze for up to 3 months.

Section 1 - Broths & Soups

Tom Yum Prawn Broth *Serves 2*

INGREDIENTS
- *2 cups rich broth*
- *250g (1 cup) prawns, shelled and deveined*
- *1 handful coriander*
- *2 red chillies, halved down the middle*
- *3 kaffir lime leaves*
- *1 stick lemongrass, tied in a knot*
- *1 large tomato, cut into wedges*
- *1 Shitake mushroom, sliced*
- *1 Tbsp. hot Thai chilli jam or paste*
- *Juice of 1 lime*
- *1 Tbsp. fish sauce*

METHOD: Set the prawns and coriander set aside. Combine all the remaining ingredients in a pot and bring to a boil. Simmer for 10 minutes, and then add the prawns and coriander. Simmer until prawns are cooked. Balance the seasoning with lime juice and fish sauce and serve.

Vegetable Broth

Serves 4

INGREDIENTS
- 4 medium leeks, white and light green parts only
- 2 Tbsp. olive oil
- 2 medium carrots, roughly chopped
- 2 celery sticks, roughly chopped
- 115g mushrooms, sliced
- 4 garlic cloves, crushed
- 4 litres water
- 4 parsley sprigs
- 5 thyme sprigs
- 2 bay leaves
- 2 tsp. table salt
- 10 peppercorns

METHOD: Cut leeks in half lengthways and wash in cold water to remove any dirt and then chop. Heat oil in a large saucepan over medium heat and add leeks, carrots, celery, mushrooms and garlic and sauté until soft but not browned, about 10 minutes. Add water, parsley, thyme, bay leaves, salt and pepper. Bring to the boil and cover and reduce heat to low and simmer 1 hour, stirring periodically. Remove from heat and strain, pressing on vegetables with a spatula or wooden spoon to release liquid. Discard solids and transfer broth to small containers; refrigerate for up to 3 days or freeze for up to 3 months.

Tip: *Vegetable Broth can also be used in place of water or chicken broth in most soup or sauce recipes.*

Section 1 - Broths & Soups

Soups

Butternut or Pumpkin Soup　　　　　　　*Serves 4*

INGREDIENTS
- *500g butternut or pumpkin, cubed*
- *2 medium onions, diced*
- *4 medium carrots, peeled and cubed*
- *2 Granny Smith apples, peeled and cubed*
- *1 tsp. butter*
- *1 tsp. olive oil*
- *½ tsp. ginger*
- *¼ tsp. cinnamon*
- *1 tsp. honey*
- *500ml water (or half water/half milk)*
- *1 chicken stock cube*
- *Cream*

METHOD: Fry onions with butter and oil until soft; add the butternut or pumpkin, carrots, apples and all seasonings and brown in the same pot, taking care not to burn them. Add the water or milk and stock cube. Simmer on low heat until tender. Liquidise, adding more water or milk if the soup gets too thick. Serve garnished with cream.

Avocado Pear Soup   Serves 4

INGREDIENTS
- *2 large ripe avocado pears (preferably those with purple skins)*
- *⅔ cup homemade chicken stock*
- *1½ Tbsp. lemon juice*
- *Black pepper*
- *Garlic chives*
- *Cream*

METHOD: Mix avocados, stock and lemon juice in a blender and refrigerate or freeze until really chilled. To serve, pour into large white soup bowls and zigzag fresh cream on top. Sprinkle garlic chives on top of soup and black pepper in the middle.

Broccoli & Coconut Milk Soup   Serves 2

INGREDIENTS
- *2 Tbsp. coconut oil*
- *1 head of broccoli, cut into florets*
- *1 onion, chopped*
- *1 bay leaf*
- *2 garlic cloves, chopped*
- *1 cup vegetable stock*
- *1 tin of coconut milk (2 cups)*
- *Salt and pepper*

METHOD: Heat the coconut oil in a saucepan over medium heat. Add the onion and garlic and cook for 7-10 minutes until soft. Add the broccoli, stock, coconut milk and bay leaf. Season to taste. Simmer for 15-20 minutes. Remove the bay leaf. Blend until smooth, using either a hand blender or blender.

Carrot and Leek Soup with Coriander *Serves 6*

INGREDIENTS
- *40g butter*
- *175g trimmed leeks, washed and sliced*
- *450g carrots, trimmed, peeled and sliced*
- *10ml ground coriander*
- *5ml almond flour*
- *1 litre vegetable stock*
- *Salt and pepper*
- *15ml natural yoghurt or sour cream*
- *Fresh coriander leaves to garnish*

METHOD: Heat the butter in a large saucepan, add the vegetables, cover and cook gently for 5-10 minutes or until the vegetables begin to soften but not colour. Stir in the ground coriander and almond flour and cook for about 1 minute. Pour in the stock and bring to the boil, stirring all the time. Season with salt and pepper, reduce the heat, cover and simmer for about 20 minutes or until all the ingredients are quite tender. Leave the soup to cool slightly and puree in a blender or with a stick blender until quite smooth. Return the soup to the pan and stir in the yoghurt or cream. Taste and adjust the seasoning if necessary. Reheat gently without boiling and serve garnished with fresh coriander leaves.

Cream of Spinach Soup Serves 4

INGREDIENTS
- 25ml butter
- 1 onion, finely chopped
- 40ml almond flour
- 500ml chicken stock
- 600g fresh spinach, washed and stems removed
- 350ml milk
- 80ml cream
- 2ml ground nutmeg
- Salt and freshly ground black pepper to taste
- Grated lemon rind and juice of ½ lemon

METHOD: Melt butter in a saucepan and sauté the onion until soft. Add the almond flour and blend to a smooth paste. Remove from the heat and slowly add the stock while stirring continuously. Bring to the boil, add the spinach and simmer for 20 minutes. Puree the soup in a food processor or with a stick blender and return to the saucepan. Put back on the heat and add the remaining ingredients except the lemon juice and rind. Bring to the boil once more and add the lemon juice and rind just before serving.

Mussel Soup Serves 4

INGREDIENTS
- 1 tin or packet of chicken soup
- 2 tins of smoked mussels
- 1 tin of tomatoes
- 350ml milk
- 250ml cream
- 2 tsp. almond flour

- *½ tsp. mixed herbs*
- *2 tsp. sherry*
- *Salt and pepper*

METHOD: Combine soup, milk and tomatoes in a saucepan and bring to the boil. In a small bowl, mix the herbs and almond flour together. Add cream and stir before adding to the soup. Add mussels, sherry, salt and pepper before serving.

Tomato & Prawn Soup *Serves 4*

INGREDIENTS
- *500g ripe tomatoes*
- *25ml butter*
- *1 large onion*
- *2 cups cauliflower*
- *10ml chopped fresh tarragon and basil*
- *1 clove garlic, minced*
- *250ml tomato juice*
- *125ml orange juice*
- *Salt and pepper*
- *5ml grated orange rind*
- *250ml cream*
- *250g prawns, peeled, deveined and blanched*

METHOD: Skin and chop tomatoes. Heat the butter in large heavy saucepan and sauté onions and cauliflower for 5 minutes. Add the tomatoes, tarragon, basil, tomato juice and garlic and simmer, covered, for 15 minutes. Purée the soup, return to the saucepan and add the orange juice. Season to taste with salt and pepper, and heat over a low heat. Stir in the orange rind, cream and prawns. Serve immediately.

Creamy Cauliflower Soup with Bacon Bits *Serves 4*

INGREDIENTS
- 1 Tbsp. coconut oil
- 2 onions, finely chopped
- 2 garlic cloves, crushed
- ¾ cup white wine
- 600g cauliflower florets
- 3 cups homemade vegetable stock
- Himalayan salt and white pepper

FOR THE HERB OIL
- 3 Tbsp. olive oil
- 5g mixed green herbs

- 250g streaky bacon, chopped

METHOD: Melt coconut oil in a pot, add onion and cook over a medium heat until soft and golden brown. Increase the heat and add garlic and wine. Cook until most of the liquid has evaporated. Add cauliflower florets and stock, cover with a lid and simmer for 20-25 minutes or until cauliflower is soft. Blend soup until smooth and creamy. Season to taste with salt and pepper.
For herb oil: Blend together olive oil and green herbs.

To serve: Fry bacon in a dry pan until crispy. Sprinkle over soup, followed by a drizzle of herb oil.

> **Crisply fried bacon rinds** make a delicious seasoning for soups and stews.

Creamy Chicken Soup with Seasonal Vegetables

Serves 4-6

INGREDIENTS
- 3 chicken fillets, cooked
- 100g sugar snap peas
- 100g broccoli
- 100g cauliflower
- 100g baby marrows
- 1 yellow pepper
- 1 red pepper
- 1 onion
- 250ml chopped fresh parsley
- 125ml chopped fresh dill
- 125ml snipped chives
- Salt and white pepper
- 500ml fresh cream
- Approx. 250ml water

METHOD: Cut the chicken up into smaller pieces and chop up all the vegetables. Place the chicken, herbs, vegetables and seasoning into a saucepan and add the cream. Bring to the boil, then reduce the heat and simmer for 15 minutes. If necessary, add water for a thinner consistency.

Cream of Tomato Soup *Serves 4*

INGREDIENTS
- *675g ripe tomatoes*
- *2 cloves garlic*
- *1 large onion*
- *2 sticks celery*
- *100g back bacon*
- *2 Tbsp. olive oil or butter*
- *Few sprigs of basil*
- *450ml vegetable stock*
- *Salt and ground black pepper*
- *2-3 Tbsp. tomato purée*
- *1 Tbsp. almond flour*
- *150ml cream*

METHOD: Place tomatoes in a bowl and cover with boiling water to remove skins. Cut tomatoes in quarters and discard the core and most of the seeds. Peel and crush garlic; peel and finely chop the onion. Wash and trim celery and chop finely. Discard any rind from the bacon and snip into pieces with scissors. Place garlic, onion, celery and bacon in a large saucepan with the oil/butter and fry gently for 5 minutes, or until onion is soft and transparent. Add the tomatoes and basil and cook gently for 5 minutes. Pour in stock and season with salt and pepper. Bring to the boil, cover and simmer gently for 15 minutes or until vegetables are soft. Allow to cool for 5 minutes, then pass through a blender and return to the heat. Mix the tomato purée with 2 Tbsp. cold water and stir into mixture, bring to just below boiling point. Blend the almond flour with 2-3 Tbsp. of cold water to form a smooth paste and stir into the soup. Stir with a wooden spoon until the soup thickens slightly and adjust seasoning if necessary.

To serve: Pour soup into a warm dish and swirl in a little cream and garnish with basil sprigs. Serve remaining cream separately, or if preferred, allow the soup to cool for about 2 minutes then stir in all the cream and serve immediately.

Italian Meatball Soup

Serves 4

INGREDIENTS
- 500g good quality beef mince
- 2 Tbsp. Parmesan cheese (optional)
- 1 can tomato purée
- 2½ tsp. dried Italian herbs
- 1 tsp. dried thyme
- 1 Tbsp. chopped garlic
- 1 medium sized brinjal, diced
- 5 medium baby marrows, diced
- 6 baby plum tomatoes, diced
- 1 onion, diced or 3 spring onion sprigs, chopped
- 1 green pepper, diced
- 4 Tbsp. coconut oil or lard
- Salt & pepper to taste (you can use garlic and celery flavoured salt)
- 2 Tbsp. Xylitol or a few Stevia drops (optional)
- 2 cups of water
- Cream and chopped chives for garnish

METHOD: Mix the Parmesan and half a teaspoon of mixed herbs into the meat and roll into prune-sized meatballs. Fry the meatballs in 2 Tbsp. coconut oil until browned on all sides. Add the tomato purée, spices and Xylitol. Let simmer on medium heat for 7-10 minutes and then add 1 cup of water. Chargrill the diced veggies in half the coconut oil under the grill, stir once or twice to get more chargrilled sides. Add ¼ cup water and give the vegetables a quick blitz in a blender or food processor, leaving a third in bigger chunks if you like a chunky, rustic soup. Purée if you like a smooth soup. Add the vegetables and ¾ cup water to the tomato and meatballs and simmer gently for about 10 minutes. Adjust liquids according to your preference. You can also use stock instead of plain water. Garnish with cream and chopped chives or parsley.

Minestrone Soup

Serves 4

INGREDIENTS
- ¼ cup olive oil
- 2 large onions, finely chopped
- 8 small carrots, peeled and finely diced
- 2 sticks celery, finely diced
- 4 cloves garlic
- 2 tsp. salt
- 6 sprigs thyme
- 2 bay leaves
- 8 small tomatoes
- 3 cups water
- 200g green beans, topped, tailed and finely sliced on the diagonal
- 6 courgettes, finely diced
- 3-6 Parmesan rinds
- 30g flat-leaf parsley, chopped

To serve:
- 4 tsp. extra-virgin olive oil
- 8 tsp. Parmesan cheese, finely grated

METHOD: Heat the oil in a large pot over medium heat, add the onions, carrots and celery and cook for 15 minutes or until tender, but without colour. Sprinkle the garlic with the salt and crush with the blade of a knife. Add the garlic to the herbs and cook for a minute or two, stirring. Cut a cross on the bottom of each tomato, cover with boiling water for one minute, drain, rinse with cold water and peel off the skins. Cut out the core and squeeze the skins and juice into a bowl. Chop the flesh and add to the soup. Strain the collected juice into the soup as well. Discard seeds and skins. Add water to the pot and bring to the boil. Add the beans, courgettes and

Parmesan rinds and simmer for 15 minutes. Season and add the parsley. Divide between four bowls; sprinkle each with one tsp. olive oil and two tsp. Parmesan cheese.

Fish, Tomato & Chorizo Soup *Serves 4*

INGREDIENTS
- 1 chorizo sausage, sliced
- 2 Tbsp. olive oil
- 1 large onion, finely chopped
- 2 Tbsp. garlic, minced
- 1 stick lemongrass, finely chopped
- 4 sticks celery, finely diced
- ½ cup white wine
- 1 tin chopped peeled tomatoes
- 4 cups fish or chicken stock
- 600g fresh fish, diced
- ½ cup parsley, finely chopped
- Juice of 1 lemon

METHOD: In a large saucepan, heat the olive oil and sauté the chorizo for 3-4 minutes. Add the onion, garlic, lemongrass and celery and continue sautéing for 3 minutes. Add the wine and reduce by half. Stir in the tomatoes and stock and simmer for 10 minutes. Add the fish and simmer for another five minutes (or until the fish is cooked). Stir in the chopped parsley, season to taste with salt, pepper and lemon juice and serve immediately.

The Low-Carb Companion

SECTION 2:

EGGS

Eating eggs makes no difference to your blood cholesterol level.

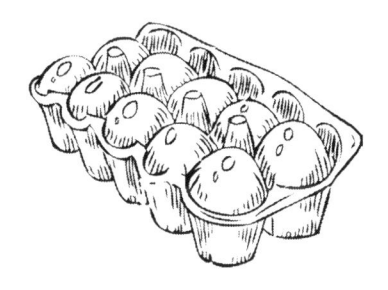

Eggs

	Page
Austin's Power Breakfast	273
Bacon, Asparagus & Soft-Boiled Eggs	273
Bacon & Spinach Frittata	274
Baked Eggs with Spinach, Yoghurt & Chilli Oil	275
Basic Breakfast Omelette	276
Cauliflower & Feta Frittata	277
Creamy Scrambled Eggs	277
Egg & Pesto Breakfast Wrap with Linseed Wrap	278
Mushroom, Egg, Chorizo & Spinach Towers	279
Olive, Ham & Vine-ripened Tomato Bake	280
Trout & Cream Cheese Omelette	281
Salmon Eggs Benedict	282
Prawn & Vegetable Foo Yung	283
Huevos Rancheros	284

Austin's 'Power Breakfast' *Serves 1-2*

INGREDIENTS

- 200g cubed fatty steak (sirloin or shin)
- 2 free-range eggs
- 100g Halloumi cheese, thickly sliced
- Coconut oil for frying
- Seasoning to taste

METHOD: Heat the frying pan and add coconut oil. Fry the steak, Halloumi cheese and eggs in hot coconut oil. Season to taste and serve.

Bacon, Asparagus & Soft-Boiled Eggs *Serves 4*

INGREDIENTS
- 250g streaky bacon
- 200g asparagus spears
- 8 eggs
- 40g butter
- Salt and black pepper

METHOD: Place a small pot of water on to boil. In a heavy-based frying pan, fry the bacon in the butter until crispy then remove from the heat. Drop the eggs into the water (4½ minutes for perfect soft-boiled eggs). Blanch the asparagus in the egg water and drop it straight into the bacon pan with the fat and butter. As the eggs come out of the water, put the bacon and asparagus pan back on the heat and allow the asparagus to colour a little. Peel the eggs under water. Serve the bacon, asparagus and pan juices with the boiled eggs broken over the top.

Bacon & Spinach Frittata

Serves 6-8

INGREDIENTS
- *10 eggs*
- *Salt and fresh ground pepper*
- *1 tsp. olive oil*
- *1 clove garlic, minced*
- *1 red pepper, diced small*
- *1 packet mushrooms, sliced*
- *One packet bacon, diced small*
- *One bag fresh baby spinach*
- *½ cup shredded Parmesan cheese, approximately*
- *Sour cream to garnish*

METHOD: Heat oven to 190° C. Beat eggs in a large bowl, season with salt and pepper and set aside. Heat large pan over medium heat and add coconut oil, garlic, red pepper and mushrooms. Cook until peppers are crisp-tender, about 5 minutes. Add bacon and spinach and cook until spinach has wilted down. Remove from heat, and add to the eggs with Parmesan and stir well. Pour into a buttered 9 x 9 casserole dish, top with a little more Parmesan and bake until set, about 20-25 minutes. Do not overcook as it will become dry. Serve topped with sour cream.

Tip: *You can make different combos, using any leftover meat.*

Note: Commercial bacon is processed meat. From a health perspective, it should be eaten infrequently. Try non-nitrated cured bacon or thinly sliced pork belly as alternatives.

Baked Eggs with Spinach, Yoghurt & Chilli Oil

Serves 2-4

INGREDIENTS
- ⅔ cup plain Greek yoghurt
- 1 garlic clove, halved
- Salt
- 2 Tbsp. unsalted butter, divided
- 2 Tbsp. olive oil
- 3 Tbsp. chopped leek, white and pale green parts only
- 2 Tbsp. chopped spring onion, white and pale green parts only
- 10 cups fresh spinach
- 1 tsp. fresh lemon juice
- 4 large eggs
- ¼ tsp. crushed red pepper flakes
- pinch of paprika
- 1 tsp. chopped fresh oregano

METHOD: Mix yoghurt, garlic and a pinch of salt in a small bowl and set aside. Preheat oven to 150°C. Melt 1 Tbsp. butter with oil in a large heavy frying pan over medium heat, add leek and spring onion and reduce heat to low. Cook until soft, about 10 minutes. Add spinach and lemon juice; season with salt and increase heat to medium-high; cook, turning frequently, until wilted, 4-5 minutes. Transfer spinach mixture to a 25cm pan, leaving any excess liquid behind. Make 4 deep indentations in the centre of the spinach and carefully break 1 egg into each hollow, taking care to keep yolks intact. Bake until egg whites are set, 10-15 minutes. Melt remaining butter in a small pan over medium-low heat and the red pepper flakes, paprika and a pinch of salt and cook until butter starts to foam and browned bits form at bottom of the pan, 1-2 minutes. Add oregano and cook a further 30 seconds. Remove garlic halves from the yoghurt and discard. Spoon yoghurt over the spinach and eggs and drizzle with spiced butter and serve.

Basic Breakfast Omelette *Serves 1*

INGREDIENTS
- *15ml coconut oil or butter*
- *2 eggs*
- *30ml heavy cream*
- *Salt and pepper*
- *Extra 15ml butter*

METHOD: Melt the oil or butter in a frying pan. Whisk the eggs and cream in a bowl and add seasoning; pour the mixture into the pan and fry over medium heat until the omelette has set. Turn over and fry the other side. Serve with extra butter on top.

VARIATIONS: **Cheese:** Make as above and when one side is ready, lay 3-4 slices Cheddar or Gouda cheese on half of the omelette. Fold over the other half and allow cheese to melt over low heat.

Bacon and Mushroom: Melt coconut oil or butter in a frying pan. Dice 2 rashers bacon and slice 2 mushrooms and fry until cooked to taste. Mix into basic omelette mix and cook as above.

Avocado, Salami and Brie cheese: Make an omelette according to the basic recipe and when one side is ready, lay 3-4 slices salami, half a sliced avocado and some pieces of Brie cheese on half of the omelette. Fold over the other half and allow the cheese to melt over low heat.

Sweet Omelette: Add cinnamon to the basic mixture and serve with whipped cream and fresh berries.

Cauliflower & Feta Frittata

Serves 2

INGREDIENTS
- 5 eggs
- 1 head cauliflower, trimmed and cut into small florets
- 1 garlic clove, peeled and finely chopped
- ½ cup feta cheese, crumbled
- 2-3 spring onions, chopped
- ¼ cup fresh parsley leaves, chopped
- 2-3 Tbsp. oil

METHOD: Heat the oil in a large frying pan on a medium heat and sauté the cauliflower florets until golden in colour, for 7-9 minutes. Add the garlic and spring onions and sauté for a further minute. Beat the eggs, and add the parsley and feta cheese to the mixture. Pour the egg mixture over the cauliflower, ensuring even coverage. Cook for 4-5 minutes until firm, and then place under a hot grill to finish off the top for 1-2 minutes.

Creamy Scrambled Eggs

Serves 1

INGREDIENTS
- 15ml coconut oil or butter
- 2 eggs
- Salt and pepper
- 30ml fresh cream

METHOD: Melt oil or butter in a pan over low heat; mix eggs, seasoning and cream together in a bowl and pour into the pan. Using a spatula, scrape the eggs towards the centre of the pan and don't overcook or they will set too firmly. Remove from the heat and serve with extra butter on top.

Egg & Pesto Breakfast Wrap

Serves 1

INGREDIENTS
- 1 linseed wrap, recipe below
- 1 Tbsp. basil pesto or sun-dried tomato pesto
- 1 hard-boiled egg, peeled and sliced thinly
- 2 thin slices tomato
- Handful of baby spinach or shredded lettuce

METHOD: If the wrap is freshly made, allow it to cool for 5 minutes. Then spread the pesto in a 5cm strip down the centre of the wrap. Place sliced egg on the pesto strip, followed by tomato slices. Top with spinach or lettuce. Roll up to serve.

Linseed Wrap

Serves 1

INGREDIENTS
- 3 Tbsp. ground linseeds
- ¼ tsp. baking powder
- ¼ tsp. onion powder
- ¼ tsp. paprika
- Pinch of fine sea salt or celery salt
- 1 Tbsp. coconut oil, melted, plus more for greasing the dishes
- 1 Tbsp. water
- 1 large egg

METHOD: Mix together the ground linseeds, baking powder, onion powder, paprika and salt in a bowl. Stir in the coconut oil. Beat in the egg and 1 Tbsp. water until blended. Grease a microwave-safe glass or plastic dish with coconut oil. Pour in the batter and spread evenly over the bottom. Microwave on high for 2-3 minutes until cooked. Let cool about 5 minutes. To remove, lift up an edge with a spatula. If it sticks, use the spatula to gently loosen from the dish. Flip the wrap over and place the desired ingredients on top. Roll up to serve.

Mushroom, Egg, Chorizo & Spinach Towers

Serves 4

INGREDIENTS
- *4 large Shitake mushrooms*
- *Olive oil*
- *1 clove garlic, chopped*
- *Himalayan salt and black pepper*
- *125g chorizo, thinly sliced*
- *4 eggs, poached*
- *Handful baby spinach*

METHOD: Preheat oven to 200°C. Drizzle mushrooms with olive oil, garlic and salt and pepper; roast until cooked. Fry chorizo and set aside in a bowl. Place the handful of baby spinach on top of each mushroom, followed by chorizo and an egg. Season and serve warm.

Olive, Ham & Vine-ripened Tomato Bake   *Serves 4*

INGREDIENTS
For the Base:
- *3 eggs, separated*
- *150g cream cheese*
- *1 Tbsp. almond flour*
- *4 sprigs fresh rosemary*

For the Topping:
- *1 Tbsp. duck fat*
- *250g button mushrooms, halved*
- *100g green olives*
- *4 slices ham, thickly cut*
- *4 balls bocconcini, halved*
- *4 eggs*
- *350g vine tomatoes, chopped*
- *Extra-virgin olive oil to drizzle*
- *Salt and black pepper*
- *Herbs to garnish*

METHOD: Preheat the oven to 180°C. **For the Base:** Whisk together eggs yolks and cream cheese until smooth. In a separate bowl, whisk egg whites until stiff peaks form. Fold the almond flour and eggs whites into the cream cheese mixture. Sprinkle over the rosemary. Spoon mixture into an oiled and lined 20 x 20cm oven dish and bake for 20-25 minutes. **For the Topping:** Heat the duck fat in a frying pan, toss in the mushrooms and sauté until soft, remove and set aside. Remove the base from the oven, top with the sautéed mushrooms, olives, ham slices and cheese. Gently press 4 hollows into the base and crack the eggs into the hollows. Top with vine tomatoes, season well and bake for 15-20 minutes or until eggs are cooked through. Slice, serve warm, drizzled with olive oil and sprinkled with fresh herbs.

Section 2 - Eggs

Trout & Cream Cheese Omelette   *Serves 4*

INGREDIENTS
- *3 eggs*
- *40g butter*
- *100g full-fat cream cheese*
- *80g smoked trout ribbons*
- *Lemon wedge*
- *Salt and pepper*
- *Fresh dill (optional)*

METHOD: Turn the oven grill to high. Add the butter to a pan over medium-high heat. Mix the eggs, salt and pepper with a fork. Break the cream cheese into large chunks and add to the egg mixture. As the butter starts bubbling, add the egg mixture and stir using a flat-edged lifter. Gently break up the omelette so the raw egg touches the base of the pan and cooks slightly. Only do this for 15 seconds. Place the omelette under the grill until the top layer of the egg is just cooked. Flip the omelette onto a plate and before folding over, cover the one side with trout, a squeeze of lemon and some dill. Fold and serve.

Option: You can use bacon and avocado in place of trout.

Tip: Smoked trout offcuts are excellent value for use in this recipe.

Tip: The trick to a perfect omelette is using a good quality pan and getting it to the right heat before you add the eggs.

Salmon Eggs Benedict   *Serves 4*

INGREDIENTS
For The English Muffins
- 1 cup coconut flour, plus extra for dusting
- ½ cup psyllium husks
- 2 tsp. baking powder
- 1 tsp. salt
- 2 large eggs, beaten
- 1 cup full cream milk
- 40g butter, melted
- ½ tsp. coconut oil for cooking

For The Hollandaise
- 3 large egg yolks
- 1 Tbsp. white balsamic vinegar
- ½ cup butter, melted
- Himalayan salt and black pepper

- 100g smoked salmon
- 4 eggs, poached
- Fresh marjoram, to garnish

METHOD: **For the English muffins:** Combine dry ingredients in a bowl. Whisk together eggs, milk and butter and add to the dry ingredients. Stir to combine, and then knead gently to form a smooth dough. Lightly dust a surface with extra coconut flour and roll out dough until 2cm thick. Cut out four 8cm rounds. Melt coconut oil in a frying pan. Cook muffins over medium heat for 8-10 minutes on each side until risen and cooked through. **For the hollandaise:** Place egg yolks and vinegar in a bowl over a bain-marie and whisk until pale. Slowly whisk in the melted butter until a thick sauce is formed, season and set aside in a warm place.

To assemble: Slice muffins in half, toast them lightly, then top with smoked salmon, poached eggs and a drizzle of hollandaise. Garnish with marjoram and serve immediately.

Prawn & Vegetable Foo Yung *Serves 4*

INGREDIENTS
- *8 eggs*
- *1 tsp. sesame oil*
- *1 Tbsp. Tamari sauce*
- *2 Tbsp. oil*
- *½ head broccoli, cut into small florets*
- *1 red pepper, deseeded and thinly sliced*
- *2 inch piece fresh ginger, peeled and cut into thin strips*
- *2 garlic cloves, peeled and chopped*
- *3 spring onions, sliced*
- *200g raw prawns or shrimp*

METHOD: Beat the eggs with the sesame oil and set aside. Heat half the oil in a large frying pan and add the broccoli, ginger, pepper, garlic and spring onions and cook for 5 minutes. Add the prawns and Tamari sauce, and cook for a further 2-3 minutes, until the prawns are pink and cooked through. Transfer to a bowl and keep warm. Heat the remaining oil and pour in half of the egg mixture, making sure the mixture is spread all over the pan. Cook for about 3 minutes until the egg is set. Flip over and cook for another 1 minute. Remove the omelette and transfer to a plate. Add the remaining egg mixture to the pan, repeating the above. Remove the omelette, place on a cutting board and cut into ribbons. To assemble, spoon the vegetables over the omelette, then scatter the omelette ribbons all over.

Huevos Rancheros

Serves 2

INGREDIENTS
- *1 Tbsp. butter or olive oil*
- *4 eggs*
- *120g coarsely torn curly endive*
- *50g sharp Cheddar cheese, grated*
- *4 Tbsp. salsa*
- *2 Tbsp. fresh coriander leaves, chopped*
- *Salt and pepper to taste*

METHOD: Add the butter or olive oil to a frying pan over medium-high heat. When hot, crack the eggs into the pan and cook for 3-4 minutes for runny yolks, more for firmer yolks. Serve the eggs over a bed of curly endive and top with cheese, salsa and coriander. Season with salt and pepper.

> **Egg yolk** will keep fresh in water in the fridge.

Section 2 - Eggs

The Low-Carb Companion

SECTION 3:

FISH

Fatty fish are rich in heart and brain-healthy Omega-3 fatty acids.

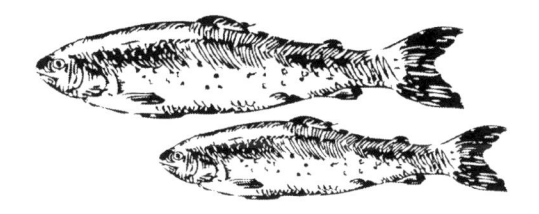

Fish

	Page
Butter-fried Salmon with Glazed Chives, Tomatoes & Coriander Cream Sauce	289
Crab Cakes	290
Fish Fingers with a Cold Herb Sauce	291
Fish Bake in Spicy Tomato Sauce	292
Fried Calamari	293
Grilled Chilli & Garlic Prawns	294
Poached Fish on Buttered Greens	295
Steamed Mussel Pot	296
White Fish with Lemon & Caper Sauce	296
Herb & Almond Crusted Baked Fish	297

Butter-fried Salmon with Glazed Chives, Tomatoes & Coriander Cream Sauce

Serves 4

INGREDIENTS
- 4 Salmon fillets
- 100g butter
- 100ml snipped garlic chives or chives
- 100ml chopped fresh coriander
- 50ml chopped fresh dill
- 800g salmon fillets
- Grated zest of ½ lemon

Coriander cream sauce
- 300ml crème fraiche
- 150ml finely chopped fresh coriander
- Salt and pepper
- Juice of ½ lemon

Tomatoes
- 50g butter
- 250g cocktail tomatoes
- 30ml snipped garlic chives or chives

METHOD: Heat the butter in a saucepan and add half the chives, coriander and dill. Place the salmon fillets in the pan and sprinkle with the rest of the herbs and the lemon zest. Fry the fish on one side over low heat for about 8 minutes and carefully turn over. Repeat with remaining salmon. Keep warm. **Coriander cream sauce:** Mix all the ingredients together and refrigerate. **Tomatoes:** Melt the butter in a saucepan and add the tomatoes. Stir in the chives and fry for a couple of minutes until glazed. Place the fish on a serving platter and spoon the tomatoes around it. Serve with the cold sauce.

Crab (or Salmon/Tuna) Cakes   *Serves 4*

INGREDIENTS
- 2 Tbsp. extra-virgin olive oil
- ½ red pepper, finely diced
- ¼ yellow onion, finely chopped
- 2 Tbsp. finely chopped fresh green chillies, or to taste
- 20 ground walnuts
- 1 large egg
- 1 ½ tsp. curry powder
- ½ tsp. ground cumin
- Fine sea salt
- 170g tinned crabmeat (or salmon/tuna), drained and flaked
- 30g ground linseeds
- 1 tsp. onion powder
- ½ tsp. garlic powder
- Baby spinach or mixed salad greens
- Homemade mayonnaise to serve (optional)

METHOD: Preheat oven to 160°C and line a baking pan with foil. Heat the oil in a large frying pan over medium heat. Add the pepper, onion and green chilli and cook until tender, 4-5 minutes. Set aside to cool. Transfer the vegetables to large bowl; stir in the walnuts, egg, curry powder, cumin and sea salt. Add the crabmeat (or salmon/tuna) to the mixture and stir well. Form into 4 patties and transfer to the baking pan. In a small bowl stir together the ground linseed, onion powder and garlic powder, then sprinkle this breading over the cakes and bake until browned and heated through (about 25 minutes). Serve on a bed of greens (spinach or salad) with homemade mayonnaise (optional).

Fish Fingers with a Cold Herb Sauce   Serves 4

INGREDIENTS

For the fish fingers
- 2 eggs
- 150g pork rind snacks
- Salt
- 100g coconut oil or butter
- 4 fish fillets

For the herb sauce
- 200ml crème fraiche
- 100ml mayonnaise
- 125ml chopped fresh herbs (parsley, dill, chives)
- Salt and pepper
- 15ml vinegar

METHOD: Beat the eggs into a bowl. Process the pork rinds in a blender so that you have a light 'flour' and add salt. Melt the oil or butter in a frying pan, cut the fish into fingers and dip each piece into egg, and then cover with pork rind 'flour'. Fry the fish for a few minutes on each side. For the sauce, mix all the ingredients together and serve as a cold dipping sauce with the fish fingers, mashed broccoli and tomatoes.

Tip: *The recipe works well with whole fillets of fish and your favourite spices can be added to the pork rind 'flour' for extra flavour.*

Fish Bake in Spicy Tomato Sauce *Serves 8*

INGREDIENTS
- 8 x 200g portions of any white fish
- Salt and pepper
- Olive oil
- 50g butter
- 2 tsp. harissa paste
- 10 pitted olives (green, black or mixed)
- 2 anchovy fillets
- 2 Tbsp. lemon zest, finely shaved
- ½ tsp. paprika
- 2 cups tomato, chopped and seeded
- 1 cup onions, chopped
- 2 Tbsp. minced garlic
- ¼ cup parsley, roughly chopped
- 2 Tbsp. fresh origanum
- 1 Tbsp. fresh thyme

METHOD: Preheat the oven to 200°C. Season both sides of the fish with salt, pepper and olive oil. To make the sauce, sauté the onions in butter until golden, add the garlic and sauté until fragrant. Add the remaining ingredients and simmer for five minutes on low heat. Pack the fish pieces tightly in a lasagne or baking dish and cover with the sauce. Bake for about 40 minutes, basting occasionally with the pan juices. Remove from the oven and allow to rest for 15 minutes. Top with some fresh herbs for garnish.

Fried Calamari

Serves 2

INGREDIENTS
- 115g calamari rings
- 2 Tbsp. coconut flour
- 1 egg
- 30ml milk
- Olive oil (for frying)
- Sea salt to taste
- Lemon wedges to serve

METHOD: Toss the calamari rings in the flour in a bowl or strong plastic bag. Beat the egg and milk together in shallow bowl. Heat the oil in a large heavy frying pan. Dip the floured calamari rings, one at a time, into the egg/milk mixture, shaking off any excess liquid. Add to the hot oil in batches and cook for 2-3 minutes each side until evenly golden all over. Drain the calamari on kitchen paper, and then sprinkle with salt. Transfer to warm plates and serve with lemon wedges.

> **Store lemon slices** in a plastic container in the freezer. This is very handy for drinks or garnishes.

Grilled Chilli & Garlic Prawns *Serves 4*

INGREDIENTS
For the sauce
- 2 red chillies, very finely chopped
- 5 cloves garlic, crushed
- ¾ cup olive oil
- ¼ cup lemon juice with the zest of each lemon

METHOD: Combine all ingredients in a small pan and simmer for 5 minutes.

For the prawns
- 24 large prawns, peeled and deveined
- 200g butter
- Olive oil
- 2 tsp. crushed garlic
- 2 Tbsp. lemon juice
- 2 Tbsp. hot chilli sauce or chopped chilli
- Salt and black pepper

METHOD: In a very large frying pan, heat the butter and a bit of olive oil before adding the garlic, lemon juice and chilli. Sauté for a minute or two to let the flavours come out, then add the prawns. Sauté the prawns for 4-5 minutes, turning until cooked. Use tongs to transfer the prawns from the pan into a warm serving dish. Add the sauce to the pan, season and mix well with the bits left in the pan, bring to a boil and simmer for a minute or so before tipping the sauce over the prawns. Serve immediately. Add a large handful of freshly chopped parsley to this for a fresh flavour.

> **Lemons** put in the microwave for 1 minute before use will yield almost twice as much juice.

Poached Fish on Buttered Greens   *Serves 2*

INGREDIENTS
- 2 x 180g oily fish (salmon, trout, mackerel or haddock)
- 1 cup white wine
- 750ml water
- 1 bay leaf
- 5 peppercorns
- 1 sprig thyme
- 1 handful parsley
- Zest of 1 lemon
- 60g fine French beans
- 60g mange tout
- 50ml cream
- 2 Tbsp. capers
- 100g butter

METHOD: Fill a small pot with the wine, water, bay leaf, peppercorns, thyme, parsley and lemon zest. Bring to a boil, simmer for about 5 minutes, then reduce the heat to an 'almost bubble'. While the stock is boiling, blanch the beans and mange tout in it and refresh them with cold water or an ice bath. Drop the fish portions into the stock and leave them for about 5 minutes. Remove them from the liquid and set aside. Using a slotted spoon, remove the solids from the water and reduce it to less than a cup. Transfer to a pan to widen the surface area. Add the cream and capers and reduce till thick. Add the butter and fish to the pan, shaking the pan continuously to emulsify the butter. Add the beans and mange tout, warm through and serve.

Steamed Mussel Pot   *Serves 4*

INGREDIENTS
- 1½ kg mussels
- ¼ cup olive oil
- 3 Tbsp. butter
- 1 medium onion, finely chopped
- 4 garlic cloves, minced
- 2 sticks celery, finely chopped
- ¼ bunch fresh thyme
- 1 cup white wine
- 200ml cream
- 1 handful basil, roughly chopped

METHOD: Rinse the mussels under cold running water. Remove the stringy mussel beards and discard any open mussels or those with broken shells. Heat two tablespoons olive oil and two tablespoons butter in a large pot over medium heat. Add the onion, garlic, celery and thyme and cook for about five minutes. Add the white wine and bring to the boil. Add the cream, bring to the boil again and add the mussels. Close the pot with a lid and steam over medium-high heat for 10 minutes, until the mussels open. Stir occasionally so that all the mussels are in contact with the heat. Season with salt and pepper; sprinkle with basil and serve immediately.

White Fish with Lemon & Caper Sauce   *Serves 2*

INGREDIENTS
- ½ lemon
- ⅓ cup almond flour
- Salt and pepper to taste

- 1 piece of white fish, such as a Sole fillet
- 2 tsp. olive oil
- 1 clove garlic, finely chopped
- ⅓ cup stock
- 1 Tbsp. capers
- 2 tsp. butter

METHOD: Remove the skin and white pith from the lemon, removing the membranes. Cut into pieces, keeping any juices in a bowl. Combine the almond flour, salt and pepper in a bowl. Coat the fish with flour on both sides. Heat the oil in a frying pan on a medium heat. Cook the fish until it is golden brown on both sides, and then transfer to a plate and keep warm. Add the garlic to the pan and fry gently for a minute, add the stock and bring to the boil, stirring. Add lemon juice, lemon pieces, capers and butter. Cook until the butter has melted. Spoon the sauce over the fish and serve.

Herb & Almond Crusted Baked Fish *Serves 2*

INGREDIENTS
- 2 white fish fillets
- 2 Tbsp. ground almonds
- 2 Tbsp. lemon thyme, chopped
- 2 spring onions, finely chopped
- 1 Tbsp. fresh parsley, chopped
- Salt and pepper

METHOD: Preheat the oven to 190°C. Mix the ground almond, onions and seasoning together in a bowl. Place the fish fillets in a lightly greased baking dish. Place the almond and herb mixture on top of the fish, covering it evenly. Bake for 20-30 minutes until the fish is cooked through.

The Low-Carb Companion

SECTION 4:

POULTRY

True free-range poultry is best. In the USA in 1950, approximately 80% of chickens were free-range; by 1980, it was only 1% and today it is about 12%.

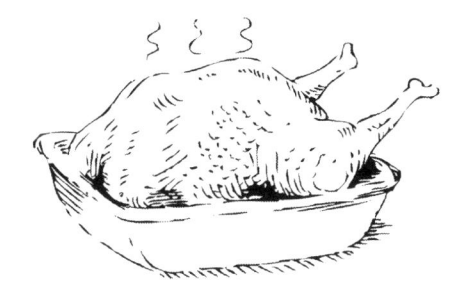

Poultry

	Page
Asian Duck Breasts With Egg Pancakes	301
Stuffed Chicken Breast In Mustard Cream with Pan-fried Vegetables	302
Chicken 'Paella'	304
Chicken & Mushroom Cauli-mash 'Pie'	305
Chicken Tikka Masala	306
Coconut Chicken Nuggets	307
Chicken With Garlic & Creamy Tarragon Asparagus	308
Creamy Chicken Livers	309
Green Chicken Curry	310
Lemon Chicken With Sweet Potatoes	312
Roast Chicken With Lime, Garlic & Roasted Vegetables	312
Spicy Chicken Wings With Blue Cheese Dip	314
Thai Chicken Stir-Fry With Ginger & Coconut	315
Turkey Cabbage Wraps & Caesar Dressing	316
Yoghurt-Marinated Chicken With Coriander Sauce	317

Asian Duck Breasts with Egg Pancakes *Serves 4*

INGREDIENTS
- 4 duck breast fillets
- Sesame oil, to drizzle
- 2 tsp. Chinese five-spice powder

For the pancakes:
- 2 Tbsp. ghee
- 6 eggs, beaten
- ½ cup water
- Big pinch Himalayan salt
- 5g fresh coriander, chopped

For the filling:
- 1 cucumber, cut into batons
- 4 spring onions, sliced
- Himalayan salt and black pepper

To serve: fresh coriander, spring onions, sesame seeds and red chilli

METHOD: Preheat the oven to 200°C. Slash each duck breast 2-3 times, drizzle with sesame oil and sprinkle with the five-spice powder. Place on a rack in a baking tin and bake for 15 minutes; during the last 2-3 minutes, turn on the grill and cook until crispy. Remove from the oven and set aside. When cool enough to handle, slice into strips. **For the Pancakes:** Brush a small frying pan with ghee; whisk together the eggs, water, salt and coriander. Place ¼ cup of the mixture into the frying pan, swirl to cover the base, cook until firm, then flip and repeat with remaining batter.
To assemble: Place the pancakes on a surface, top with sliced duck, cucumber and roll up. Repeat with remaining ingredients. Serve garnished with fresh coriander, spring onions, sesame seeds and chilli.

Stuffed Chicken Breast in Mustard Cream with Pan-fried Vegetables

Serves 4

INGREDIENTS
- 4 chicken breasts, skin on, deboned
- 6-8 rashers of bacon, chopped
- ½ green or red pepper, chopped
- 4 tsp. pesto
- 4 Tbsp. cream cheese or grated Cheddar cheese
- Herbed salt in grinder or salt and pepper to taste
- Coconut oil for frying

Vegetables:
- Baby marrows, sliced
- Plum tomatoes, halved
- Herbed salt in grinder or salt and pepper to taste
- Coconut oil for frying

METHOD: In a pan on medium to high heat, cook the bacon rashers in a bit of coconut oil. As soon as the rashers start to cook through, add the chopped peppers and sauté in the bacon fat along with the bacon. As soon as the peppers are soft, remove from heat. Cut a pocket into the chicken breasts and stuff them with a tablespoon layer of cream cheese or Cheddar cheese, a teaspoon of pesto, and a quarter of the bacon mix. Tuck the skin as tightly as you can to close the pockets. Secure with a toothpick. In the bacon pan, on medium to high heat, add a bit of coconut oil to the leftover bacon fat. Sear the breasts on both sides until brown (about 1-2 minutes on each side), sprinkle with salt and pepper, and turn heat down to medium to low. Add the chopped vegetables all around the chicken pieces and allow to gently sauté in the pan juices. Put a lid on the pan and cook for 6-8 minutes (times may vary according to fillet size). The inside of the filling must ooze and the chicken must be warm throughout when poked with a knife in the thickest part. Remove the chicken from the pan, put it aside for a minute while you quickly allow the vegetables in the pan to caramelise on high heat.

Mustard cream sauce
- *1 Tbsp. Dijon mustard*
- *1 cup cream*
- *3 Tbsp. butter*
- *Salt to taste*
- *1 tsp. Xylitol*
- *A grind of black pepper*
- *A squeeze of lemon juice*

METHOD: In a saucepan over medium heat, melt the butter. Add the rest of the ingredients and allow the sauce to simmer on medium heat for 2-3 minutes and reduce to a creamy consistency. This recipe make approximately 4 Tbsp. of sauce. Smother the chicken breast with warm mustard sauce. Serve with a salad.

> **Sprinkle a little salt** in the pan before frying food to stop explosions.

Chicken 'Paella' — Serves 6

INGREDIENTS
- 3 chicken drumsticks
- 3 chicken wings
- 2 Tbsp. duck fat or coconut oil
- 2 cloves garlic, crushed
- 1 onion, finely chopped
- 1 red pepper, sliced
- 1 head cauliflower, roughly blended
- Big pinch of saffron in a little hot water
- 1 cup homemade chicken stock
- 2 bay leaves
- 3 large red tomatoes, diced
- Himalayan salt and black pepper
- 500g mussels in their shells, cleaned
- 10g fresh thyme
- Homemade mayonnaise, to serve

METHOD: Heat a griddle pan and char grill chicken pieces until dark golden and cooked through. Heat a large frying pan or paella pan, add duck fat (or coconut oil) and toss in garlic, onion and pepper. Sauté until golden; add the cauliflower rice and cook for 2 minutes. Pour in the saffron, stock, bay leaf and tomato, bring to a boil, and then simmer for 5 minutes to reduce. Season. Add the chicken pieces and mussels to the pan and cover with a lid or foil and cook over a low heat for 10 minutes. Remove lid and stir in the thyme. Serve with homemade low-carb mayonnaise.

Chicken & Mushroom Cauli-mash 'Pie'   *Serves 4*

INGREDIENTS
- *1 whole medium-sized chicken*
- *1 onion, chopped*
- *4 bacon rashers, chopped*
- *1 tsp. chicken spice*
- *Salt & freshly ground black pepper*
- *2 tsp. white vinegar*
- *1 tsp. Worcestershire sauce*
- *1 can (430g) of asparagus*
- *Punnet of button mushrooms, fried in a little oil*
- *250ml cream*
- *2 eggs*
- *100ml grated cheese*
- *450g cauliflower, cooked and mashed*

METHOD: Place the whole chicken, onion and bacon in a pressure cooker or deep pot, season with chicken spice, salt and pepper. Add the vinegar, Worcestershire sauce and about 400ml water, cover and simmer until the chicken is cooked and tender. Remove the meat from the bone and cut into small pieces and set aside. Drain the asparagus. Heat the cream and beat in the eggs to form a thick sauce – do not boil. Season with salt and pepper and add half the grated cheese. Put a layer of chicken meat and mushrooms into a greased ovenproof dish and spoon over some of the sauce. Add the remaining meat as another layer and arrange the asparagus over the top before covering with the remaining sauce. Spoon the cauli-mash on top, sprinkle remaining cheese over and bake in a preheated oven to 180°C for 20-30 minutes until heated through and the top is golden brown. Serve with a mixed salad.

Chicken Tikka Masala *Serves 4*

INGREDIENTS
- *500g boneless, skinless chicken thighs*
- *1 cup extra-thick yoghurt*
- *1 Tbsp. fresh ginger, grated*
- *3 cloves garlic, minced*
- *Salt and pepper*

METHOD: Mix the yoghurt, ginger and garlic and season to taste. Add chicken and marinate for at least 30 minutes.

For the sauce
- *3 Tbsp. butter*
- *2 tsp. olive oil*
- *2 cloves garlic, minced*
- *1 ½ Tbsp. ginger, peeled and minced*
- *1 red chilli, minced (remove seeds if you don't want it spicy)*
- *2 Tbsp. tomato paste*
- *2 tsp. paprika*
- *1 tsp. garam masala*
- *7 Roma tomatoes, diced or 1 tin chopped, peeled tomatoes*
- *1 ½ tsp. salt*
- *2 cups water*
- *½ cup cream*
- *1 handful fresh coriander, roughly chopped*

METHOD: Place a large pan on medium heat and add the butter and olive oil. When the butter has melted, add the garlic, ginger and chilli and sauté until lightly browned. Add the tomato paste and cook until the tomato has darkened in colour, about 3 minutes. Add the paprika and garam masala and sauté for another minute. Add the tomatoes, salt and water. Bring the sauce to the boil and then turn down to a simmer and cover. Cook for 20 minutes, take the pan off the heat and allow the sauce to cool for 5 minutes. Meanwhile, preheat your grill and cover a roasting tray with foil. Remove the chicken thigh chunks from the marinade and place on the tray; put under the grill and cook for about 5 minutes each side, until lightly charred and almost cooked through. Use a blender or food processor to blend the sauce until smooth. Pour back into the pan, bring sauce back up to a boil and add the chicken. Reduce heat to simmer and cook, covered, for about 10 minutes. Add cream and fresh coriander, stir through and serve.

Coconut Chicken Nuggets   *Serves 4*

INGREDIENTS
- 500g minced chicken
- 1 egg yolk
- ¼ tsp. garlic powder
- ¼ cup plus ½ cup almond flour
- ½ cup unsweetened desiccated coconut
- 1 Tbsp. dried onion
- Salt and pepper
- 2-3 Tbsp. oil

METHOD: In a shallow bowl, mix the ¼ cup almond flour and desiccated coconut. Season to taste. In another bowl, mix the chicken, ½ cup almond flour, dried onion, garlic powder, egg yolk and mix thoroughly. Make small balls of the meat mix and toss them in the flour and coconut mix. Cook the chicken nuggets in the frying pan until golden brown on all sides.

Chicken With Garlic & Creamy Tarragon Asparagus

Serves 4

INGREDIENTS

For the chicken
- 1 whole chicken
- 45g butter, softened
- Himalayan salt and black pepper
- 1 lemon, quartered
- 5g fresh thyme
- 1 bulb garlic, halved
- 6 celery sticks
- 1 onion, quartered

For the asparagus
- 1 tsp. ghee
- 2 shallots, finely sliced
- 1 cup cream
- ½ tsp. nutmeg
- ½ tsp. white pepper
- 1 Tbsp. fresh tarragon, chopped
- 300g asparagus spears
- 400g exotic mushrooms, sliced if large

METHOD: Preheat oven to 180°C degrees. Rub chicken with butter. Season the skin and cavity well. Stuff the lemon and thyme into the cavity. Tie legs with string and place the chicken on a roasting tray with garlic, celery and onion. Roast for 1-1 ½ hours, or until chicken is cooked and golden.

Melt ghee for the asparagus and fry shallots until golden. Add cream, nutmeg and pepper and simmer for 5 minutes or until reduced by a third.

Add the remaining ingredients and simmer for 2 minutes or until tender. Season to taste.

To serve: Carve the chicken and serve with the creamy asparagus and mushroom mixture.

Creamy Chicken Livers *Serves 2*

INGREDIENTS
- 1 small tub of chicken livers
- ½ cup of cream
- 1 tsp. garlic
- 1 tsp. Dijon mustard
- 1 tsp. turmeric
- A squeeze of lemon juice
- Salt & black pepper
- 2 sprigs chopped spring onion
- 6 chopped mushrooms
- 6 cherry tomatoes (optional)
- 1 Tbsp. coconut oil

METHOD: Fry the chicken livers and spices in the coconut oil until brown and almost caramelised. Sauté the vegetables with the livers for a few minutes. Add a tablespoon of water to get all the components to infuse. Add the rest of the ingredients, turn down the heat and simmer for a few minutes until thick and saucy. You can add spicy peri peri or curry to add to the flavour combination.

Green Chicken Curry   *Serves 2*

INGREDIENTS
- 2 tsp. olive oil for frying
- 2 tins coconut milk
- 200g chicken breast, sliced
- 1 handful fresh or frozen garden peas
- 1 tin bamboo shoots, drained and other vegetables of your choice, thinly sliced
- 2 tsp. fish sauce
- 1 tsp. Xylitol
- 4 lime leaves, torn
- 1 handful of basil leaves
- 2 long red chillies, diagonally sliced
- 2 tsp. green curry paste (see recipe below)

METHOD: Heat the oil in a pot and fry 2 tsp. of green curry paste until fragrant; pour in coconut milk and bring to simmer. Add the sliced chicken breasts, garden peas, bamboo shoots and other thinly sliced vegetables of your choice; bring back to simmer until the chicken is tender. Add fish sauce, Xylitol and the torn lime leaves and simmer for another minute. Remove from the heat and let rest for 10 minutes before serving. Just before serving, add one handful of basil leaves and garnish with the sliced red chillies.

Green Curry Paste

INGREDIENTS
- 2 tsp. de-seeded green chilli
- Large pinch salt
- 1 tsp. chopped ginger
- 2 tsp. chopped lemongrass stalk
- ½ tsp. lime zest
- 1 tsp. scraped and chopped coriander root
- 1 tsp. fresh turmeric, scraped and chopped
- 3 tsp. chopped shallots
- 2 anchovy fillets (optional)
- 10 white peppercorns
- ½ tsp. toasted coriander seeds
- ½ tsp. toasted cumin seeds

METHOD: In the food processor, mix all ingredients to a fine paste, adding a little olive oil to moisten if ingredients stick to the sides. At this stage, the paste can be stored with a little oil in a sealed jar in the fridge or used straight away.

Lemon Chicken with Sweet Potatoes *Serves 4*

INGREDIENTS
- 1kg sweet potatoes, cut into 3cm cubes
- 3 Tbsp. olive oil
- 8 crushed garlic cloves
- 3 sprigs rosemary
- 4 chicken quarters
- ½ lemon, cut into slices

METHOD: Preheat the oven to 200°C. Put the potatoes in a pan of cold water and bring to the boil; simmer for 5 minutes. Drain and tip the potatoes into a large roasting tin. Add the olive oil, garlic and rosemary and combine and season well. Place the chicken pieces on top of the potatoes, squeeze the lemon over the chicken and potatoes, and drop the squeezed slices into the tin. Roast for one hour or until the sweet potatoes are golden and the chicken is cooked through.

Roast Chicken with Lime, Garlic & Roasted Vegetables *Serves 4*

INGREDIENTS
- 100g coconut oil or butter
- 1 whole chicken
- 2 limes
- 30ml dried tarragon
- 6 cloves garlic, peeled
- 5ml cayenne pepper

- *5 ml paprika*
- *5ml ground sea salt*

Vegetables
- *4-6 broccoli florets*
- *1 carrot*
- *1 baby marrow*
- *1 onion*
- *100ml coconut oil (heated slightly to liquefy)*
- *1 clove garlic, crushed*
- *Salt and pepper*

METHOD: Pre-heat oven to 180°C. Grease an ovenproof dish or baking tray with half the oil or butter. Rinse and dry the chicken. Cut limes into wedges and squeeze juice into a glass. Place the tarragon, garlic and lime wedges inside the chicken cavity. Rub chicken with the remaining oil or butter and sprinkle with the cayenne pepper, paprika, salt and lime juice. Place chicken in the prepared dish. Cut up the vegetables and place them in a small freezer bag, adding the oil, garlic and seasonings. Close the bag and shake until the vegetables are coated with oil. Remove from the bag and place them all around the chicken. Roast for 45-70 minutes, depending on your oven and the size of the chicken. Near the end of the cooking time, set the oven on grill function and grill the chicken until golden and crisp.

> **Fresh ginger** can be scrubbed and finely sliced, unpeeled, placed in a jar and covered with sherry or wine vinegar to keep it fresh for months.

Spicy Chicken Wings with Blue Cheese Dip   *Serves 6*

INGREDIENTS
For the blue cheese dipping sauce
- 50g blue cheese
- 50g cream cheese
- 200ml buttermilk
- 1 handful parsley, chopped
- 1 small bunch chives, roughly chopped
- Salt and pepper

METHOD: Combine all ingredients and puree with a stick blender or food processor.

For the chicken wings
- 24 wings, tips removed and drumettes and flats separated
- 250g butter, melted
- 1 cup Parmesan cheese, grated
- 1 tsp. dried origanum
- 1 tsp. dried chilli flakes
- 2 tsp. paprika
- 2 tsp. dried parsley
- 1 tsp. salt
- 1 tsp. ground black pepper

METHOD: Preheat oven to 180°C. In a bowl, mix the Parmesan, origanum, chilli, paprika, parsley, salt and pepper. Dip each leg in melted butter, then into the seasoning mixture and place on a foiled tray. Roast the wings until dark and crispy (roughly 40 minutes), and serve hot with dipping sauce.

Thai Chicken Stir-Fry with Ginger & Coconut

Serves 4

INGREDIENTS
- 50g coconut oil or butter
- 5 mushrooms, chopped
- ⅓ head cauliflower, broken into florets
- ½ head broccoli, broken into florets
- 1 onion sliced
- 1 leek, sliced
- 15ml green curry paste
- 400g chicken breasts
- 400ml coconut cream
- 200ml fresh cream
- Salt and pepper
- 4 cloves garlic
- 45ml grated fresh ginger
- Grated zest and juice of 1 lime
- 45ml cream cheese
- 1 red pepper, sliced into rings
- 15ml chopped fresh coriander

METHOD: Melt the coconut oil or butter in a wok and stir-fry the mushrooms, cauliflower and broccoli until cooked but still crisp. Remove the vegetables from the pan and set aside. Add the onion, leek and curry paste to the wok and stir-fry for a couple of minutes. Cut up the chicken and add to the onion and curry paste. Add the coconut cream, fresh cream, seasoning, garlic, ginger and lime. Stir-fry for a couple of minutes until the chicken is cooked. Add the cream cheese and stir well. Add the fried vegetables and top with red pepper rings. Serve garnished with fresh coriander.

Turkey Cabbage Wraps & Caesar Dressing *Serves 4*

INGREDIENTS
For the dressing
- 6 cloves of garlic, minced
- 1 Tbsp. Dijon mustard
- 2 Tbsp. mayonnaise
- ½ cup olive oil
- Juice of 1 lemon
- 2 Tbsp. anchovy fillets, minced

METHOD: Combine all ingredients using a stick blender. Season to taste with salt and pepper.

For the wraps
- 600g cooked turkey breast
- 4 large cabbage leaves (white or red)
- ½ cup cream cheese
- 2 cups lettuce mix
- ½ cup mange tout and spring onions, shredded
- ½ cup cherry tomatoes, cut into quarters
- ½ avocado, sliced
- 100g dried cranberries
- Salt and pepper

METHOD: Blanch the cabbage leaves in boiling water for 30 seconds and pat dry. Top each leaf with half a cup of lettuce and place 150g sliced turkey on top. Sprinkle a Tbsp. of shredded vegetables and tomatoes on the turkey; add the avocado and berries. Drizzle with Caesar dressing and season with salt and pepper. Roll the leaves, starting at the edge where you placed the turkey and other ingredients. Using a serrated knife, cut the wraps in half, on the diagonal. Arrange on a plate to serve.

Yoghurt-Marinated Chicken with Coriander Sauce

Serves 4

INGREDIENTS

For the Marinade
- *1 cup thick yoghurt*
- *2 tsp. paprika*
- *1 tsp. turmeric*
- *2 tsp. garam masala*
- *Juice of one lemon*
- *2 Tbsp. ghee, melted*
- *Himalayan salt and black pepper*
- *3 stalks celery*
- *1 red onion, cut into wedges*
- *1 whole chicken*

For the Sauce
- *30g coriander leaves and stems*
- *½ cup thick yoghurt*
- *½ cup desiccated coconut*
- *A squeeze of fresh lemon*

METHOD: Mix together the marinade ingredients and season. Arrange celery and onion in a roasting dish and top with chicken; cover the chicken with marinade and allow to stand for 30-60 minutes. Preheat the oven to 180°C. Roast the chicken for 1 hour 15 minutes or until cooked through. Remove and set aside.

For the sauce
METHOD: Place all the ingredients in a blender and blend until smooth.
To serve: Carve the chicken into portions and top with the sauce.

SECTION 5:

BEEF

Free-range, grass-fed, fatty beef is best.

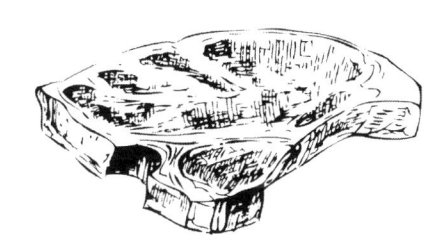

Beef

	Page
Fillet Steak with Chunky Mushroom Wine Sauce	321
Bacon Beef Burgers with Bacon, Onion & Balsamic Jam	322
Carpaccio	323
Beef & Cauli-Mash Cottage Pie	324
Steak 'Sandwiches'	325
Beef Chilli Con Carne with Crispy Aubergine	326
Low-Carb Bobotie	327
Beef Lasagne	328
Peppered Fillet with Rocket Salsa Verde	330
Rustic Meat Loaf With Eggs	331
Skewered Beef Koftas with Mixed Tomato & Cucumber Pickle	332
Steak & Kidney 'Pie'	333
Beef Steak with Horseradish Crème Fraiche & Roasted Tomato Salsa	334
Sticky Beef Short Ribs	335

Fillet Steak with Chunky Mushroom Wine Sauce

Serves 4

INGREDIENTS
- 600g fillet of beef
- Crushed garlic
- Coarsely ground black pepper
- 30ml olive oil
- 10ml butter

For the sauce:
- 125ml red wine
- 4-6 spring onions, chopped
- 125g white mushrooms, chopped
- 125g English cucumber, chopped
- 250ml beef stock
- 15ml soy sauce
- 30ml fresh cream
- 30g butter

METHOD: **For the sauce:** Fry the onions, mushrooms and cucumber in the butter and add the red wine and beef stock; reduce until thick and glossy. Add the cream and soy sauce and keep warm.

For the steaks: Slice the beef into steaks about 4cm thick; sprinkle the garlic and pepper on both sides and press in with the heel of your palm, taking care not to flatten them. Heat the oil and butter in a heavy pan and cook the steak until done to taste. Remove to a serving platter and keep warm. Add the sauce to the pan and stir until thick and glossy. Check the seasoning and pour over the steaks. Serve immediately.

Bacon Beef Burgers with Bacon, Onion & Balsamic Jam

Serves 4

INGREDIENTS

For the jam
- 4 thick slices bacon, cut crosswise into 1.5cm strips
- 1 large red onion, halved and thinly sliced
- Salt and freshly ground black pepper
- ⅓ cup balsamic vinegar
- ½ tsp. Dijon mustard

For the burgers
- 2 thick slices bacon
- 500-750g minced beef
- ½ tsp. Worcestershire sauce
- Salt and freshly ground black pepper

METHOD: For the Jam: In a heavy-duty pan, cook the bacon until well browned, about 8 minutes and transfer to paper towels to drain. Pour off all but 2-3 Tbsp. of bacon fat from the pan. Add the onion to the skillet, season with salt and pepper, cover the pan, and cook for 2 minutes. Uncover, add a splash of water, and scrape up any browned bits from the bottom of the skillet. Cover, and continue to cook, stirring occasionally, until the onions are soft and beginning to colour, about 10 minutes. Add the vinegar, mustard, and ⅓ cup water. Return the bacon to the skillet and bring the mixture to a simmer. Simmer, uncovered, until the liquid has thickened and most of it has been absorbed, 2-4 minutes. Transfer to a small bowl and let cool slightly. Cover with plastic wrap and leave at room temperature for up to 2 hours, or refrigerate for up to 2 days and gently reheat before serving.

For the burgers: With a sharp knife or food processor, mince the bacon. Transfer to a large mixing bowl, and add the minced beef, Worcestershire,

1 tsp. salt, and ½ tsp. pepper. Using a fork, gently toss until well mixed but not overworked. Form into 4 equal patties, each ¾ to 1 inch thick. Press your thumb in the centre of each patty to create a deep depression.

Tip: Making an indentation in the centre of each burger keeps them from swelling up on the grill.

Grill the burgers over medium temperature and direct heat until grill marks form on them, 4-5 minutes (move them to indirect heat if any flare-ups occur). Flip the burgers and cook for 4-5 minutes more for medium (a faintly pink centre). For well-done meat, cook an additional minute.

Carpaccio

Serves 4

INGREDIENTS
- *400g beef fillet*
- *Crystal salt and black pepper*
- *2 large lemons*
- *80g Parmesan cheese, finely grated*
- *4 Tbsp. capers, drained*
- *30g wild rocket*
- *Olive oil*

METHOD: Season the fillet liberally with the salt and pepper. In a smoking-hot pan, grill the fillet just enough to give it a little colour on each side, then cool quickly. Slice the beef as thinly as possible (use a meat slicer if you have one) and lay each slice slightly overlapping the next on a large platter (you can put it in the fridge if you are serving later). Generously squeeze lemon juice over the meat. Season it very well with crystal salt and cracked black pepper. Evenly scatter with grated Parmesan and capers, top with rocket and a liberal sprinkling of olive oil.

Beef & Cauli-Mash Cottage Pie   *Serves 4*

INGREDIENTS
For the mince
- 400g beef mince
- 125g streaky bacon, chopped
- 40g butter
- 1 large onion, finely chopped
- 4 celery sticks, roughly chopped
- 2-3 cloves garlic, minced
- 50g tomato paste
- 1 cup beef stock
- 3 large sprigs thyme, chopped
- 200g button mushrooms, sliced
- 1 tin chopped tomatoes
- 3 large sprigs fresh origanum, chopped
- Salt and pepper

For the Cauli-Mash
- 1 cauliflower head, broken into florets
- 100g butter
- 2 egg yolks
- Ground nutmeg

METHOD: In a medium-sized, heavy-based frying pan, sauté the mince and bacon in the butter until golden brown. Remove the meat from the pan and leave the fat in the pan. Add the onion and celery and sauté until golden. Add garlic and sauté until aromatic. Return meat to the pan, add the tomato paste and stir until dark sediment collects on the base of the pot – this gives the mince an amazing roasted flavour. Add the beef stock, thyme, mushrooms and tinned tomato and simmer on a low heat for about an hour to cook and reduce. Add the origanum and season to taste with salt and pepper. **For the Cauli-mash:** Steam the cauliflower until mushy. Place in a food processor and puree until smooth. While blender is running, add the egg yolks. Add in the butter, one knob at a time until it has melted and the mixture looks smooth. Season with nutmeg to taste. **To make the Cottage Pie:** Fill a pie dish with the mince. Top it with the cauliflower puree and press the classic fork pattern into the top. Place it under the grill for 15 minutes until golden brown. If you need extra fat, cover the top with a generous coating of grated cheese.

Steak 'Sandwiches'

INGREDIENTS
- *Precooked steak*
- *Cream cheese or grated cheese*
- *Tomato*
- *Rocket*
- *Mustard*
- *Homemade mayonnaise*

METHOD: Slice precooked steak into thinner palm-sized pieces; two of these will form the 'sandwich' slices. For the 'sandwich' filling, use low-carb mustard, mayonnaise, rocket, tomato, grated cheese or cream cheese and a dash of hot sauce for adults.

Beef Chilli Con Carne with Crispy Aubergine

Serves 4

INGREDIENTS

For the Chilli
- 2 Tbsp. beef tallow
- 2 garlic cloves, minced
- 1 onion, finely diced
- 2-3 green chillies, finely sliced
- 1 tsp. ground cumin
- 1 tsp. ground coriander
- 600g beef mince
- 2 Tbsp. tomato paste
- 1 x 400g tin chopped tomatoes
- 2 tsp. Xylitol
- 1 cup homemade beef stock
- Himalayan salt and black pepper

For the Aubergine Rounds
- ¾ cup coconut oil, for frying
- 1 aubergine, thinly sliced
- 1 tsp. ground coriander
- 1 tsp. ground cumin

To serve: Guacamole, chopped tomato, fresh coriander and lime wedges

METHOD: For the chilli: Heat the tallow in a pan, add the garlic, onion, chilli and spices, sauté for 3 minutes or until the onion is soft and golden. Add the beef mince and cook until browned; add tomato paste and cook for another minute, then stir through the remaining ingredients. Bring to the boil, reduce heat and simmer for 15 minutes. Season. **For the aubergines:** Heat coconut oil in a small saucepan. Fry aubergine slices until golden and

crisp. Toss together the spices and sprinkle over the hot aubergine rounds.
To serve: Place the mince in four bowls and serve with aubergine rounds, guacamole, tomato, fresh coriander and lime leaves.

Low-Carb Bobotie

Serves 4

INGREDIENTS
- *50g coconut oil or butter*
- *1 onion, chopped*
- *Salt and pepper*
- *Pinch of cayenne pepper*
- *10ml curry powder*
- *½ tsp. ground cinnamon*
- *500g minced beef or lamb*
- *½ apple, finely chopped*
- *2 dried apricots, finely chopped*
- *1 tomato, peeled and diced*
- *75ml flaked almonds*
- *60ml desiccated coconut*
- *150ml fresh cream*
- *45ml balsamic vinegar*

For the topping
- *4 eggs*
- *200ml fresh cream*

METHOD: Preheat the oven to 180°C. Heat the oil or butter in a large frying pan and fry the onion with rest of the spices. Add the meat and fry until browned. Add the rest of the ingredients and fry for a few minutes. Spoon the meat mixture into an ovenproof dish. Beat the eggs and cream together for the topping and pour over the meat. Bake for 20-30 minutes until the egg mixture has set and the bobotie has a golden colour. Serve with a salad.

Beef Lasagne

Serves 6

You can use either homemade carb-free pasta or sliced raw aubergine or courgettes as pasta sheets.

INGREDIENTS

For the mince:
- 250g streaky bacon, chopped
- 400g fatty beef mince
- 40g butter
- 2 large onions, finely chopped
- 2-3 cloves garlic, minced
- 50g tomato paste
- ½ cup red wine
- 1 cup beef stock
- 3 large springs fresh thyme, chopped
- 1 tin chopped tomatoes
- 1 Tbsp. Worcestershire sauce
- 3 large sprigs fresh origanum, chopped
- Salt and pepper

For the cheese sauce:
- 2 cups cream
- 4 cups grated cheese (Cheddar or Parmesan)
- Salt and pepper
- Pinch grated nutmeg
- Grated cheese for the top

METHOD: In a medium-sized, heavy-based frying pan, sauté the bacon and mince in the butter until golden brown. Once the mince is brown, remove the meat, leave the fat in the pan, and add the onions. Sauté the onions in the fat until golden brown. Add the garlic and sauté until aromatic. Add back the mince along with the tomato paste and stir until dark sediment collects on the base of the pot. Once good sediment has collected, add the red wine and reduce by half. Add the beef stock, thyme and tinned tomatoes and simmer on a low heat for about an hour. Add the Worcestershire sauce and origanum and season to taste with salt and pepper. **For the cheese sauce:** Bring the cream to the boil, then add the cheese and reduce the heat. Stir continuously until the cheese has melted and the sauce is a good cheesy consistency. Season with salt, pepper and nutmeg.

To make the lasagne: Lay sheets of carb-free 'pasta' or aubergines/courgettes on the base of a lasagne dish. Cover this with ⅓ of the mince, and then cover with a layer of 'pasta'. Add another layer of mince, then 'pasta'. Add the final layer of mince and top with the cheese sauce and a layer of grated cheese on top. Bake in the oven at 180°C for 30 minutes.

> **To remove burnt-on food from a pan,** add a drop of dishwasher and enough water to cover the pan and bring to the boil.

Peppered Fillet with Rocket Salsa Verde *Serves 4-6*

INGREDIENTS
- 1½ kg beef fillet
- 1 Tbsp. melted beef tallow
- Salt and black pepper
- ⅓ cup Dijon mustard
- 3 Tbsp. pink peppercorns, lightly crushed

For rocket salsa verde
- 30g rocket, chopped
- 30g dill, chopped
- 30g basil leaves, chopped
- 2 anchovies, chopped
- 1 tsp. Dijon mustard
- 1 Tbsp. capers, chopped
- Juice of ½ lemon
- ½ cup extra virgin olive oil
- Salt and black pepper

METHOD: Preheat oven to 200°C. Brush fillet with melted tallow and season well. Place a large frying pan over a high heat, sear the fillet on all sides until browned, then remove and set aside. Brush fillet with mustard and roll in pink peppercorns; place on a lined baking tray and roast for 20 minutes. Remove and let stand for 20 minutes before slicing.

For the rocket salsa verde: Mix together the rocket, dill, basil, anchovies, Dijon mustard and capers. Stir in the lemon juice and olive oil and season. Slice the fillet and serve with salsa verde.

Rustic Meat Loaf with Eggs

Serves 6

INGREDIENTS
- 400g rindless pork rashers, chopped
- 2 garlic cloves, crushed
- 2 tsp. dried rosemary
- 1 red onion, finely chopped
- 1 Tbsp. Dijon mustard
- 600g beef mince
- 1 tsp. smoked paprika
- Himalayan salt and black pepper
- 3 soft-boiled eggs, peeled
- 250g streaky bacon
- Coleslaw, to serve
- Fresh origanum sprigs, to garnish

METHOD: Preheat oven to 180°C. Heat a frying pan, add chopped pork and cook over a medium heat until pork is golden and all the fat has rendered out. Add the garlic, rosemary and onion and sauté until golden. Remove from heat. Place in a bowl and add the mustard, mince, paprika and seasoning; stir well to combine. Make ⅓ of the mince into an oblong shape on a baking tray. Place the whole boiled eggs in a row down the middle, then use the remaining mince to form a loaf shape around the eggs. Cover the loaf with bacon strips arranged at an angle. Place in the oven and bake for 30-40 minutes. Remove from oven and allow to cool slightly before slicing.

To serve: Place slices on serving plates with a spoonful of coleslaw, garnish with origanum sprigs and serve immediately.

Skewered Beef Koftas with Mixed Tomato & Cucumber Pickle

Serves 4

INGREDIENTS

For the Koftas
- 400g beef mince
- 2 garlic cloves, crushed
- 1 Tbsp. ground coriander
- 1 Tbsp. ground cumin
- 1 red chilli, seeded and finely chopped
- 3 Tbsp. each fresh oregano and coriander, chopped
- Himalayan salt and freshly ground black pepper
- 1 Tbsp. beef tallow, for frying

For the Pickle
- 400g mixed exotic tomatoes, quartered
- 3 Israeli cucumbers, finely sliced
- ½ red onion, finely sliced
- ¼ cup white balsamic vinegar
- 1 Tbsp. Xylitol
- 2 Tbsp. water
- 8 fresh bay leaves to garnish

METHOD: **For the Koftas:** Place all kofta ingredients in a bowl and mix until combined. Season well. Roll the mixture into about 8 x 50g balls, thread onto pre-soaked wooden skewers and shape into a long oval on the skewer. Heat tallow in a large frying pan and cook koftas for 3-4 minutes on each side or until brown and cooked through. Set aside and keep warm.

For the pickle: Toss all ingredients together in a bowl and season well. Marinate for at least 3 hours before serving. Store in an airtight container in the fridge. **To Serve:** Place the warm koftas on serving plates and top with the pickle and fresh bay leaves.

Steak & Kidney 'Pie' *Serves 6*

INGREDIENTS
- *300g beef ox kidneys, fat removed and chopped*
- *1½ kg beef chuck steak, chopped*
- *2 medium onions, sliced*
- *1 cup beef stock*
- *1 Tbsp. soy sauce*
- *Bay leaf*
- *½ tsp. thyme*
- *3 Tbsp. olive oil*
- *100ml cream mixed with 2 tsp. Worcestershire sauce*
- *500g cauliflower*
- *1 egg, beaten*
- *2 Tbsp. cream*
- *salt and pepper*
- *100 ml grated cheese for topping*

METHOD: Heat olive oil in a heavy-based frying pan and fry the kidneys, beef and onions until browned. Add the stock, herbs and soy sauce; cover the pan and simmer for approximately 1 hour or until the beef is tender. A crock-pot or pressure cooker can be used. Transfer the meat into an ovenproof dish and stir in the cream mixture to thicken and check the seasoning, adding salt and pepper if necessary. Break the cauliflower into small florets and steam until tender. Mash the cauliflower with the beaten egg and cream and season to taste. Spread the mixture on top of the cooked meat, cover with grated cheese and bake in the oven at 180°C to brown the topping and heat through, about 15 minutes.

Beef Steak with Horseradish Crème Fraiche & Roasted Tomato Salsa

Serves 2

INGREDIENTS

For the horseradish crème fraiche:
- ⅓ cup horseradish
- ⅓ cup crème fraiche or soured cream

For the roasted tomato salsa:
- 5 Roma tomatoes
- ⅓ cup chopped fresh basil
- 2 cloves garlic, minced
- 1 Tbsp. fresh lime juice
- 1 Tbsp. balsamic vinegar
- 2 tsp. salt
- ½ tsp. cracked black pepper
- 4 Tbsp. olive oil

For the steak:
- 2 x 300g thick-cut steak (rump or sirloin)
- Salt & freshly ground black pepper
- 1 tsp. coriander seeds, toasted and crushed
- Olive oil for searing

METHOD: **For the horseradish crème fraiche**: Mix together ⅓ cup horseradish and ⅓ cup crème fraiche or soured cream in a bowl and leave in the fridge till needed. **For the salsa:** Under a hot grill, roast the tomatoes until the skin is blackened. Remove charred bits, dice and place in a bowl. Cover and leave to cool for 15 minutes. Add the basil, garlic and lime juice and marinate for 10 minutes. Add the vinegar, salt and pepper; slowly whisk in the oil. **For the steak:** Preheat the oven to 220°C. Season the beef with salt, pepper and coriander and brush with olive oil. Heat a griddle pan until smoking and sear the steaks until they are brown all over. Transfer steaks to a tray and cook them in the oven until medium-rare. Set aside to rest for 10 minutes. Re-sear the steak in the pan. Plate with a tablespoon of horseradish mix on top and serve salsa on the side.

Sticky Beef Short Ribs   *Serves 4*

INGREDIENTS
- *1 kg beef short ribs, on the bone*
- *2 bay leaves*
- *1 onion, quartered*
- *2 tsp. black peppercorns*

For the Marinade
- *1 Tbsp. apple cider vinegar*
- *1 Tbsp. Xylitol*
- *Juice of 1 lemon*
- *1 cup homemade beef stock*
- *¼ cup tomato paste*
- *2 Tbsp. Dijon mustard*
- *1 cinnamon stick*
- *3 star anise*
- *Himalayan salt and black pepper*

To serve: Coleslaw

METHOD: Preheat the oven to 200°C. Place the ribs in a pot, cover with water and add the bay leaves, onion and peppercorns. Bring to a boil and simmer for 20 minutes. Remove, drain and place in an ovenproof dish. In a small bowl, add the marinade ingredients, stir to combine and pour over the beef ribs. Roast ribs for 30 minutes, then turn on the grill and cook until golden and crispy.
To Serve: Place hot on a plate with coleslaw.

The Low-Carb Companion

SECTION 6:

LAMB

'A writer need not devour a whole sheep in order to know what mutton tastes like, but he must at least eat a chop. Unless he gets his facts right, his imagination will lead him into all kinds of nonsense, and the facts he is most likely to get right are the facts of his own experience'.
W. Somerset Maugham

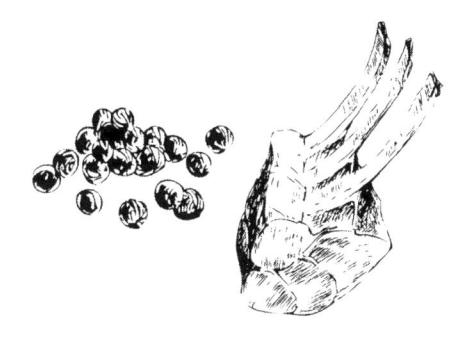

Lamb

	Page
Lamb Curry	339
Aubergine & Lamb Involtini with Yoghurt Sauce	340
Roast Lamb Chops with Butternut & Lemon	341
Lamb Shanks	342
Spicy Double Lamb Patties On Low-Carb Wraps	343

Lamb Curry

Serves 6

INGREDIENTS
- 2½ kg leg of lamb meat, cubed
- ½ tsp. salt
- 1 Tbsp. mild curry paste
- 1 tsp. chilli powder
- 1 clove garlic, crushed
- ¼ cup brown vinegar
- ¼ tsp. turmeric
- 60g ghee or butter
- 2 onions
- 3 cloves garlic, crushed (extra)
- 1 tsp. fresh ginger, grated
- 1 tsp. coriander
- 1 tsp. cumin
- 3 cups water
- 2 beef stock cubes
- 1 Tbsp. tomato paste

METHOD: Place cubed meat into a bowl and add salt, curry paste, chilli powder, crushed garlic, vinegar, turmeric and stir until meat is coated. Cover and stand for 30 minutes. Melt half the ghee or butter in a pan and when hot, add half the meat and stir until well browned. Repeat with the other half of the butter and meat and return all meat to the pan. Add sliced onions, extra crushed garlic, ginger, coriander and cumin, and cook while stirring over medium heat for 2 minutes. Pour into an ovenproof dish, add water, stock cubes and tomato paste, cover and bake at 180°C for one hour. Serve with cauli-rice and sambals.

Aubergine & Lamb Involtini with Yoghurt Sauce

Serves 4

INGREDIENTS
- 2 aubergines, finely sliced
- Coarse salt, to sprinkle
- Coconut oil, to brush

For the filling:
- 1 Tbsp. ghee
- 1 onion, finely chopped
- 2 garlic cloves, crushed
- 1 tsp. fennel seeds
- 1 tsp. cumin seeds
- 1 tsp. ground cinnamon
- 600g lamb mince
- 2 cups homemade vegetable or beef stock
- Himalayan salt and black pepper
- 50g pine nuts, toasted
- 10g fresh parsley, chopped

For the sauce:
- ½ cup double-cream yoghurt
- 5g fresh mint, chopped

METHOD: Sprinkle the aubergine slices with coarse salt, place in a colander and leave for 30 minutes. Rinse off the salt and pat dry. Preheat the oven grill, brush the aubergine slices on both sides with oil and grill until golden. **For the filling:** Heat the ghee; add the onion, garlic and spices and sauté until golden. Toss in the mince and the stock; simmer until the stock has been absorbed. Remove from heat, season and stir through the nuts and parsley. **For the sauce:** Mix together the yoghurt and mint. Place dollops of the filling on to the aubergine and roll up; secure with a toothpick. Divide between 4 plates and serve topped with yoghurt sauce.

Roast Lamb Chops with Butternut & Lemon

Serves 4

INGREDIENTS
- *8 lamb chops*
- *60ml olive oil*
- *1 kg butternut or pumpkin, peeled, seeded and cubed*
- *2 onions, sliced into wedges*
- *8 unpeeled garlic cloves*
- *2 tsp. Xylitol*
- *15 ml fresh thyme, chopped*
- *Juice of 1 lemon*
- *1 small lemon, thinly sliced*
- *Salt and freshly ground black pepper to taste*
- *Fresh thyme sprigs to garnish*

METHOD: Preheat the oven to 200°C and heat the oil in a large pan. Add the butternut or pumpkin, onion, garlic and Xylitol and stir-fry for 5 minutes over high heat or until the vegetables just begin to soften and caramelise. Transfer the vegetables to a large roasting pan and add the chopped thyme, lemon juice and slices. Season with salt and pepper. Place the chops on top of the vegetables and sprinkle over the whole thyme sprigs. Roast for 25-30 minutes or until the meat is done and the butternut or pumpkin is cooked.

> **Mushrooms** plunged into boiling water for a few minutes before cooking will not shrink.

Lamb Shanks

Serves 4

INGREDIENTS
- 4 lamb shanks
- Salt and ground pepper
- 1 tsp. coriander seeds
- 2 tsp. fresh chilli, chopped
- 1 tsp. fresh rosemary
- 1 tsp. dried oregano
- 1 Tbsp. olive oil
- ⅓ cup fresh basil, chopped
- ⅓ cup fresh marjoram, chopped
- ⅓ cup fresh parsley, chopped
- 1 clove garlic, chopped
- 1 large carrot, finely sliced
- 6 sticks celery, chopped
- 2 Tbsp. balsamic vinegar
- 170ml white wine
- 6 anchovy fillets (optional)
- 2 tins tomatoes

METHOD: Preheat oven to 180°C. Season lamb with salt and pepper. Crush coriander seeds and chilli and mix with chopped rosemary and dried oregano. Roll the lamb in this mixture, pressing it into the meat. Heat a thick-bottomed casserole pot, add the oil and brown the meat on all sides and remove from the pan. Add garlic, carrot, celery, onions and a pinch of salt and sweat until soft. Add balsamic vinegar and reduce liquid to a syrup. Pour in white wine and simmer for a couple of minutes. Add anchovies if using them. Add tinned tomatoes. Return lamb to the pot, bring to the boil, put the lid on and simmer in the oven for about 2 hours. Remove lid and cook for ½ hour longer. Season. Stir in mixed herbs and serve with cauli-mash.

Spicy Double Lamb Patties On Low-Carb Wraps

Serves 4

INGREDIENTS

For The Patties
- 600g lamb mince
- 2 green chillies, seeded and chopped
- 2 garlic cloves, crushed
- 70g Feta cheese, crumbled
- 10g fresh coriander leaves, chopped
- 1 Tbsp. ground coriander
- Himalayan salt and black pepper
- 2 Tbsp. beef or lamb tallow, for frying

For The Pickled Onions
- 1 Tbsp. vinegar
- 2 tsp. Xylitol
- 1 red onion, finely sliced

To Serve: Low-carb wraps, lettuce, sliced tomatoes, double-cream yoghurt and fresh herbs

METHOD: For the patties: Place all the ingredients except the tallow in a bowl, season well and stir to combine. Divide mixture into 8 patties. Heat tallow in a frying pan and cook patties until done to your liking. Remove and set aside, keep warm. **For the pickled onions:** In a small bowl, mix together the vinegar and Xylitol, add 2 Tbsp. water and toss in the onion. Allow to stand for 10 minutes. **To assemble:** Heat the wraps, top with lettuce, tomato, two patties per wrap and pickled onion.

To serve: Serve immediately with a dollop of double-cream yoghurt and fresh herbs.

The Low-Carb Companion

SECTION 7:

PORK

Historically and today, pork is the most widely eaten meat in the world. Avoid eating excessive amounts of processed pork products.

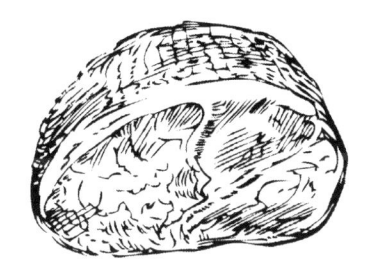

Pork

	Page
Pork Chops With Mushrooms & Cheese	347
Pork Fillet Stir-Fry With Green Chilli Paste & Coconut Milk	348
Roast Pork Belly With Crisp Crackling	349
Cheesy Bacon & Egg Slice	350
Sweet Potato & Bacon Bake	350
No Bread Crumbed Pork Chops	351

Pork Chops with Mushrooms & Cheese   *Serves 4*

INGREDIENTS
- 4 thick pork chops
- 2 Tbsp. almond or coconut flour
- Salt and pepper
- 4 Tbsp. butter
- 350-450g button mushrooms
- 2 Tbsp. lemon juice or dry white wine
- 100ml stock
- 200ml double cream
- 2 egg yolks
- 3 Tbsp. grated Cheddar cheese

METHOD: Preheat the oven to 180°C. Beat chops lightly with your hand or a rolling pin and score along the fatty edge of chop to prevent them curling up during frying. Dip in seasoned almond or coconut flour. Fry for 6-8 minutes on either side in half the butter. Place chops in an ovenproof dish, deglaze the pan with stock and pour the juices over the chops. Clean the mushrooms, one by one, under cold running water and drain in a colander. Slice and cook for 1 minute in 2 Tbsp. butter over high heat. Turn the heat to low and stir in the lemon juice or wine and half the double cream. Simmer for 2-3 minutes, stirring continuously. Mix the egg yolks with the remaining cream and stir into the mushroom sauce, turning off the heat. Season to taste and pour the sauce over the chops and sprinkle with a thin layer of grated cheese. Bake in the bottom of the preheated oven until cheese melts. Sprinkle with parsley before serving with mashed sweet potatoes or cauli-rice and a salad.

Pork Fillet Stir-Fry with Green Chilli Paste & Coconut Milk

Serves 4

INGREDIENTS
- 400g pork fillet, thinly sliced
- 3 tsp. Thai green curry paste
- 3 cloves garlic, finely chopped
- ¼ cup coriander, chopped
- 1 Tbsp. coconut oil
- 2 Tbsp. oyster sauce
- 1 Tbsp. fish sauce
- ½ cup chicken stock
- 200ml coconut milk
- ½ cup carrot, shredded
- ½ cup spring onions, shredded
- ½ cup mange tout, shredded
- ⅓ cup basil leaves, thinly sliced

METHOD: Combine the green curry paste, garlic and coriander in a small bowl and mix well. Heat oil in a wok, swirling to coat the surface. Add the curry mixture and stir-fry until garlic is aromatic, about 1 minute. Add the pork and stir-fry, stirring often, until meat is cooked, about 5 minutes. Add the oyster sauce, fish sauce, chicken stock and coconut milk and stir to combine and heat thoroughly. Add the shredded vegetables and toss for one minute. Stir in the basil leaves and serve immediately.

> **Soak fresh pork** in apple cider vinegar in the refrigerator for up to 24 hours before cooking to enhance its health benefits.

Roast Pork Belly With Crisp Crackling *Serves 6-8*

INGREDIENTS
- *1½kg pork belly, unrolled*
- *2 Tbsp. Himalayan salt flakes*
- *2 cloves garlic, crushed*
- *2 Tbsp. parsley, chopped*
- *Ground black pepper*
- *1 red onion, sliced into eighths*
- *100g baby leeks*
- *4 long stalks celery*
- *5g fresh sage leaves*
- *1½ cups homemade vegetable stock or white wine*
- *Roasted baby savoy cabbages and red onions, to serve*

METHOD: Preheat oven to 220°C. Pat the skin of the pork belly with paper towel to dry; never wash the pork under running water. Once the skin is as dry as possible, rub it with plenty of salt and refrigerate for a couple of hours. Combine garlic, chopped parsley and sage and rub over the underside of the meat; season with a little salt and pepper. Arrange the onion, leeks and celery in a roasting pan and top with the pork belly, skin side up. Scatter over sage leaves. Roast for 35 minutes, or until the crackling begins to blister and turn golden. Add stock or wine and reduce heat to 190°C. Roast for a further 1-1½ hours or until the crackling is crisp and the meat is tender.

To serve: Slice pork and serve with roasted cabbage and vegetables.

Cheesy Bacon & Egg Slice　　　　　　*Serves 6*

INGREDIENTS
- 400g cauliflower florets, partly cooked
- 125g grated Cheddar cheese
- 5 rashers bacon
- 3 spring onions, chopped
- 1 small green pepper, chopped
- 6 eggs
- 2 cups milk
- 1 tsp. dry mustard
- 1 tsp. Worcestershire sauce
- 1 Tbsp. homemade low-carb mayonnaise
- Pepper
- ½ tsp. dried basil leaves
- 1 small red pepper, chopped

METHOD: Preheat oven to 180°C. Place cauliflower in a single layer in an ovenproof pie dish and sprinkle with the grated cheese. Cut bacon into 2½ cm pieces; fry the bacon until crisp and brown and drain. Place over the cheese; top with onions and chopped green pepper. Whisk eggs with a fork; add the milk, mustard, Worcestershire sauce, mayonnaise, pepper and basil. Pour over the mixture in the dish, top with chopped red pepper and bake in a moderate oven for 50-60 minutes.

Sweet Potato & Bacon Bake　　　　　　*Serves 4*

INGREDIENTS
- 250g bacon rashers, chopped into pieces
- 2 large eggs
- 250ml fresh cream
- ½ cup grated Cheddar cheese

- 4 large sweet potatoes
- 1 large onion, chopped
- 1 Tbsp. chopped parsley
- 2 tomatoes, sliced
- Olive oil to fry

METHOD: Preheat oven to 200°C. Fry the onion in a little oil and add the bacon and fry for 5 minutes. Cut potatoes into thin slices and place half on the base of an ovenproof dish. Place half the bacon on top of the potatoes; continue to layer the rest of the potatoes and bacon. Cover with rings of peeled, sliced tomatoes. Beat eggs, cream, parsley, salt and pepper in a small bowl. Pour egg mixture over the dish. Sprinkle cheese on top and place in the oven for 45 minutes or until potatoes are soft and the top is golden brown.

No Bread Crumbed Pork Chops   *Serves 2*

INGREDIENTS
- 2 pork chops
- 2 Tbsp. almond or coconut flour
- 1 Tbsp. grated Parmesan cheese

For the dipping sauce
- 1 egg, beaten
- ¼ tsp. dried oregano
- Salt & pepper
- ½ tsp. Dijon or English mustard

METHOD: Preheat the oven to 200°C. Mix all dipping sauce ingredients together. Mix the flour and Parmesan cheese in a shallow dish. Beat the pork chops with a meat hammer or rolling pin until fairly flat. Dip the chops into the sauce and then into the Parmesan cheese crumbs. Bake in the oven for 20 minutes.

SECTION 8:

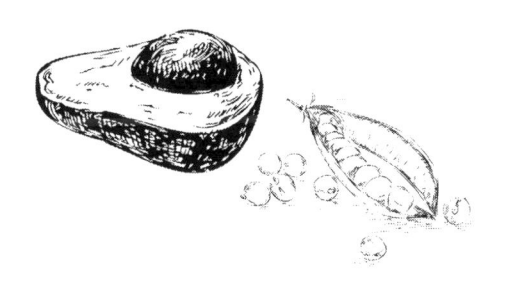

SIDES, SALADS & VEGETABLES

There is a funny story about the chef who stayed up late making a rotisserie chicken with a salad to go with it and then spent the whole night tossing and turning.

Sides, Salads & Vegetables

	Page
Avocado, Snow Pea & Mint Salad With Poppy Seed Dressing	355
Asparagus & Feta Fritters	356
Broccoli & Avocado Salad With Roasted Almond Dressing	356
Aubergine, Tomato & Mozzarella Stacks	357
Crunchy Cabbage Salad With Creamy Red Curry Dressing	358
Cauliflower Cheese	359
Cauliflower Rice (Cauli-Rice)	360
Creamy Guacamole	360
Green Beans With Toasted Almonds & Lemon Butter	361
Herb & Baby Leaf Salad	361
Herby Cream Cheese Spread	362
Lettuce Cups With Prawn Salad	362
Mixed Tomato Salad With Mozzarella & Crispy Chorizo	363
Shitake Mushroom, Bok Choi & Mange Tout Stir Fry	364
Spicy Roast Butternut or Pumpkin, Feta & Olive Salad	365
Spinach & Mushroom Salad	366
Stuffed Avocado	366
Zucchini Fritters	367
Pumpkin Hummus	368
Strawberry & Macadamia Nut Chicken Salad	368

Avocado, Snow Pea & Mint Salad with Poppy Seed Dressing
Serves 2

INGREDIENTS

For the dressing
- Juice of 1 lemon (25ml)
- 2 Tbsp. red wine vinegar
- 1 tsp. Dijon mustard
- 1 clove garlic, minced
- 4 Tbsp. poppy seeds, toasted
- 150ml extra-virgin olive oil
- Salt and pepper

For the salad
- 1 large ripe avocado, cut into chunks
- 200g snow peas (sugar snaps or mange tout)
- 1 bunch spring onions, thinly sliced
- 1 head butter lettuce, washed and torn
- 1 handful of mint leaves

METHOD: **For the dressing:** Combine the lemon juice, vinegar, mustard, garlic and poppy seeds in a mixing bowl. While whisking continuously, pour in the olive oil until emulsified. Season to taste. **For the salad:** Cut the sugar snaps in half lengthways on the diagonal. Lay the lettuce leaves on a platter. Layer with snow peas, avocado, mint and spring onions and cover with the dressing and serve immediately. Add any nut or seed to give this salad more of a crunch.

Asparagus & Feta Fritters   *Serves 4*

INGREDIENTS
- 1 bunch asparagus, cleaned and stalks removed
- ⅓ cup fresh dill, finely chopped
- 2 spring onions, finely chopped
- ½ cup Feta cheese, crumbled
- 1 egg, beaten
- ⅓ cup coconut flour
- Salt and pepper
- 2 Tbsp. coconut oil (or other oil to fry)

METHOD: Grate the asparagus. Add the remaining ingredients, except the oil, and season to taste. Meld into patties. Heat the oil in a pan. Gently fry the patties until golden on each side.

Broccoli & Avocado Salad with Roasted Almond Dressing   *Serves 4*

INGREDIENTS
For the dressing
- ½ cups whole almonds
- 1 Tbsp. lemon juice
- 1 Tbsp. wholegrain mustard
- 4 Tbsp. crème fraiche
- 100ml milk

For the salad
- 400g broccoli florets
- 2 ripe avocados, pitted and cut into chunks

- 1 bunch spring onion, finely sliced
- 1 small packet wild rocket

METHOD: **For the dressing:** Roast the nuts in the oven at 180°C or under the grill until they are golden brown, and roughly chop them. Add the remaining ingredients and half the nuts to a tall, narrow container and blend using a stick blender. Stir in the remaining nuts and season to taste. **For the salad:** In a small pot of boiling salted water, blanch the broccoli until al dente and refresh it in cold water. Combine the broccoli, avocados, spring onion and wild rocket; mix gently and spread over a platter. Pour over the dressing and serve.

Aubergine, Tomato & Mozzarella Stacks

INGREDIENTS
- 2 medium aubergines (eggplant)
- 2 beefsteak tomatoes
- 1 ball of Buffalo mozzarella
- Handful of basil leaves
- 2-3 Tbsp. olive oil
- Salt and pepper to taste

METHOD: Cut the ends off the aubergines. Slice into circles of about 1 cm thick. Repeat with the tomatoes. Heat the olive oil on a griddle pan on a medium heat. Fry the aubergines until golden brown on each side. Place on a plate and keep warm. Fry the tomatoes on both sides until cooked. In the meantime, slice the mozzarella. **To assemble:** Place the aubergine on a plate, followed by a slice of mozzarella and then a few basil leaves. Place the tomatoes on top, season with salt and pepper, and then top with a piece of aubergine.

Crunchy Cabbage Salad with Creamy Red Curry Dressing

Serves 4

INGREDIENTS

For the dressing
- 1 Tbsp. good-quality red Thai curry paste
- 1 Tbsp. lime juice
- 1 Tbsp. fish sauce
- 150ml coconut cream
- 2 Tbsp. macadamia nut butter
- 1 handful fresh coriander, roughly chopped

For the salad
- ½ white cabbage, shredded
- 1½ cups bean sprouts
- 1 bunch spring onions
- 1 cup toasted macadamia nuts (other nuts can be substituted, just be aware of the carb count)

METHOD: For the dressing: Place all ingredients in a small saucepan and bring to the boil. Set aside and leave to cool.

To serve: Combine all the ingredients in a mixing bowl and pour the dressing over. Mix together and serve immediately.

> **Cabbage** is improved in colour and flavour by adding a few sprigs of mint to the cooking water, or by cooking it in a little butter and garlic for a few minutes before adding 2 Tbsp. stock to the pan. Switch off the heat, cover and leave to steam.

Cauliflower Cheese

Serves 4

INGREDIENTS
- *1½ cups cream*
- *1½ cups homemade vegetable stock*
- *2 garlic cloves, crushed*
- *2 bay leaves*
- *5 peppercorns*
- *3 sprigs thyme*
- *1 Tbsp. arrowroot, mixed with 3 Tbsp. water*
- *½ cup grated Parmesan cheese*
- *½ cup white Cheddar cheese*
- *Himalayan salt and black pepper*
- *900g cauliflower florets*

METHOD: Preheat oven to 170°C. Place cream, stock, garlic, bay leaves, peppercorns and thyme in a saucepan and bring to the boil. Strain mixture through a sieve and return to the pot. Add arrowroot and whisk over low heat for about 5 minutes until sauce is thickened. Add Parmesan and half the Cheddar; whisk until smooth and then season. Arrange cauliflower in a baking dish, pour over sauce, scatter over remaining Cheddar and bake for 30-40 minutes until cooked.

Cauliflower Rice (Cauli-rice)   *Serves 6*

INGREDIENTS
- *1 cauliflower*
- *1 onion*
- *100 g butter or coconut oil*

METHOD: In a food processor, pulse the cauliflower until you reach couscous consistency. Melt the butter or oil in a heavy-based frying pan and sauté the onion until soft. Add the cauliflower and mix through the onion. Leave the heat on low or medium and place the lid on top of the pan. Cook for 5-8 minutes and either set aside or serve immediately. **Note:** You can add just about anything to cauli-rice, but you will need to adjust the water content if you are reading off a rice recipe as cauli-rice needs no water to cook. It does not hold its texture well over long cooking periods, so dishes like paella or risotto will need the rice added at the end rather than the beginning.

Creamy Guacamole   *Makes about 2 Cups*

INGREDIENTS
- *200ml fresh cream*
- *1 large avocado, mashed*
- *½ onion, finely chopped*
- *15ml finely chopped red pepper*
- *1 clove garlic, crushed*
- *100ml crème fraiche*

METHOD: Whip the cream; stir the mashed avocado, onion, red pepper and garlic in and then add the crème fraiche. Stir well.

Green Beans with Toasted Almonds & Lemon Butter
Serves 4

INGREDIENTS
- *400g green beans, topped and tailed*
- *60g butter*
- *3 Tbsp. almond slithers, toasted in a dry pan*
- *Juice of 1 lemon*
- *Salt and pepper*

METHOD: In a small pot, bring some water to a boil and blanch the beans for 2 minutes. Refresh them in cold or iced water so they keep their colour and texture. In a large pan or wok, melt the butter until just before it turns brown, and then add the beans. Toss the beans until they are warmed through; add the almonds and lemon juice. Season with salt and pepper and serve.

Herb & Baby Leaf Salad
Serves 4

INGREDIENTS
- *4 large handfuls baby leaves and herb leaves*
- *Garlic chive flowers*

For the dressing
- *1 clove garlic, minced*
- *1 generous pinch of salt*
- *1 Tbsp. red wine vinegar*
- *2 Tbsp. extra virgin olive oil*

METHOD: Whisk together dressing ingredients. Dress the leaves just before serving and scatter the garlic chive flowers over the top.

Herby Cream Cheese Spread   *Makes about 1½ Cups*

INGREDIENTS
- 2 gherkins, chopped
- 2 Tbsp. parsley, chopped
- 2 Tbsp. chives, chopped
- 2 Tbsp. mint, chopped
- 250g cream cheese
- Lemon juice
- Salt and pepper

METHOD: Stir together gherkins, chives, parsley and mint into the cream cheese. Place in a food processor and blitz until well combined. Add lemon juice to taste and season.

Lettuce Cups with Prawn Salad   *Serves 4*

INGREDIENTS
- 2-3 baby gem lettuces, washed and leaves separated
- 200g prawns, cleaned
- 6 red salad onions, finely chopped
- 3 cucumbers, finely chopped
- Juice and zest of 1 lime
- ⅓ cup homemade mayonnaise
- Salt and black pepper
- Fresh coriander and mint, to garnish
- Lime wedges and extra homemade mayonnaise to serve

METHOD: Fry the prawns in hot olive oil for 1 minute on each side and set aside to cool. Place the lettuce cups on a surface. In a large bowl, combine the prawns, red salad onions, cucumber, lime juice and zest, and mayonnaise, stir well to combine and season. Spoon dollops of the mixture into the lettuce cups, garnish with coriander and mint and serve with lime wedges and extra mayonnaise.

Mixed Tomato Salad with Mozzarella & Crispy Chorizo

Serves 4

INGREDIENTS
- *600g sliced tomatoes*
- *2 Tbsp. coconut oil*
- *Fresh bay leaves*
- *50g chorizo, sliced*
- *2 balls fresh mozzarella, torn into pieces*
- *Salt and black pepper*
- *Extra virgin olive oil and balsamic vinegar to drizzle*
- *Salad leaves to serve*

METHOD: Preheat oven to 160°C. Place tomatoes in a small roasting tin, drizzle over coconut oil, scatter over bay leaves, season and roast in the oven for 10-15 minutes. Remove and set aside to cool. Heat a frying pan, toss in the chorizo and cook until crispy. Drain on paper towel and set aside. **To assemble:** Place the mozzarella and chorizo on a platter, top with the tomatoes and drizzle liberally with extra virgin olive oil and balsamic vinegar. Serve with seed crackers, lots of black pepper and salad leaves.

Shitake Mushroom, Bok Choi & Mange Tout Stir Fry

Serves 4

INGREDIENTS
- *1 Tbsp. coconut oil*
- *2 cloves garlic, minced*
- *5cm piece of ginger, peeled and grated*
- *1 small chilli, minced*
- *1 bunch spring onions, finely sliced*
- *150g fresh shiitake mushrooms, sliced*
- *200g mange tout, halved lengthwise*
- *200g baby bok choi, thickly sliced*
- *1 Tbsp. fish sauce*
- *2 Tbsp. mirin*
- *Juice of 1 lime*
- *1 large handful basil, roughly chopped*
- *2 Tbsp. sesame seeds, toasted*

METHOD: In a wok, heat the coconut oil over high heat. As the oil begins to smoke, add the garlic, ginger, chilli and spring onion and stir. Before the garlic starts to colour, add the mushrooms and sauté for about 2 minutes. Once they are cooked, add the mange tout and sauté until bright green. Add the bok choi and cook until wilted. Season with fish sauce, mirin and lime juice. Mix through the basil leaves and sesame seeds and serve.

Spicy Roast Butternut or Pumpkin, Feta & Olive Salad

Serves 4

INGREDIENTS
- 3 Tbsp. olive oil
- ½ tsp. ground cumin
- ½ tsp. coriander
- ½ tsp. ginger
- ½ tsp. cinnamon
- ½ tsp. cayenne pepper
- 1 clove garlic, crushed
- Sea salt
- Freshly ground black pepper
- 800g butternut or pumpkin, cut into 2cm cubes
- 100g mixed lettuce and rocket
- 150g marinated Feta cheese, drained and crumbled or cubed
- 20 calamata olives

For the Dressing
- 1 Tbsp. red wine vinegar
- 60ml olive oil
- 1 small onion, finely sliced

METHOD: Whisk all dressing ingredients together. Preheat the oven to 200°C. Place olive oil, garlic and spices in a bowl and mix; add butternut or pumpkin and stir to coat. Transfer to a roasting tin and bake for 30 minutes or until the butternut or pumpkin is tender and slightly caramelised. Put the lettuce and rocket leaves on a platter and scatter the butternut, Feta cheese and olives on top. Drizzle with dressing.

Spinach & Mushroom Salad *Serves 2*

INGREDIENTS
- 240g baby spinach leaves
- 140g sliced mushrooms
- ½ yellow or red pepper, chopped
- 50g chopped spring onions or 80g chopped red onion
- 2 hard-boiled eggs, sliced
- 50g walnut halves
- 170g cubed Feta cheese
- Homemade mayonnaise

METHOD: Toss together the spinach, mushrooms, spring onions, eggs, walnuts and Feta in a large bowl. Toss with mayonnaise dressing just before serving. **Variations:** Add herbs such as basil and coriander. Substitute Goat's cheese, creamy Gouda or Emmental for the Feta. Add whole pitted olives.

Stuffed Avocado *Serves 2*

INGREDIENTS
- 1 avocado
- 30-45ml cream cheese, softened
- Salami, sliced
- Marinated sun-dried tomatoes
- Chopped chives
- Lemon wedges, to serve
- Tabasco sauce, to serve

METHOD: Halve the avocado and dollop cream cheese into each hollow. Drape with a few slices of salami and sun-dried tomatoes. Scatter with chives and serve with lemon wedges and Tabasco sauce.

Zucchini Fritters

Serves 2

INGREDIENTS
- *1 punnet of baby marrows, grated*
- *1 egg, beaten*
- *1 small onion, thinly sliced*
- *1 small piece of fresh ginger, grated (optional)*
- *½ tsp. cayenne pepper*
- *Black pepper & salt*
- *¼ cup coconut flour, sifted*
- *1 tsp. psyllium husks*
- *1 Tbsp. water (if needed)*
- *Coconut oil*
- *Fresh parsley, chopped*

METHOD: Put the grated baby marrows in a colander in the sink and sprinkle some salt over to draw out most of the moisture. Leave it for about 10 minutes. Meanwhile, put some coconut oil in a pan and cook the onions until soft; add the grated ginger and cayenne pepper. Squeeze out all the moisture in the baby marrows (they will not hold together if you don't do this properly). In a dry bowl, mix the dry baby marrows, the onion mix, some black pepper and salt, a beaten egg, a sprinkling of parsley, coconut flour and psyllium husks. Add a Tbsp. of water if necessary. Let the mixture stand for around 5 minutes to bind nicely. Add about 2 Tbsp. of coconut oil to a pan and put on medium-high heat. Squeeze together to make balls using your hands. Place them into the heated pan and use the back of a spatula to flatten. Turn when brown; keep turning them until cooked through. Add more coconut oil as needed. **Variation:** Bulk the fritters up with cooked cauliflower rice and bits of bacon for a chunkier patty.

Pumpkin Hummus

Makes about 1½ Cups

INGREDIENTS
- 1 cup cooked pumpkin, mashed
- 2-3 Tbsp. tahini
- 1 clove garlic, minced
- 1 tsp. ground cumin
- Lemon juice
- Pumpkin seeds, toasted
- Salt and pepper
- Olive oil

METHOD: Mix mashed pumpkin with tahini, garlic and cumin. Season and add lemon juice to taste.
To serve: Drizzle with olive oil and scattered pumpkin seeds.

Strawberry & Macadamia Nut Chicken Salad

Serves 4

INGREDIENTS
- 500g chicken breast
- 1 tsp. macadamia nut oil, or oil of choice
- Few pinches of salt and pepper
- 1½-2 cups strawberries, chopped
- ½ cup macadamia nuts, chopped
- ½ cup celery, diced
- 3 Tbsp. mayonnaise, preferably homemade
- 2 Tbsp. julienned basil
- 1 Tbsp. lemon juice

METHOD: Preheat oven to 180°C. Place chicken breasts on sheet tray, drizzle with oil and a pinch of salt and pepper. Bake for about 35 minutes until cooked through. Remove from oven and let cool. In a large bowl, shred chicken. Add strawberries, nuts, celery, basil, mayonnaise, lemon juice, and a pinch of salt and pepper. Gently stir until combined.

> **Celery** wrapped in aluminium foil will keep in the fridge for weeks.

The Low-Carb Companion

SECTION 9:

SALAD DRESSINGS, SAUCES, DIPS, MARINADES & RUBS

Commercial salad dressings and sauces are processed foods containing unhealthy vegetable oils and sugar. Make your own delicious and healthy low-carb dressings and sauces.

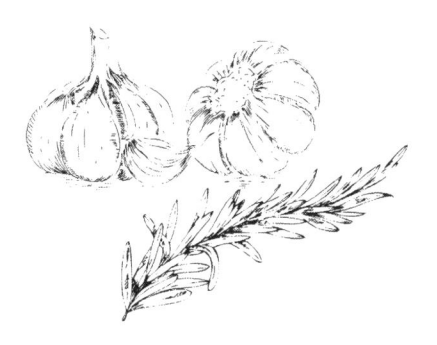

Salad Dressings, Sauces, Dips, Marinades & Rubs

SALAD DRESSINGS

	Page
Blue Cheese Dressing	374
Sun-dried Tomato Pesto	374
Greek Vinaigrette	375
Homemade Low-Carb Mayonnaise	376
Italian Dressing	376
Caesar Salad Dressing	377
Ranch Dressing	378
French Dressing	378

SAUCES

Blue Cheese Sauce	379
Garlic Sauce	379
Béchamel Sauce	380
Mushroom Gravy	380
Mushroom Sauce	381
Mustard-Cream Sauce	382
Tartar Sauce	382
Homemade Tomato Sauce	383

DIPS

Chutney Dip	384
Herb Dip	384
Pesto with Pecan Nuts	385
Tomato & Macadamia Dip	385

Section 9 - Salad Dressings, Sauces, Dips, Marinades & Rubs

MARINADES   Page
Asian Marinade   386
Cajun Marinade   386
Mediterranean Marinade   387
Hearty Red Wine Marinade   388
Latin Marinade   388
Chutney & Tomato Braai Marinade   389
Chilli & Garlic Marinade   390
Spicy Yoghurt Marinade   390

RUBS
BBQ Rub   391
Cajun Rub   391

Salad Dressings

Blue Cheese Dressing

INGREDIENTS
- 115g blue cheese, crumbled
- 115g mayonnaise
- 115g soured cream
- 75ml double cream
- 1 Tbsp. fresh lemon juice
- ½ tsp. Dijon mustard
- ½ tsp. pepper

METHOD: Combine blue cheese, mayonnaise, soured cream, double cream, lemon juice, mustard and pepper in a medium bowl, mashing with a fork to break up the cheese. Use straight away or refrigerate in an airtight container for up to 3 days. Drizzle this thick and creamy dressing over iceberg lettuce or other salad leaves. Serve as a dip for fresh vegetables or chicken wings or on top of cold roast beef. If you can, make the dressing a day ahead to let the flavours develop. Homemade mayonnaise produces scrumptious results.

Sun-dried Tomato Pesto

INGREDIENTS
- 40g sun-dried tomatoes (not packed in oil)
- 475ml boiling water
- 60ml water
- 175ml extra virgin olive oil
- 15g basil leaves
- 40g pine nuts, toasted

- 3 Tbsp. grated Pecorino Romano
- 1 garlic clove

METHOD: Combine sun-dried tomatoes and boiling water in a bowl; leave until tomatoes are pliable, about 10 minutes. Drain and squeeze out excess liquid. Combine tomatoes, water, oil, basil, pine nuts, Pecorino Romano and garlic in a blender and pulse until fairly smooth. Serve immediately or refrigerate in an airtight container for up to 2 days or freeze for up to 1 week.

Tip: This is a tasty twist on the classic Basil Pesto and can be mixed with soured cream or cream cheese for a delicious dip. Dry-packed sun-dried tomatoes are much less expensive and fresher tasting than oil-packed ones.

Greek Vinaigrette

INGREDIENTS
- 90ml extra virgin olive oil
- 1 garlic clove, finely chopped
- ½ tsp. dried oregano, crumbled
- ½ tsp. salt
- ¼ tsp. pepper
- 2 Tbsp. fresh lemon juice
- 1 tsp. red wine vinegar

METHOD: Whisk together oil, garlic, oregano, salt and pepper in a small bowl; whisk in lemon juice and vinegar. Use straight away or refrigerate in an airtight container for up to 2 days.

Tip: Serve this tangy lemon-garlic dressing on iceberg lettuce with some black olives, red onions, tomatoes, cucumbers and Feta cheese for a Greek salad. Add grilled prawns to turn it into a hearty supper salad.

Homemade Low-Carb Mayonnaise   *Makes 400ml*

INGREDIENTS
- 1 whole egg
- 2 egg yolks
- 1 Tbsp. Dijon mustard
- Juice of 1 lemon
- ½ cup coconut oil
- ½ cup quality olive oil
- 1 Tbsp. double thick Greek yoghurt
- Salt and pepper

METHOD: Combine the egg, egg yolks, mustard and lemon juice in a food processor. Melt the coconut oil in a small pot until it turns to liquid; avoid heating it too much or it will make the eggs curdle. Turn the processor to a fast speed and slowly pour the oil mixture into the egg mix. Once the mayonnaise has emulsified, add the yoghurt and season to taste. This mayonnaise will keep up to a week in the fridge. You can add extra yoghurt to bulk it up.

Italian Dressing

INGREDIENTS
- 175ml extra virgin olive oil
- 60ml red wine vinegar
- 2 Tbsp. fresh lemon juice
- 2 garlic cloves, pressed
- 3 Tbsp. fresh parsley, finely chopped
- 1 Tbsp. fresh basil, finely chopped
- 1 tsp. dried oregano

- ½ tsp. chilli flakes
- ¼ tsp. salt
- ¼ tsp. pepper
- ½ tsp. Xylitol

METHOD: Combine oil, vinegar, lemon juice, garlic, parsley, basil, oregano, chilli flakes, salt, pepper and Xylitol in a jar with a tight-fitting lid and shake vigorously. This can also be done in a blender. Use straight away or refrigerate in an airtight container for up to 3 days. This traditional favourite combines the perfect ratio of oil to vinegar. If you don't have a garlic press, crush the cloves with the flat side of a knife and then mince them very finely.

Caesar Salad Dressing

INGREDIENTS
- *55g mayonnaise*
- *3 Tbsp. grated Parmesan*
- *1 Tbsp. anchovy paste*
- *1 Tbsp. lemon juice*
- *2 garlic cloves, finely chopped*
- *2 tsp. extra virgin olive oil*
- *1 tsp. Worcestershire sauce*
- *1 tsp. Dijon mustard*
- *½ tsp. pepper*
- *Hot pepper sauce*

METHOD: Combine mayonnaise, Parmesan, anchovy paste, lemon juice, garlic, oil, Worcestershire sauce, mustard, pepper and hot sauce in a small bowl. Use straight away or refrigerate in an airtight container for up to 2 days.

Ranch Dressing

INGREDIENTS
- 175g mayonnaise
- 120ml double cream
- 2 Tbsp. fresh parsley, chopped
- 2 Tbsp. chives, chopped
- 2 tsp. fresh lemon juice
- 2 tsp. Dijon mustard
- 1 garlic clove, finely chopped
- 1 tsp. fresh dill, chopped
- ½ tsp. salt
- ¼ tsp. pepper

METHOD: Whisk mayonnaise, cream, parsley, chives, lemon juice, mustard, garlic, dill, salt and pepper in a small bowl. Use straight away or refrigerate in an airtight container for up to 3 days.

French Dressing

INGREDIENTS
- 120g low-carb tomato ketchup
- 120ml olive oil
- 60ml cider vinegar
- 1 Tbsp. Xylitol
- ½ tsp. salt
- ¼ tsp. garlic powder or 1 clove garlic, crushed
- Pinch cayenne pepper

METHOD: Whisk tomato ketchup, oil, vinegar, Xylitol, salt, garlic powder and cayenne pepper in a medium bowl. Use straight away or refrigerate in an airtight container for up to 3 days.
Tip: Try this classic salad dressing with crisp pieces of iceberg lettuce and wedges of sweet ripe tomatoes.

Sauces

Blue Cheese Sauce

INGREDIENTS
- 50g butter
- 1 onion, finely chopped
- 1 leek, finely chopped
- 1 stalk celery, finely chopped
- 5ml finely chopped garlic
- 100g crumbled blue cheese
- 250ml fresh cream

METHOD: Heat the butter and sauté the vegetables until transparent. Add the cheese and cream. Stirring continuously, simmer for about 2 minutes, or until thick and creamy. Serve with steak, chicken or low-carb pasta.

Garlic Sauce

INGREDIENTS
- 1 onion, finely chopped
- 5 cloves garlic, crushed
- 1 Tbsp. olive oil
- 125ml fresh cream
- 125ml milk
- 60ml red wine
- Salt and freshly ground black pepper to taste

METHOD: Sauté the onion and garlic in the heated oil until soft. Add the cream, milk and wine. Heat until the sauce comes to the boil and simmer until flavoursome and slightly thickened. Add seasoning to taste.

Béchamel Sauce

INGREDIENTS
- 225ml double cream
- 225ml water
- ½ small onion, chopped
- 1 tsp. salt
- ¼ tsp. pepper
- Pinch of ground nutmeg
- 1 Tbsp. psyllium husks
- 1 Tbsp. butter

METHOD: Combine cream, water, onion, salt, pepper and nutmeg in a small saucepan over medium heat and bring to a simmer. Remove from heat; let stand 15 minutes. Strain cream mixture and return to saucepan over medium heat. Whisk in psyllium husks and cook until sauce thickens, about 3 minutes. Remove from heat, swirl in butter until melted and use straight away.

Mushroom Gravy

INGREDIENTS
- 55g butter, divided
- 1 small onion, chopped finely
- ¼ tsp. salt
- ⅛ tsp. pepper
- 175g mixed mushrooms, sliced
- 2 cloves garlic, finely chopped
- 2 tsp. soya sauce
- 1 tsp. red wine vinegar
- 475ml chicken broth

- *1½ tsp. psyllium husks*
- *2 tsp. fresh thyme, chopped*

METHOD: Melt 15g of butter in a non-stick frying pan over medium-high heat. Add onion and seasoning and sauté until soft, about 3 minutes. Add mushrooms and sauté until golden brown, about 8 minutes. Add garlic and sauté until fragrant, about 30 seconds. Add broth and boil until mixture is reduced by one third, about 10 minutes. Stir in psyllium husks and thyme and simmer until sauce thickens, about 2 minutes. Remove from heat, swirl in remaining butter until melted and serve warm.

Tip: *This low-carb gravy gets its rich flavour from sautéed mushrooms rather than from pan drippings. For a vegetarian version, replace the chicken broth with vegetable broth.*

Mushroom Sauce

INGREDIENTS
- *25ml butter*
- *1 small onion, finely chopped*
- *250g button mushrooms, sliced*
- *30ml mushroom soup powder*
- *300ml fresh cream*
- *Salt to taste*
- *Few drops of Tabasco sauce or freshly ground black pepper*

METHOD: Heat the butter in a saucepan over medium heat and brown the onion and mushrooms. Add the mushroom soup powder and sauté for 1 minute. Gradually stir in the cream and simmer, stirring continuously, until the sauce has thickened. Add more cream if a thinner sauce is needed. Season with salt and Tabasco sauce or pepper.

Mustard-Cream Sauce

INGREDIENTS
- 120ml double cream
- 1 spring onion, chopped
- 1½ Tbsp. coarse-grained mustard
- ¼ tsp. pepper
- ¼ tsp. salt

METHOD: Pour cream into a small frying pan and bring to the boil over high heat. Stir in spring onion and cook, stirring frequently until cream thickens slightly, about 4 minutes. Remove from heat and stir in mustard and seasoning.

Tip: Serve this savoury sauce over chicken, pork or veal cutlets or poached salmon or chicken breasts.

> **Make cream go further** by adding half its volume of milk and beating well.

Tartar Sauce

INGREDIENTS
- 120ml mayonnaise
- 4 Tbsp. dill pickle gherkins, finely chopped
- 2 Tbsp. onion, finely chopped
- 1 Tbsp. drained capers, chopped
- 2 tsp. Dijon mustard
- ½ tsp. Xylitol

METHOD: Combine mayonnaise, gherkins, onion, capers, mustard and Xylitol in a small bowl. Serve immediately or refrigerate in an airtight container for up to 5 days.

Homemade Tomato Sauce

INGREDIENTS

- *60ml extra virgin olive oil*
- *1 medium onion, finely chopped*
- *½ medium celery stick, finely chopped*
- *2 garlic cloves, chopped*
- *1 tsp. dried basil*
- *800g tinned crushed tomatoes*
- *Salt and pepper to taste*

METHOD: Heat oil in a medium saucepan over medium heat. Add onion, celery and garlic and sauté until vegetables are very soft, about 6 minutes. Add basil and cook, stirring continuously, for about 30 seconds. Stir in tomatoes. Bring to the boil; reduce heat to medium-low and simmer, partially covered, until thickened, about 30 minutes. Season with salt and pepper and serve hot.

> **Spray Tupperware** with non-stick cooking spray before pouring in tomato-based sauces to avoid staining.

Dips

Chutney Dip

INGREDIENTS
- *2 Tbsp. chutney*
- *2 Tbsp. chives, chopped*
- *1 tub cream cheese*
- *1 Tbsp. homemade mayonnaise*

METHOD: Mix all ingredients together until smooth and serve when chilled.

Herb Dip

INGREDIENTS
- *1 tub cream cheese*
- *1 Tbsp. homemade mayonnaise*
- *1 clove garlic, crushed*
- *2 Tbsp. mixed fresh herbs (basil, chives, parsley, coriander), finely chopped*

METHOD: Mix together in a bowl and serve with nutty crackers or vegetable batons.

Pesto with Pecan Nuts

INGREDIENTS
- 1½ cups rocket, chopped
- ½ cup olive oil
- 2 cups pecan nuts, toasted
- 2 Tbsp. lemon juice
- 1 tsp. garlic
- ½ cup Parmesan cheese

METHOD: Put all the ingredients in a blender and whizz until smooth. Place in a bowl and garnish with extra pecan nuts and rocket.

Tomato & Macadamia Dip

INGREDIENTS
- 1 cup olive oil
- 200g macadamia nuts
- ½ onion
- 1 tsp. garlic
- ½ tsp. salt
- 1 tsp. Xylitol
- 4 Tbsp. tomato paste
- 1 cup sun-dried tomatoes
- 1 cup fresh basil leaves

METHOD: Put all ingredients in a blender and whizz until smooth. Put in a bowl and garnish with fresh basil.

Marinades

Asian Marinade

INGREDIENTS
- 120ml soya sauce
- 2 Tbsp. unseasoned rice wine vinegar
- 2 Tbsp. Xylitol
- 1 Tbsp. peeled ginger, grated
- 2 garlic cloves, finely chopped
- 2 tsp. dark sesame oil
- 2 Tbsp. olive oil

METHOD: Combine soya sauce, vinegar, Xylitol, ginger, garlic and sesame oil in a bowl. Slowly whisk in olive oil until combined.

Tip: Discard marinades after soaking food as it may contain harmful bacteria. If you wish to use marinade as a basting sauce or gravy, reserve some before adding to food, or make a fresh batch. Try this marinade with chicken kebabs, salmon or tuna steaks, pork chops or beef fillet. Marinate chicken and meat for up to 24 hours, and fish for up to 2 hours.

Cajun Marinade

INGREDIENTS
- 1 Tbsp. ground allspice
- 1 Tbsp. cayenne pepper
- 1 Tbsp. black peppercorns, crushed
- 2 tsp. ground cinnamon

- 100ml tomato puree
- 100ml olive oil
- 15ml balsamic vinegar
- 2 cloves garlic, crushed

METHOD: Mix all the ingredients together and pour into an airtight container. Store in the fridge for up to 2 weeks. Use this marinade for fish, prawns, chicken, lamb and beef.

Mediterranean Marinade

INGREDIENTS
- 2 Tbsp. Dijon mustard
- 1 Tbsp. fresh rosemary leaves, chopped
- 3 garlic cloves, peeled
- 1 tsp. grated lemon zest
- ½ tsp. ground fennel
- ½ tsp. pepper
- 1 tsp. salt
- 120ml extra virgin olive oil

METHOD: Combine mustard, rosemary, garlic, lemon zest, fennel, pepper and salt in a blender. With motor running, slowly drizzle in oil until incorporated.

Tip: This marinade is great on all grills, sautés or roasts, especially on chicken, veal chops, aubergine slices, and mild flavoured fish such as snapper, bass and scallops. As this mixture is low in acid, even fish and shellfish can be marinated in it for up to 24 hours.

Hearty Red Wine Marinade

INGREDIENTS
- 120ml dry red wine
- 60ml extra virgin olive oil
- 2 Tbsp. red wine vinegar
- 1 medium shallot, chopped
- 2 tsp. Xylitol
- 10 juniper berries (optional)
- 2 tsp. fresh rosemary leaves, chopped
- ¼ tsp. coarsely ground black pepper
- ¾ tsp. salt

METHOD: Combine wine, oil, vinegar, shallot, garlic, Xylitol, juniper berries, rosemary, pepper and salt in a bowl and mix well.

Tip: This marinade is good with steaks, venison or other game, thick onion slices and summer squash. Substitute a small onion for the shallot if desired.

Latin Marinade

INGREDIENTS
- 5 garlic cloves, peeled
- 60ml fresh lemon juice
- 2 Tbsp. fresh lime juice
- 2 Tbsp. coriander leaves, chopped
- ½ small onion, chopped
- 1½ tsp. grated orange zest
- ¾ tsp. dried oregano
- 1½ tsp. salt
- 175ml rapeseed oil

METHOD: Combine garlic, lemon juice, lime juice, coriander, onion, orange zest, oregano and salt in a blender; blend until smooth. Add the oil and pulse to combine.

Tip: *Many of the ingredients in marinades and rubs contain carbs, but since you usually discard the marinade, you will actually consume only negligible amounts. The garlic and lime flavour this marinade is particularly good with all cuts of pork and chicken (marinate at least 2 hours and up to 24 hours), fish and shellfish (marinate for no longer than 20 minutes).*

Chutney & Tomato Braai Marinade

INGREDIENTS
- *125ml olive or coconut oil*
- *60ml tomato puree*
- *60ml chutney, preferably diabetic*
- *1 tsp. curry powder*
- *½ tsp. turmeric*
- *30ml diabetic apricot jam*
- *1 tsp. Xylitol*

METHOD: Mix all ingredients well and pour into an airtight container and store in the fridge for up to 2 weeks.

Chilli & Garlic Marinade

INGREDIENTS
- 1 Tbsp. crushed chilli
- 1 Tbsp. garlic, crushed
- 2 Tbsp. lemon juice
- 2 Tbsp. olive oil
- 1 tsp. salt

METHOD: Mix all the ingredients together and refrigerate. Baste any braai meat or fish with this tasty sauce that gets hotter the longer you keep it!

Spicy Yoghurt Marinade

INGREDIENTS
- 250ml plain yoghurt
- 2 cloves garlic, crushed
- 2cm piece fresh ginger, peeled and finely grated
- Juice of ½ lemon
- 1 tsp. ground cumin
- 1 tsp. ground coriander
- ½ tsp. cayenne pepper
- ½ tsp. salt
- 45ml fresh mint, chopped

METHOD: Mix all the ingredients together and pour into an airtight container. Store in the fridge for up to a week.

Rubs

BBQ Rub

INGREDIENTS

- 2 Tbsp. ground cumin
- 2 Tbsp. garlic powder
- 2 Tbsp. onion powder
- 2 Tbsp. Xylitol
- 1½ Tbsp. chilli powder
- 1½ Tbsp. pepper
- 1 Tbsp. salt
- 1 tsp. powdered mustard
- 1 tsp. ground mixed spice

METHOD: Combine cumin, garlic powder, onion powder, Xylitol, chilli powder, pepper, salt, mustard and mixed spice in a bowl and mix well.

Tip: Use this rub to spice up meats before grilling or roasting. Rub this on ribs before cooking and then baste ribs with the sauce during the last 10-20 minutes of grilling. Extra spice rub can be stored in an airtight container in a cool place for up to 2 months.

Cajun Rub

INGREDIENTS

- 2 Tbsp. plus 2 tsp. paprika
- 2 Tbsp. dried oregano
- 1 Tbsp. garlic powder
- 1 Tbsp. salt
- 1 tsp. dried thyme
- 1 tsp. cayenne pepper

METHOD: Combine paprika, oregano, garlic powder, salt, thyme and cayenne pepper in a bowl and mix well.

Tip: This is a classic 'blackening' rub for fish steaks such as tuna or swordfish, or fillets such as catfish and snapper, but it also works well for poultry and pork chops.

SECTION 10:

BREAD

'The hunger for love is much more difficult to remove than the hunger for bread'.
Mother Theresa

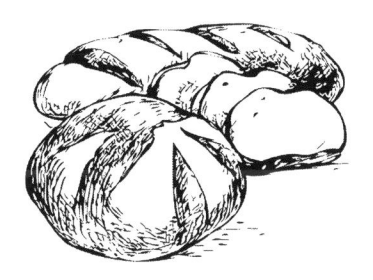

Bread

	Page
Bread Sticks	395
Breakfast Bread in Two Minutes	395
Buttermilk Bread Loaf	396
Carb-Free Bagels	396
Carb-Free Bread	397
Low-Carb Bread	398
Nutty Courgette Loaf	398

Bread Sticks

Makes 6 sticks

INGREDIENTS
- 1 cup Parmesan cheese, grated
- 1 cup almond flour
- 1 egg, beaten
- 2 Tbsp. melted butter
- ½ tsp. garlic powder (optional)

METHOD: Mix all ingredients well and chill in the refrigerator for 30 minutes. Preheat the oven to 180°C. Roll out little fingers of the mixture into 6 sticks and flatten them out. Place on a baking tray covered with parchment paper. Bake for 10 minutes, turning them over halfway through cooking to brown on both sides.
Tip: You can add ½ cup grated Mozzarella cheese, 1 Tbsp. flax meal and 1 tsp. dried oregano for a variation.

Breakfast Bread in Two Minutes

Makes 2 mini loaves

INGREDIENTS
- 1 egg
- 100ml almond flour
- Pinch of salt
- 25ml melted butter

METHOD: Beat the egg in a bowl, add the almond flour and salt and mix well. Add melted butter to the mixture. Divide mixture into two equal amounts and pour into two small bowls or dishes. Place the dishes in the microwave at 100% power for 2 minutes or until you see that the 'bread' is becoming firm and sponge-like. Remove from the microwave and place 'breads' on a plate.

Buttermilk Bread Loaf

Makes 1 loaf

INGREDIENTS
- 1 cup almond meal
- 1½ cup desiccated coconut, fine
- ½ cup flax meal
- 2 Tbsp. Xylitol
- 2 eggs, beaten
- 2 tsp. baking powder
- 2 tsp. psyllium husk
- 300ml buttermilk/amasi/lacto
- 75g melted butter

METHOD: Preheat the oven to 180°C. Add the dry ingredients to a mixing bowl and mix through so the psyllium and baking powder are mixed into the flours. Beat the Xylitol and butter together and then add the eggs and buttermilk or amasi (lacto); mix into the dry ingredients and pour into a greased loaf pan. Bake for 40-50 minutes until the bread is browned, firm and slightly pulls away from the edges. Allow to cool. Slice bread and store needed portions in plastic bags. Portion bags can be refrigerated for 3-5 days or frozen for later use. Yields 14-16 slices.

Carb-Free Bagels

INGREDIENTS
- 3 Tbsp. ground flaxseed
- 2 Tbsp. coconut flour
- ¼ tsp. baking powder
- 4 eggs, separated
- 1 tsp. dried onion
- 1 tsp. garlic powder

METHOD: Preheat the oven to 170°C. Grease a doughnut pan with butter or non-stick oil. Mix the flaxseed, coconut flour, baking powder and dried onion. Whisk the egg whites until soft peaks form. Slowly add the yolks then add the dried mixture. Allow the batter to sit for 5-10 minutes to thicken. Spoon into the doughnut pan. Sprinkle additional dried onion on top of each bagel. Bake for 30 minutes until bagels are golden brown (if baking mini-bagels, the cooking time is 15-20 minutes).

Carb-Free Bread

Makes 1 loaf

INGREDIENTS
- 2 cups flaxseed, milled
- 5 egg whites
- 2 whole eggs
- 5 Tbsp. coconut oil or olive oil
- 1 tsp. baking powder
- 1 tsp. salt
- ½ cup water
- 3g Stevia

METHOD: Preheat oven to 180°C. In a food processor, blend the dry ingredients together. Add the wet ingredients to the food processor and blend them together until a batter is formed. Pour the mixture into greased loaf tin and bake until it is cooked through the middle. You can use a skewer to test this, but it usually takes 30 minutes. Tip it out onto a cooking rack and use as needed. Allow to cool before slicing. This bread does not keep very long and it is preferable to slice and store in the freezer.

Tip: *To this basic 'dough' recipe you can add any flavouring you like along with cheese or vegetables. For example, blue cheese and butternut go really well in this bread. The whole loaf has only 47g of carbs!*

Low-Carb Bread

Makes 1 loaf

INGREDIENTS
- 100g flaxseed, milled
- 100g sunflower or pumpkin seeds, milled
- 30g psyllium husk
- 200g almond or coconut flour, or a mix of both flours
- 10g baking powder
- 5g salt
- Pinch of Stevia (about 2 sachets) or Xylitol
- 6 eggs, beaten
- 250ml Greek yoghurt

METHOD: Mix wet ingredients together and combine with dry ingredients. Bake in a loaf tin for 50 minutes at 180°C degrees. Sprinkle the top with poppy and sesame seeds if desired.

Nutty Courgette Loaf

Makes 1 loaf

INGREDIENTS
- 5 eggs, beaten
- ½ cup coconut oil, melted
- Zest and juice of ½ lemon
- 1 garlic clove, crushed
- 2½ cups grated courgette
- 50g desiccated coconut
- 1½ tsp. baking powder
- ½ tsp. salt
- ¾ cup pumpkin seeds
- ½ cup sunflower seeds

- 50g pecan nuts, toasted
- 1 tsp. fresh rosemary, chopped
- 80g Feta cheese, crumbled

For the topping:
- ¼ cup pumpkin seeds
- 2 Tbsp. sunflower seeds
- 15g pecan nuts
- 20g Feta cheese, crumbled

METHOD: Preheat the oven to 180°C. Line a one-litre loaf tin. Place all loaf ingredients in a large bowl and stir until well combined. In a separate bowl, mix together the topping ingredients. Spoon the loaf mixture into the prepared tin and sprinkle with the topping; bake for 1 hour. Allow to cool. Remove from the tin and cool completely on a rack before slicing. Slice and serve spread with butter or cream cheese.

The Low-Carb Companion

SECTION 11:

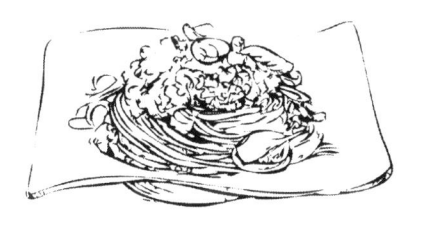

PIZZA, QUICHES & PASTA

Believe it or not, there is pizza and pasta in the 'low-carb world'!

Pizza, Quiches & Pasta

	Page
Broccoli & Blue Cheese Quiche	403
Low-Carb Pasta	404
Flour-Free Pizza (cauliflower base)	404
Courgette Noodles	406
Quick Low-carb Pizza	406
Spinach Quiche	407
Chicken & Mushroom Pasta	408

Pasta Sauces

Bacon & Tomato Sauce	409
Carbonara Sauce	410
Mushroom, Basil & Cream Sauce	410
Tomato & Garlic Sauce	411

Some Handy, Budget Nut Flour Substitutes:

Pumpkin seed meal (Pumpkin seeds ground in your coffee grinder)

Coconut meal (Desiccated coconut ground in your coffee grinder)

Flax meal (Flax seed ground in your coffee grinder) – must be used quickly as it goes rancid

You can substitute almost any recipe with these nut alternatives. Almonds, in particular, have a very neutral taste, and the above meals might add a bit of a different flavour to the palette. Pumpkin meal has a very subtle taste, too.

Broccoli & Blue Cheese Quiche   *Serves 6-8*

INGREDIENTS

For the Base
- 2½ cups almond flour
- ½ cup ground golden flaxseed
- ¼ cup coconut flour
- 1 Tbsp. psyllium powder
- 2 tsp. baking soda
- 120g butter, softened at room temperature

For the Filling
- 10 eggs
- 500g broccoli florets
- 125g blue cheese
- ½ tsp. salt
- ½ tsp. pepper

METHOD: Preheat the oven to 200°C. Place all the base ingredients into a bowl and work the butter into the dried ingredients until dough-like mixture is obtained (add a drop of water if too dry). Grease a pie dish with butter and place the dough into the dish, spreading it out evenly with your hands across the bottom and up along the sides. Bake for 20 minutes. Whilst the 'crust' is cooking, place the broccoli florets into a saucepan, bring to the boil, cover and simmer for 10-12 minutes until tender. Drain and wash in cold water to stop the cooking process. After removing the pie dish from the oven, reduce the temperature to 180°C. Whisk the eggs and add the seasoning. Place the broccoli in the pie dish; scatter the blue cheese around it. Pour over the egg mixture. Bake for 45 minutes until firm.

Low-Carb Pasta   *Serves 4*

INGREDIENTS
- 4 eggs
- 125g cream cheese
- ½ cup psyllium husks
- Coconut flour for dusting

METHOD: In a food processor, blend all the ingredients and leave the mixture to thicken for 10 minutes. Dust the pasta with coconut flour, place between greaseproof paper and roll into pasta sheets. Cut into small strips and set aside. The pasta can be left between greaseproof paper and frozen or cooked immediately. Cook in boiling water for 2-3 minutes but take note that it cooks very quickly. Low-carb pasta is very filling and the quantity eaten will be far less than conventional pasta.

Flour-Free Pizza   *Serves 4-6*

INGREDIENTS
- 1 head cauliflower, cut into pieces 2.5-5cm in size
- 180ml extra-virgin olive oil
- 2 large eggs
- 335g grated Mozzarella cheese

Choice of meat toppings
- 225g sausage, pepperoni, beef, turkey or pork mince
- 350ml pizza sauce

Choice of vegetable toppings
- Chopped peppers
- Sun-dried tomatoes

- *Chopped onions or spring onions*
- *Finely chopped garlic*
- *Fresh spinach*
- *Olives*
- *Chopped or sliced mushrooms*
- *Diced broccoli or asparagus*
- *Fresh or dried basil*
- *Fresh or dried oregano*
- *Black pepper*
- *25g Parmesan cheese, grated*

METHOD: In a large pot of boiling water or in a vegetable steamer, cook the cauliflower until soft, about 20 minutes. Drain the cauliflower and transfer to a large bowl. Mash until it is the consistency of mashed potatoes with few chunks and add 60ml of the oil, the eggs and 110g of the mozzarella cheese and mix well. Preheat the oven to 180°C and lightly coat a pizza pan or large rimmed baking tin with about 1 Tbsp. olive oil. Pour the cauliflower mixture onto the pizza pan and press the 'dough' into a flat, pizza-like shape no more than 1.5 cm thick, mounding it up higher at the edges. Bake for 20 minutes. If using mince, brown in a frying pan until cooked through. Remove the pizza crust from the oven (leave the oven on) and spread it with pizza sauce or tomato paste, the remaining 2 cups Mozzarella, vegetable and meat toppings, basil, oregano and pepper. Drizzle with remaining olive oil and sprinkle with the Parmesan. Bake until the Mozzarella melts, about 10-15 minutes. Cut the pizza into wedges and use a spatula to transfer to plates.

Courgette Noodles   *Serves 2*

INGREDIENTS
- 400g large courgettes (the bigger they are, the easier they are to slice)
- 2 tsp. fine salt
- 1 Tbsp. coconut oil

METHOD: Using a knife, a mandolin, a shredder/peeler or a Chinese slicer, cut the courgettes into noodles. Mix with salt and leave in a colander in the sink for about 20 minutes to drain any excess moisture. Warm the coconut oil in a large pan and add the courgettes. Sauté for a few minutes until they are just cooked.

Tip: *These can be used as a substitute for any pasta with sauce, in any Asian broth, in a stir-fry or on their own as a light side with some grilled chicken or fish.*

Quick Low-carb Pizza   *Makes 1 serving*

INGREDIENTS
For the base
- 2 eggs
- 200ml grated hard cheese (like Cheddar or Gouda)
- 25ml tomato puree

Toppings
- A selection of your favourite toppings (e.g. mushrooms, bacon, ham, olives, tomatoes, peppers, salami, pepperoni)
- 200ml grated cheese (Cheddar or Mozzarella)

METHOD: Preheat oven to 200°C. Whisk eggs and add the grated cheese. Spread the mixture in a circle on a greased baking sheet. Bake the pizza base for 10 minutes. Remove from the oven when crisp and golden brown. Spread the tomato puree over the pizza base; add your favourite toppings, sprinkle over the grated cheese and place back in the oven for about 10 minutes until the cheese has melted.

Spinach Quiche   *Serves 6*

INGREDIENTS
- 250g Cheddar cheese
- ⅓ block Feta cheese, crumbled
- 2 cups spinach
- 1 onion
- 6 eggs
- 100ml almond flour, sifted with 2 tsp. baking powder
- 1 cup black pitted olives
- Cherry tomatoes
- White pepper
- Pinch of salt
- Olive oil

METHOD: Grate the cheese and spread on the bottom of greased pie dish, keeping a handful to sprinkle on top. Boil spinach for 5 minutes; drain off as much water as possible. Chop up onion and fry in olive oil until transparent. Place eggs, flour mixture, white pepper, salt, spinach and cooked onion in food processor and blend. Pour mixture over the cheese in the prepared dish. Scatter chopped feta cheese and submerge. Insert black pitted olives, chopped into halves and submerge. Place halved cherry tomatoes, cut side facing upwards, on the surface. Sprinkle remaining Cheddar cheese over the top and bake at 180°C for 30 minutes.

Chicken & Mushroom Pasta   *Serves 4*

INGREDIENTS
- *8 chicken legs and thighs*
- *1 litre water*
- *1 chicken stock cube*
- *1 cup chopped cabbage*
- *½ cup celery, chopped*
- *½ cup onion, chopped*
- *½ cup carrots, chopped*
- *Salt and pepper to taste*
- *6 cloves garlic*
- *low-carb pasta*

For the sauce:
- *900g tomato puree*
- *3 onions, chopped*
- *6 cloves garlic, crushed*
- *2 green peppers, chopped*
- *1 tsp. sweet chilli sauce*
- *2 chicken stock cubes*
- *Salt and pepper*
- *4 tsp. chopped sweet basil*
- *1 cup strained stock*
- *2 tins chopped mushrooms*
- *½ cup cream*

METHOD: Simmer the first 9 ingredients together and when the chicken is cooked, remove from the stock and cool. Take the meat from the bones and put in a covered dish. Put the bones back into the stock and simmer until reduced by half. Strain the stock. **For the sauce**: Fry onions, peppers and garlic in olive oil or butter; add all the other ingredients except the mushrooms and cream and simmer for approximately 10 minutes. Add the chicken pieces, chopped mushrooms and cream. Serve with low-carb pasta, sweet potatoes or wild rice.

Pasta Sauces

Bacon & Tomato Sauce *Serves 4*

INGREDIENTS
- *6 rashers bacon, chopped*
- *1 onion, chopped*
- *1 tin tomatoes*
- *250ml white wine*
- *2 Tbsp. fresh basil, chopped*
- *250ml cream*
- *5 tsp. capers*
- *1 Tbsp. olive oil*
- *Grated Parmesan cheese to serve*

METHOD: Sauté the onion in the oil, add the bacon and fry until browned. Add the tinned tomatoes and wine, season and cook until the sauce is reduced. Add the basil, capers and cream and stir until combined. Serve with freshly grated Parmesan cheese over low-carb pasta.

Mushroom, Basil & Cream Sauce *Serves 4*

INGREDIENTS
- 250g brown mushrooms, wiped and chopped
- 2 cloves garlic, crushed
- 1 leek, chopped
- 60ml sherry
- 125ml cream
- 125ml cultured sour milk or crème fraiche
- 2ml salt
- 1 egg, beaten
- 125ml fresh basil leaves, chopped
- Chopped walnuts or pecans
- Freshly grated Parmesan cheese and ground black pepper to serve

METHOD: Place all ingredients except half the basil and the nuts in the top of a double boiler and cook, covered, over simmering water for 30 minutes, stirring occasionally. Add the remaining basil and nuts. Toss with your choice of low-carb pasta and serve with grated Parmesan and black pepper.

Tomato & Garlic Sauce *Serves 4*

INGREDIENTS
- 1 tin tomatoes or 8 fresh, ripe peeled tomatoes and a sprig of parsley
- 10 or more peeled garlic cloves
- Olive oil
- Salt and pepper for seasoning

METHOD: Chop the peeled garlic and put into a pan with some olive oil. When garlic is just about to turn black (i.e. very brown and oil is smoking), throw in the tomatoes, which have been chopped quite small. Be ready to cover the pot as it can be a bit fiery. Cook on medium for 20 minutes and serve with your choice of low-carb pasta or wild rice.

Carbonara Sauce   *Serves 4*

INGREDIENTS
- *8 rashers streaky bacon*
- *4 large eggs*
- *25g grated Parmesan or Cheddar cheese*
- *Salt and pepper to taste*
- *Low-carb pasta*

METHOD: Remove the bacon rind and fry until the fat begins to run. Chop the bacon into small pieces and fry with the rinds for 5-8 minutes until they are cooked, but not crisp. Whisk the eggs in a bowl and season with plenty of salt and pepper. Put the low-carb pasta, drained, into a pan and pour on the eggs, tossing so that the eggs cook with its heat. Drain the bacon pieces on kitchen paper, add to the pan, toss well and turn on to a serving dish and sprinkle with the cheese. Serve immediately.

The Low-Carb Companion

SECTION 12:

PANCAKES & MUFFINS

Keeping St Patrick happy.

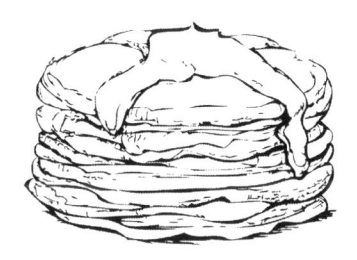

Pancakes & Muffins

	Page
1 Minute Flax Muffin in a Mug	415
Cream Cheese Muffins	415
Basic Pancakes	416
Cocoa Crêpes with Cream Cheese & Raspberries	416
Simple Savoury Egg Muffins	417
Coconut Batter Pancakes / Waffles	418
Pumpkin Spice Muffins	419

1 Minute Flax Muffin in a Mug *Makes 1 muffin*

INGREDIENTS
- 1 tsp. butter
- 1 egg, beaten well
- ¼ cup ground flax meal
- 1 tsp. ground cinnamon
- ½ tsp. baking powder
- 1 tsp. Stevia or Xylitol
- Other flavourings of choice (optional): blueberries and coconut

METHOD: Lightly grease the inside of a mug with a dab of butter. Add the tsp. of butter to the mug and microwave for a few seconds to melt it. Remove the mug from the microwave, add the remaining ingredients and mix well. Put the mug back into the microwave and cook for about 45 seconds to a minute or more, depending upon your microwave. When the muffin is done, turn it out onto a plate.

Cream Cheese Muffins *Makes 10-12 muffins*

INGREDIENTS
- 500g cream cheese
- 2 eggs
- ¼ cup Xylitol
- ½ tsp. vanilla
- 1 tsp. cinnamon

METHOD: Preheat the oven to 180°C. Mix the cream cheese, eggs, Xylitol and vanilla together until very soft. Place the mixture into muffin or cupcake cases. Sprinkle cinnamon on top. Bake for 20 minutes. Remove and cool.

Basic Pancakes

Makes 4-6 crêpes

INGREDIENTS
- 110g coconut flour
- Pinch of salt
- 2 large eggs
- 200ml milk mixed with 80ml water
- 2 Tbsp. butter, melted
- Extra butter for frying

METHOD: Sift the flour and salt into a large mixing bowl, make a well in the centre and add eggs, milk and water mixture. Whisk by hand or with an electric beater and when you are ready to cook, add 2 tsp. butter and stir in. Heat a small knob of butter in a non-stick frying pan. Pour in enough mixture to coat and fry until first side is cooked; flip over and cook until second side is golden brown and remove. Continue till all mixture is used up. To serve as a dessert, fill with fresh berries and cream. For savoury pancakes, fill with a mixture of meat, vegetables, fish, etc. The latter can be put in an ovenproof dish, covered with grated cheese and reheated in the oven.

Cocoa Crêpes with Cream Cheese & Raspberries

Serves 4

INGREDIENTS
- 4 eggs
- ¼ cup water
- Big pinch salt
- ¼ tsp. bicarb
- 2 tsp. Xylitol
- 1 Tbsp. cocoa powder dissolved in 1 Tbsp. water

- *30g coconut flour*
- *Butter for greasing*

For the filling:
- *150g cream cheese, softened*
- *2 tsp. Xylitol*
- *100g raspberries and strawberries*
- *2 Tbsp. desiccated coconut, toasted*

METHOD: Place the eggs in a bowl with the water, salt, bicarb, Xylitol and cocoa powder. Whisk until smooth. Add the coconut flour and whisk until combined. Grease a 12cm frying pan with a little butter, add some of the batter to the pan and swirl until the batter covers the base in a thin layer. Cook the crepe for 2-3 minutes on each side or until firm. Repeat until you have 8 crepes. For the filling, mix the cream cheese with the Xylitol, spread onto the crêpes, top with a few berries and fold up; repeat with all the remaining crêpes. Serve immediately, sprinkled with coconut.

Simple Savoury Egg Muffins   *Makes 6-8 muffins*

INGREDIENTS
- *4 eggs*
- *1 cup vegetables: spinach/onions/peppers/tomatoes/ or veggie of choice, finely chopped*
- *½ cup cheese: Feta/Cheddar/Parmesan, grated*
- *Salt and pepper to taste*

METHOD: Heat the oven to 200°C. If you are using spinach or onions, cook them in a frying pan gently until cooked. Beat the eggs then add the vegetables and cheese. Pour into greased muffin tins (or small mini bread tins). Cook for 15-20 minutes until they are golden brown and firm.

Coconut Batter Pancakes / Waffles *Serves 4*

INGREDIENTS
- ¼ cup coconut flour
- 1 tsp. cinnamon
- 1 tsp. baking powder
- Salt
- 4 extra-large eggs
- 1 tsp. vanilla essence
- ¼ cup melted butter
- 2-3 Tbsp. milk

METHOD: Mix the coconut flour, cinnamon and baking powder together and add a pinch of salt. Whisk the eggs, vanilla essence and melted butter together. Beat wet ingredients with dry ingredients and add the milk until a smooth batter forms (add more flour or liquid if needed). Fry dollops of batter in a lightly greased pan until golden. Great served with Greek yoghurt and berries.

Tip: This coconut batter can also be used to make waffles in a preheated greased waffle machine; use ¼ of batter per waffle.

> **To freshen cream or milk that** has just turned, add a pinch of bicarbonate of soda and some sweetener.

Pumpkin Spice Muffins

Makes 12 small muffins

INGREDIENTS
- 200g ground almonds
- 120g chopped walnuts
- 30g ground flaxseed
- ½ cup Xylitol
- 2 tsp. ground cinnamon
- 1 tsp. ground allspice
- 1 tsp. grated nutmeg
- 1 tsp. baking powder
- Pinch of fine sea salt
- 425g tinned unsweetened pumpkin puree or fresh
- 120ml soured cream or coconut milk
- 2 large eggs
- 60ml walnut oil, melted coconut oil or extra-light olive oil

METHOD: Preheat oven to 160°C and grease a 12-muffin tin with oil. Stir together the ground almonds, walnuts, ground flaxseed, Xylitol, cinnamon, allspice, nutmeg, baking powder and salt in a large bowl. Stir together the pumpkin, soured cream or coconut milk, eggs and oil in another large bowl. Stir the pumpkin mix into the almond mix and mix thoroughly. Spoon the batter into muffin holes, filling about halfway. Bake until a cocktail stick inserted in a muffin comes out dry, about 45 minutes. Leave to cool in the tin for 10-15 minutes then turn out onto a rack to cool completely.

SECTION 13:

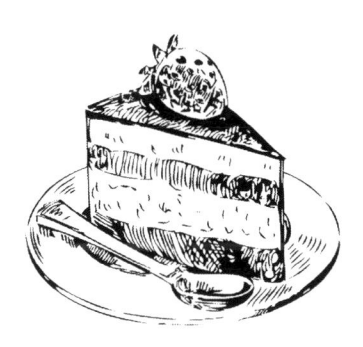

CUPCAKES, CAKES & COOKIES

You can have your (low-carb) cake and eat it, too!

Cupcakes, Cakes & Cookies

	Page
Chocolate Cupcakes	423
Carrot Cake	424
Lemon & Lime Cake With Coconut Flour	425
Choc-Coconut Creams	426
Classic Low-Carb Cheesecake	427
Coconut Cake	428
Lemon Yoghurt Poppy Seed Cake	429
Quick Mocha Icing	430
Quickie 10-Minute Chocolate Cake	430

Chocolate Cupcakes

Makes 8 cupcakes

INGREDIENTS
- ¼ cup cocoa powder
- ¼ cup coconut flour
- 1½ tsp. baking powder
- ½ tsp. cinnamon
- Pinch of salt
- 4 eggs, beaten
- 2 Tbsp. honey (optional)
- 1 tsp. vanilla essence
- ¼ cup of coconut oil or melted butter
- 70-85% dark chocolate blocks, chopped up (optional)

METHOD: Preheat oven to 160°C. Combine dry ingredients first, and then the wet ingredients. Add chocolate bits if using. Mix well. Spoon into 8 cupcake moulds and bake for 30 minutes or until cooked through. (Smaller cupcakes take 20 minutes.)

3 options for the ganache topping:
1. 300g cocoa powder + 150ml full fat yoghurt or cream
2. 250g cream cheese + little bit of lemon zest + a squeeze of the juice + bit of vanilla essence + honey to taste
3. 1 heaped Tbsp. macadamia nut butter + 1 tsp. honey + 1 tsp. cocoa powder + 2 Tbsp. hot water

Mix chosen ganache ingredients together and spread on cooled cupcakes. Cut a little hole in the top of the cupcake to fit more topping in, or slice the cupcakes in half and spread the topping so that you have a nice layer in the middle.

Carrot Cake *Serves 16*

INGREDIENTS
For the Cake
- 2 Tbsp. butter at room temperature
- 5 Tbsp. Xylitol
- 4 eggs
- ½ cup butter, melted
- 1½ cups nut meal (almond or pecan)
- ¾ cup coconut meal
- 2 tsp. baking powder
- 1 tsp. ground cinnamon
- 1 tsp. ground ginger
- ¼ tsp. bicarbonate of soda
- ½ cup roughly chopped pecan nuts
- ½ cup grated carrots
- 1 cup grated pumpkin
- 1 cup grated yellow patty pans

For the Icing
- 7 Tbsp. butter at room temperature
- 115g block cream cheese
- 2 tsp. lemon juice
- 2 Tbsp. Xylitol

METHOD: For the cake: Preheat oven to 180°C. Use an electric mixer to cream the butter and Xylitol together. Add the eggs and melted butter and mix well. In a separate bowl, mix the nut meal, coconut meal, baking powder, cinnamon, ginger, bicarbonate of soda and pecans together. Pour in the egg mixture and add grated veggies, then fold in the dry ingredients. Divide the batter between 2 buttered loaf pans and bake for 30 minutes, or until cakes are fairly browned and firm to the touch. Allow to cool in tins and then turn out. **For the icing:** Use an electric mixer to blend all the ingredients together until smooth. Spread over carrot cakes.

> **When substituting with coconut meal**, it is always good to add liquids like an extra egg, yoghurt or milk to the batter.

Lemon & Lime Cake with Coconut Flour

Serves 4-6 (About 10 slices)

INGREDIENTS
- *1 lemon*
- *1 lime*
- *6 eggs*
- *½ cup Xylitol*
- *¾ cup coconut flour*
- *150g butter, melted*
- *2 tsp. baking powder*

METHOD: Place the lemon and lime in a small saucepan and cover with water. Bring to the boil, cover and simmer for an hour. Preheat the oven to 170°C. Place the lemon and lime in a food processor or blender and blitz well. Add the eggs and butter to the mixture and blend. Add the remaining ingredients and continue to blend. Pour into a greased cake tin and bake for 35-40 minutes. Cool, decorate and eat.

Choc-Coconut Creams

Serves 18

INGREDIENTS

For the Cookies
- ¾ cup fine desiccated coconut
- 1½ cups medium desiccated coconut
- ¾ cup almond flour
- 2 Tbsp. cocoa powder
- 1 tsp. baking powder
- 7 Tbsp. butter at room temperature
- 4 Tbsp. Xylitol
- 1 egg, beaten
- ½ cup boiling water

For the filling
- ½ cup fresh cream
- 2 Tbsp. cocoa powder
- 1 Tbsp. Xylitol
- 2 tsp. psyllium husk powder

METHOD: **For the cookies:** Preheat oven to 180°C. Mix the coconut, almond flour, cocoa powder and baking powder together in a mixing bowl. In a separate bowl, mix the butter and Xylitol together until creamy. Add the egg. Add the egg mixture to the dry ingredients; add the boiling water and mix well. Roll the dough into giant lollipop-sized balls. Arrange on a buttered baking tray, press down slightly with 2 fingers and bake for about 20 minutes until golden brown. Cool on a wire rack. **For the filling:** Combine all ingredients in a saucepan on medium heat and stir until it reaches a thick custard-like consistency. Cool for a minute before sandwiching the cookies together with the filling. Store in an airtight container.

Section 13 - Cupcakes, Cakes & Cookies

Classic Low-Carb Cheesecake *Makes 6-8 servings*

INGREDIENTS

For the Base
- 120g ground pecan nuts
- 3 Tbsp. Xylitol
- 1½ tsp. ground cinnamon
- 85g unsalted butter, melted and cooled
- 1 large egg, lightly beaten
- 1 tsp. vanilla extract

For the Filling
- 450g cream cheese, at room temperature
- 180ml soured cream
- 3 Tbsp. Xylitol
- Pinch of fine sea salt
- 3 large eggs, beaten
- Juice of 1 small lemon
- 1 Tbsp. grated lemon zest
- 2 tsp. pure vanilla extract

METHOD: Preheat oven to 160°C. **For the base:** Combine the ground pecans, Xylitol and cinnamon in a bowl; stir in the melted butter, egg and vanilla and mix thoroughly. Press the mixture into the bottom and 4-5cm up the side of a 24cm cake tin. **For the filling:** Combine the cream cheese, soured cream, Xylitol and salt in a bowl. Using an electric beater, mix at low sped to blend; beat in the eggs, lemon juice, zest and vanilla and beat at medium speed for 1 minute. Pour the filling into the base and bake until nearly firm in the centre, about 50 minutes. Leave the cheesecake to cool on a rack and refrigerate to chill before serving.

Variations: The filling can be modified by adding 45g unsweetened cocoa powder and top with shavings of plain chocolate, substitute lime juice and zest for the lemon, or top with berries, mint leaves and whipped cream.

Coconut Cake

Serves 10-12

INGREDIENTS
- 200g cream cheese
- 6 eggs, separated
- 80g Xylitol
- 1 tsp. vanilla extract
- 220g coconut flour, lightly toasted
- 1 Tbsp. baking powder
- Pinch Himalayan salt

For the filling
- 1 cup chilled coconut cream, whipped to stiff peaks, or double-cream yoghurt
- 100g strawberries
- 25g desiccated coconut, toasted
- 100g raspberries

METHOD: Preheat oven to 170°C and line 3 x 20cm cake tins with baking paper. Whisk together cream cheese, egg yolks, Xylitol and vanilla. Fold through coconut flour, baking powder and salt. Whisk egg whites to stiff peak stage and fold through the coconut mixture. Pour into prepared tins and bake for 20 minutes or until firm to the touch. Layer the cakes with whipped coconut cream, strawberries and a little sprinkling of coconut.
To Serve: Place onto a serving platter and top with toasted coconut and fresh raspberries.

Lemon Yoghurt Poppy Seed Cake *Makes 1 loaf*

INGREDIENTS
- *200g butter*
- *100g Xylitol*
- *4 eggs, separated, at room temperature*
- *2 tsp. poppy seeds, soaked in 2 Tbsp. milk for 30 minutes*
- *200g almonds, ground*
- *70g coconut flour*
- *1 tsp. baking powder*
- *1 cup double-cream yoghurt*
- *Grated zest and juice of 1 lemon*

For the topping:
- *Double-cream yoghurt and pomegranate rubies*

METHOD: Preheat the oven to 170°C; line a 1-litre loaf tin. Place the butter and Xylitol in a bowl and beat until light and fluffy; add the egg yolks and continue to beat until combined. Whisk the egg whites in a separate bowl until stiff. Add half the poppy seeds, almonds, coconut flour and baking powder to the mixture and then add half the yoghurt and all the lemon juice. Add the remaining dry ingredients and then the remaining yoghurt. Fold in the egg whites. Pour the mixture into the prepared loaf tin and bake for 40 minutes. Remove from the oven and allow to cool completely. Serve cake sliced with yoghurt and rubies.

> **The juice of one lemon** is equal to about ten drops of lemon essence.

Quick Mocha Icing

INGREDIENTS
- 2 Tbsp. cream cheese, at room temperature
- 2 Tbsp. finely ground Xylitol (grind regular Xylitol in your coffee grinder to make powdered xylitol)
- ½ tsp. instant coffee, mixed in 1 Tbsp. warm water
- 1½ Tbsp. cocoa
- ¼ cup cream

METHOD: Mix all the ingredients together in a mixing bowl with an electric mixer until light and fluffy.

Quickie 10-Minute Chocolate Cake   *Serves 6-8*

INGREDIENTS
For The Cake
- 1 cup almond flour or pumpkin seed meal
- 4 Tbsp. fine desiccated coconut
- 2 tsp. baking powder
- 2 Tbsp. cocoa powder
- 2 Tbsp. Xylitol
- Pinch of salt
- 2 Tbsp. melted butter
- 2 eggs
- ½ cup amasi or full-cream milk

Quick Caramel Syrup
- 2 Tbsp. butter

Section 13 - Cupcakes, Cakes & Cookies

- 1½ Tbsp. Xylitol
- ½ cup fresh cream
- 1 tsp. vanilla extract

METHOD: **For the cake:** Mix all the dry ingredients in a microwave-safe mixing bowl. Add the wet ingredients and stir well using a fork. Cook in the microwave on high for 5-6 minutes. Check progress around 4 minutes. The cake is ready when it is spongy, firm and pulls away from the side of the bowl. (You want this cake to be moist rather than dry). **For the caramel syrup:** Melt the butter in a small saucepan on medium to high heat. Add the Xylitol and stir until dissolved completely. Add the cream and stir for a minute. Allow the sauce to boil, forming big bubbles, then adjust the heat to medium and allow the sauce to simmer gently and reduce for 2-3 minutes. The sauce will turn a lovely caramel colour. Tip the cake onto a serving plate and pour over the syrup.

> **Cooking Chocolate substitute:**
> 3 Tbsp. cocoa and 30g butter
> mixed well together.

SECTION 14:

DESSERTS

The 'sweet-tooth' can be satiated and the '3 course meal' completed with low-carb dessert options.

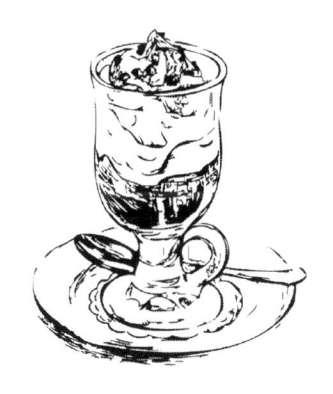

Desserts

	Page
Nut, Berry & Seed Clusters	435
Chocolate Mousse	435
Chocolate Brownies	436
Almond Butter Ice Cream	437
Lemon Ice Cream	437
Coconut Ice Cream	438
Panna Cotta	438
Nutty Chocolate & Coconut Shards	439

Section 14 - Desserts

Nut, Berry & Seed Clusters   *Serves 6*

INGREDIENTS
- ¼ cup desiccated coconut
- ¼ cup ground almonds
- ½ cup sunflower seeds
- ½ cup raw almonds, chopped
- 2 Tbsp. dried, unsweetened cranberries or goji berries
- ⅓ cup coconut oil
- Himalayan salt

METHOD: Combine the coconut, sunflower seeds, ground and chopped almonds. Place in a dry pan and toast under the grill until golden. Put this toasted seed and nut mix into a bowl and then mix in the cranberries, coconut oil and a pinch of salt. Press the mixture into a silicone mould to set and thereafter break it up into 'granola' size clusters. Serve with fresh fruit, yoghurt or cream.

Chocolate Mousse   *Serves 4*

INGREDIENTS
- 100g dark chocolate
- 30g butter
- 1 egg, separated

METHOD: Break up the chocolate and butter and put them into a bowl over a pot of boiling water and melt. Beat egg yolk with a fork and add it to the melted chocolate mixture off the heat. Add one tsp. of warm water. Whip the egg white until stiff, and fold into the mixture with a metal spoon so you don't lose the air in the egg white. Spoon it into individual cups and refrigerate until set.

Chocolate Brownies

Serves 8-10

INGREDIENTS
- *1 cup nut meal or flour (almond or pecan)*
- *½ cup cocoa powder*
- *1 tsp. baking powder*
- *½ tsp. bicarbonate of soda*
- *3 Tbsp. Xylitol*
- *2 free-range eggs, beaten*
- *7 Tbsp. fresh cream*
- *4 Tbsp. melted butter*

METHOD: Preheat oven to 180°C. Mix together all the dry ingredients in a mixing bowl; in a separate bowl whisk all the wet ingredients together. Add the wet ingredients to the dry ingredients and mix well. Pour the batter into a greased square brownie pan or silicone muffin tray. Bake for 8-10 minutes until cracks appear on the surface. If you like a moist 'gooey' brownie, 8 minutes is fine. For a fluffy brownie, bake for 10-12 minutes. Serve with chocolate, berry or caramel mousse, quick ice cream, chocolate ganache or any icing.

Waffle Option

This recipe makes a lovely waffle mix for a waffle machine. Separate the eggs; add the yolks when you mix the wet ingredients, and then fold in stiffly beaten egg whites after the batter is mixed.

Almond Butter Ice Cream

Serves 8-10

INGREDIENTS
- *Macadamia oil*
- *2 x 410g tins coconut cream, chilled*
- *80g Xylitol*
- *½ cup almond butter*
- *100g toasted almonds, chopped*
- *1 tsp. salt*
- *Mixed berries to serve*

METHOD: Oil an 18cm Bundt tin or a 2-litre loaf tin. Place the chilled coconut cream in a large bowl and beat until stiff; add the Xylitol and continue to whip for 2 minutes. Mix together the almond butter, chopped almonds and salt; stir well to combine. Stir this mixture through the coconut cream and pour into the oiled tin. Place the tin in the freezer for at least 4 hours or until completely set. **To serve:** Unmould onto a serving platter, slice and serve garnished with mixed berries.

Lemon Ice Cream

Serves 4

INGREDIENTS
- *300ml fresh cream*
- *3 eggs, separated*
- *2 tsp. Xylitol*
- *Rind and juice of 1 large lemon*

METHOD: Whisk the three egg whites until stiff. Beat the egg yolks and Xylitol until pale and creamy. Whisk the cream until stiff, then fold into the egg yolk mixture. Fold the lemon juice and rind and the egg whites into this mixture and freeze, stirring at intervals to break up the ice crystals.

Coconut Ice Cream

Serves 6

INGREDIENTS
- 2 tins coconut milk
- 1 tsp. vanilla essence
- ½ cup Xylitol

METHOD: Put the cans of the coconut milk in the fridge overnight. Take the coconut milk cans out of the fridge and tip over vertically on the opposite end it was stored (this will allow you to pour off the liquid part of the coconut milk leaving only the milk fat). Pour the liquid out of the can into one bowl, and into another bowl, scrape the thick cream left behind (this is what you use for the ice cream). Place the thick coconut cream in a bowl, add the vanilla essence and Xylitol and whisk until blended. Pour the mixture into a large bowl with a large surface area. Cover and place in the fridge. Remove from the fridge about every 30-40 minutes; whisk thoroughly to distribute the icy mixture for about 4-5 hours until you get the desired consistency of ice cream.

Panna Cotta

Serves 6

INGREDIENTS

- 500ml fresh cream
- 15ml coconut oil
- 200ml desiccated coconut
- Seeds from 1 vanilla pod
- 5ml or 2 sheets gelatine
- Berries and/or coconut for decoration

METHOD: Pour the cream and coconut oil into a saucepan and bring to the boil; add the coconut and vanilla. Stir and remove from heat. Prepare the gelatine according to the package instructions and add to the mixture, stirring continuously. Pour the Panna Cotta into small glasses or a large bowl, and put in the fridge for at least 2 hours or until it's time to serve. Decorate with berries and/or coconut flakes.

Nutty Chocolate & Coconut Shards *Serves 4-6*

INGREDIENTS
- *50g 85% dark chocolate*
- *50g coconut oil*
- *20ml cocoa powder*
- *1 Tbsp. Xylitol*
- *200g hazelnuts*
- *1 cup coconut shavings*

METHOD: Melt chocolate and coconut oil over a pot of boiling water. Stir in cocoa powder and sweeten with Xylitol. Place hazelnuts and coconut shavings in 15cm square dish lined with baking paper. Pour over chocolate mixture and refrigerate to set. Slice into chunks and serve.

> **Egg Whites** can be frozen in ice trays for future use.

The Low-Carb Companion

SECTION 15: SMOOTHIES & SHAKES

Healthy quick low-carb liquid meals and snacks.

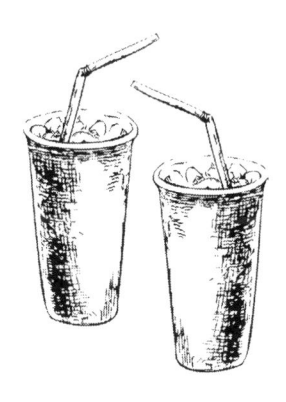

Smoothies and Shakes

	Page
Avocado & Raspberry Shake	443
Berry Coconut Smoothie	443
Chocolate Fat Shake	444
Yoghurt, Almond & Strawberry Smoothie	444
Egg Milk	445
Mango & Ginger Smoothie	445

Avocado & Raspberry Shake *Serves 1*

INGREDIENTS
- ½ ripe avocado, pitted and peeled
- 100g frozen raspberries
- 100g extra-thick Greek yoghurt
- Squeeze of lemon juice
- ½ cup ice blocks

METHOD: Combine all ingredients in a blender and blitz.

Berry Coconut Smoothie *Serves 1*

INGREDIENTS
- 120ml coconut milk
- 120ml low-fat plain yoghurt
- 40g blueberries, blackberries, strawberries or other berries
- 50g unflavoured or vanilla whey protein powder
- 1 Tbsp. ground linseeds
- ½ tsp. coconut extract
- 4 ice cubes

METHOD: Combine the coconut milk, yoghurt, berries, whey protein, linseed, coconut extract and ice cubes in a blender. Blend until smooth. Serve immediately.

Chocolate Fat Shake   *Serves 1*

INGREDIENTS
- 150ml full-cream milk
- 50g butter
- 50ml cream
- 200ml coconut cream
- 1 Tbsp. sugar-free hot chocolate (or a good chunk of 80% dark chocolate or 1 Tbsp. cocoa powder)
- ¼ tsp. salt

METHOD: For the hot version, warm all the ingredients in a small saucepan and then blend with a stick blender. For a cold shake, simply blend all ingredients and enjoy.

Yoghurt, Almond & Strawberry Smoothie   *Serves 1*

INGREDIENTS
- 1 Tbsp. almond butter
- 150ml double-cream or full-cream Greek yoghurt
- 100g frozen strawberries
- 10 blocks of ice

METHOD: Place all ingredients in a blender and blitz.

Section 15 - Smoothies & Shakes

Egg Milk
Serves 1

INGREDIENTS
- 2 eggs
- 50g butter or coconut oil
- 300ml boiling water

METHOD: Mix the eggs, butter or oil and water in a large mug or jug. Add a pinch of ground cinnamon or a dash of vanilla for extra flavour.

Variations: For hot chocolate, add 5ml cocoa powder and seeds from ½ vanilla pod or melt 20g dark chocolate. Add 100ml fresh cream and use only 200ml boiling water. This is a great pre or post-exercise workout protein and fat drink.

Mango & Ginger Smoothie
Serves 2

INGREDIENTS
- 1 mango, pitted and peeled
- 1 cup full-cream Greek yoghurt
- 2 Tbsp. Xylitol to taste
- 1 tsp. finely grated ginger
- ¼ tsp. ground cinnamon
- 5 ice cubes
- 60ml coconut milk

METHOD: Place the mango in a blender. Add the yoghurt and Xylitol, then the ginger and cinnamon. Add the ice and coconut milk. Blend until smooth, adding a little bit more coconut milk if the smoothie is too thick. Serve immediately.

The Low-Carb Companion

SECTION 16:

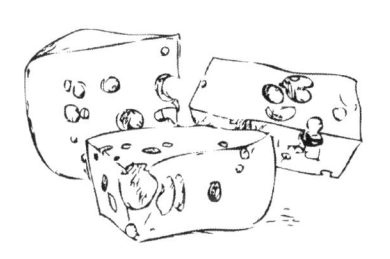

SNACKS & MISCELLANEOUS

The little things that keep the big thing going.

Snacks and Miscellaneous

	Page
Blue Cheese Mousse	449
Cheese Chips	450
Cheesy Almond Crackers	450
Chicken Liver Pâté	451
Chocolate Balls	452
Low-Carb Cold Drink/Juice Concentrate	452
Homemade Low-Carb Muesli	453
Low-Carb Yorkshire Puddings	454
Nut Granola	454
Spicy Cashew & Red Pepper Hummus	455
Savoury Crackers	456
Seed Clusters	457
Spicy Bacon Nuts	458
Stuffed Mushrooms With Creamy Bacon	458
Pastry-Free Sausage 'Rolls'	459

Blue Cheese Mousse

Makes approx. 3 cups

INGREDIENTS
- 125g creamy blue cheese, crumbled
- 250ml thick plain yoghurt
- 3 sticks celery, trimmed and finely chopped
- 2 tsp. chopped fresh chives
- Salt to taste
- Freshly ground black pepper
- 1 tsp. gelatine
- 4 tsp. water
- 250ml whipping cream
- Watercress to garnish

METHOD: Pulse cheese and yoghurt in a blender until combined; add garlic, celery, chives and seasoning and mix well. Sprinkle gelatine over water and leave until it forms a sponge. Soften the sponge in the microwave on medium for 1 minute, or alternatively stand in a bowl over a pan of hot water. With the food processor running, pour the softened gelatine through the feed tube in a thin stream into the blue cheese mixture. Whip cream until slightly thickened and fold gently into the mixture. Pour into a wet mould, cover and refrigerate overnight or until set. Turn out and garnish. Serve with low-carb crackers.

Cheese Chips

Makes approx. 20 chips

INGREDIENTS
- 80g Cheddar, Parmesan or any other hard cheese

METHOD: Heat the oven to 200°C. Slice the cheese with a cheese slicer, fold double and arrange on a baking sheet or tray. Separate the slices so they don't melt together. Place on the top shelf of the oven and cook for about 3-7 minutes, watching that the cheese becomes crisp but does not burn.

Tip: Alternatively, these can be cooked in the microwave at 100% power for 3-5 minutes, again watching that the cheese does not burn.

Cheesy Almond Crackers

Makes 1 tray of crackers

INGREDIENTS:
- 1 cup Cheddar cheese
- 1 cup almond flour or almond meal
- ¼ tsp. salt
- ¼ tsp. garlic powder
- 2-3 Tbsp. of water to bind the mixture

METHOD: Heat the oven to 180°C. Blend all the ingredients together and then add water to make dough. Place the dough onto a greaseproof paper lined baking tray. Cover with another piece of greaseproof paper and use a roller to flatten out the mixture, avoiding rolling it too thin. Remove the top layer of greaseproof paper. Score the dough into squares and then triangles. Place in the oven and cook for about 15 minutes. Watch that the mixture does not get too dark. Turn the mixture over for another five minutes. Remove and break into cracker shapes. Serve with dips.

Chicken Liver Pâté

Makes approx. 2 cups

INGREDIENTS
- 175g chicken livers
- 125g soft butter
- ½ small onion, chopped
- ¼ clove garlic, crushed
- 1 bay leaf
- A few sprigs of parsley leaves
- A tiny sprig of thyme without stalk
- 2 juniper berries, crushed
- 1 Tbsp. gin
- Salt and pepper

METHOD: Pick over the livers, carefully removing all threads and green-tinged flesh. Melt 50g butter and gently fry the chopped onion, crushed juniper berries and bay leaf until the onion softens. Add the chicken livers and sauté briskly over high heat until sealed and lightly browned. Stir in the crushed garlic, herbs and seasoning; cover with a lid and cook gently for 3-5 minutes (the livers should still be just pink inside). Remove the bay leaf and cool the livers a little. In a food processor, blend the livers until smooth before adding the gin and, with the motor running, add the soft butter, bit by bit, to make a smooth pâté mixture. Add seasoning and turn out into a serving dish. Serve at room temperature.

Chocolate Balls *Makes approx. 24 medium sized balls*

INGREDIENTS
- *100ml coconut cream*
- *75g butter*
- *75g coconut oil*
- *100ml raw mixed nuts, finely chopped*
- *100ml desiccated coconut*
- *2 egg yolks*
- *30ml cocoa powder*
- *Seeds from 1 vanilla pod*
- *Extra chopped nuts or coconut for coating*

METHOD: Separate the thick, creamy part of the coconut cream from the liquid (it is usually in a lump). Only use the thick cream. Add the rest of the ingredients and mix well. Using your hands, roll the mixture into balls of any size. Roll the balls in chopped nuts or coconut to coat.

Low-carb cold drink/juice concentrate *Makes 1 litre*

INGREDIENTS
- *700ml water*
- *1 cinnamon stick*
- *1 vanilla pod, split lengthways*
- *Juice from 1 orange*
- *700ml mixed berries (blackberries, strawberries, blueberries, mulberries)*

METHOD: Pour the water into a saucepan and add the cinnamon, seeds from the vanilla pod and the orange juice. Add all the berries, bring to the boil, then reduce the heat and simmer for 15 minutes. If it is very thick, add a little water. Remove the saucepan from the heat and leave to draw for 3 hours or overnight. Strain the cold drink through a clean cloth or tea towel and pour into a bottle. Refrigerate. Add water to taste.

Homemade Low-Carb Muesli *Makes 1kg*

INGREDIENTS
- *150ml sesame seeds*
- *150ml flaxseeds*
- *100ml pumpkin seeds*
- *100ml sunflower seeds*
- *200ml chopped mixed raw nuts*
- *100ml desiccated coconut*
- *150ml coconut shavings*
- *1 tsp. cinnamon*
- *1 tsp. vanilla essence*
- *100ml water*
- *5 Tbsp. coconut oil*

METHOD: Mix all ingredients together and let stand for 15 minutes. Heat oven to 200°C. Spread your mixture on a baking tray and bake for around 15-20 minutes (depending on how crunchy you like it.) Serve with milk, yoghurt or coconut cream. Add fruit, if desired.

> **Nuts can be cracked more easily** if heated in the oven for a few minutes.

Low-Carb Yorkshire Puddings *Makes 6*

INGREDIENTS
- 1 cup milk
- 1 cup almond flour (this must be fine almond flour, not ground almonds)
- 3 eggs
- ¼ tsp. salt
- 1 tsp. baking powder
- ½ cup cold water

METHOD: Mix salt, flour and baking powder. Add milk and eggs and beat until light and foamy. Place in the fridge for an hour. Take a square pan or muffin pan and cover the bottom with very hot fat from the roast if possible, or heated olive oil. Put the pan in the oven and get the oil sizzling hot. Add the cold water to the mixture and beat together. Pour the batter into the pan. Place in the oven at 230°C and bake for 20-30 minutes. Serve with a roast beef meal.

Nut Granola *Makes 500g granola*

INGREDIENTS
- 100g sunflower seeds
- 200g chopped mixed nuts (walnuts / hazelnuts / pecans / macadamia nuts)
- 100g almond flakes
- 3 Tbsp. coconut oil
- 2 tsp. cinnamon
- 2 tsp. ginger
- ½ tsp. nutmeg

METHOD: Preheat oven to 160°C. Chop the nut roughly and mix them together. In a large pan, fry the spices in the coconut oil and then add the nuts and toast them briefly. Tip the nuts onto an oven tray and bake for 10 minutes. Cool before storing in airtight container.

Spicy Cashew & Red Pepper Hummus

Makes approx. 2 cups

INGREDIENTS
- 1 cup cashew nuts (soaked in water for 2 hours)
- ¼ cup tahini
- Juice of half a lemon
- 2 cloves of garlic, crushed
- 1 tsp. salt
- 4 Tbsp. olive oil
- ½ cup water
- 3 red peppers
- 1 Jalapeño chilli, deseeded and chopped
- 1 dash of chipotle sauce/spice (or chopped chipotle chilli, de-seeded)
- Pepper and salt

METHOD: Preheat the oven to 200°C. Cut the peppers in half, remove the seeds and place on a baking tray. Splash over half the olive oil and season. Roast for 30-40 minutes until the skins are charred. Cool, remove skins and stalks. Drain the cashew nuts from the water. Put the remaining ingredients into a food processor; add the red peppers and blend until smooth. You may want to add a bit more water for a smoother consistency.

Savoury Crackers

Makes approx. 32 crackers

INGREDIENTS
- 2 cups nut flour (almond, macadamia or pecan)
- ¼ cup sesame seed
- ¼ cup sunflower seeds
- 50g grated Parmesan
- 1 tsp. dried thyme
- 3 tsp. gelatine powder
- 3 Tbsp. psyllium husk fibre
- 3 tsp. baking powder
- Herbed salts or pepper blend to season
- 4 Tbsp. cold butter
- 1 egg
- 3 Tbsp. apple cider vinegar
- ⅓ cup boiling water

METHOD: Mix all the dry ingredients and gelatine powder in a bowl. Rub the cold butter into the mix until it forms a breadcrumb consistency. Mix the egg into the batter thoroughly and then quickly mix in boiling water and the apple cider vinegar to form a dough ball. Place the dough ball onto cling wrap and roll into a sausage shape of about 5cm in diameter. Wrap the dough in cling wrap and place in the refrigerator for 10 minutes. Remove from the fridge, cut into 1cm slices and place them onto a buttered flat pan. Bake at 180°C for about 20-25 minutes. For nice crispy crackers, you need to bake them just long enough that they snap when broken in half.

Tip: Bake in batches, the dough will keep in the refrigerator for 2-3 days.

Section 16 - Snacks & Miscellaneous

Seed Clusters   *makes 12 clusters*

INGREDIENTS
- *100g coconut flakes or ¾ cup desiccated coconut*
- *50g butter*
- *2 Tbsp. cocoa*
- *2 Tbsp. Xylitol*
- *2 Tbsp. boiling water*
- *4 Tbsp. coconut cream*
- *4 Tbsp. sunflower seeds*
- *4 Tbsp. desiccated fine coconut*
- *4 Tbsp. pumpkin seeds*
- *2 Tbsp. grated orange peel (optional)*

METHOD: In a dry pan, toast seeds and coconut flakes slightly on medium heat till brown colour starts to show. Remove from heat. In a medium saucepan over medium-high heat, melt the butter, then add Xylitol and mix. Dissolve the cocoa in the boiling water and add coconut cream, then add this to the saucepan. Stir the sauce, allowing it to bubble and thicken for 2 minutes. Remove from heat and allow cool for 1-2 minutes. Add all the seeds and coconut and stir into the chocolate sauce. Spoon into a 12-hole tiny cupcake latex mould or into small cupcake liners. (An alternative is to line an egg carton with cling wrap and mould little clusters in the oval moulds). If you don't use the coconut chips, you can just roll the batter into 12 balls. Allow to cool and set for at least 2-3 hours until they are firm.

Tip: *You can use chopped nuts instead of seeds.*

Spicy Bacon Nuts *Makes 800g*

INGREDIENTS
- 250g streaky bacon rashers
- 4 cups assorted nuts (almonds, hazelnuts, pecan, Brazil, macadamia and cashew nuts)
- ½ tsp. ground cumin
- ¼ tsp. cayenne pepper
- 1 large pinch ground nutmeg
- 2 tsp. unsalted butter
- 1 tsp. salt

METHOD: Grill the bacon on a greased tray until crispy. Remove from the fat and cut the rashers into small pieces. Keep the bacon fat. Toast the nuts in a large, heavy-based dry pan until golden. Add the bacon fat and butter and cook until the nuts begin to darken. Add the spices and fry them in the butter until they become fragrant. Add a teaspoon of water and mix in the bacon. Tip the nuts back onto a lined oven tray and cook them in the oven for another 5 minutes at 160°C to dry out properly. Tip out onto a paper towel to cool. Store in an airtight container.

Stuffed Mushrooms with Creamy Bacon *Serves 4*

INGREDIENTS
- 16 large flat (e.g. portobellini) mushrooms
- 2 Tbsp. butter (or ghee or duck fat)
- Himalayan salt and black pepper
- 200g bacon, chopped
- 2 tsp. dried rosemary
- 1 cup cultured cream (crème fraiche)
- 5 spring onions, finely sliced

METHOD: Preheat the oven to 200°C. Remove the mushroom stems and chop the stems into small pieces. Place the mushrooms on a baking tray, dot with butter and season. Bake for 20 minutes, tossing the tray at intervals; remove from the heat and set aside. Heat a small frying pan and fry the bacon and chopped mushroom stems for 3 minutes. Add the rosemary, season and cook until golden and crisp. Remove from heat and allow to cool. Set aside 2 Tbsp. cooked bacon pieces. When cooled, combine the remaining bacon mix with the cultured cream, spring onions and season with salt and pepper. **To assemble:** Place the mushrooms on a platter, top with dollops of the bacon mix and sprinkle with the reserved bacon. Serve immediately with fresh herbs.

Pastry-Free Sausage 'Rolls'

Makes approx. 24 rolls

INGREDIENTS
- *500g sausage meat*
- *1 tsp. Italian seasoning*
- *1 tsp. sage*
- *1 medium onion, grated*

METHOD: Mix sausage meat with onion, Italian seasoning and sage and roll into small balls. Bake in the oven at 180°C for 15-20 minutes, or fry in coconut oil.

The Low-Carb Companion

SECTION 17:

CONVERSION CHARTS & OVEN TEMPERATURES

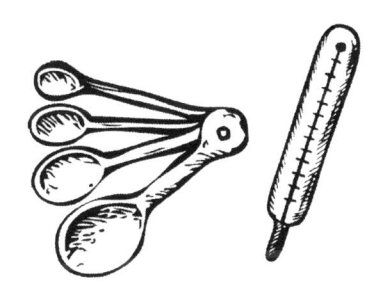

CONVERSION CHARTS

Volume / Measure

Metric	Standard
5ml	1 teaspoon (tsp.)
15ml	1 Tablespoon (Tbsp.)
60ml	4 Tbsp. or ¼ cup
80ml	⅓ cup
125ml	½ cup
160ml	⅔ cup
180ml	¾ cup
250ml	1 cup
300ml	1¼ cups
375ml	1½ cups
400ml	1⅔ cups
450ml	1¾ cups
500ml	2 cups
600ml	2½ cups
750ml	3 cups

Weight

Metric	Standard
15g	½ oz
30g	1 oz
60g	2 oz
90g	3 oz
125g	4 oz
175g	6 oz
250g	8 oz
300g	10 oz
375g	12 oz
400g	13 oz
425g	14 oz
500g	1 lb
750g	1½ lb
1kg	2 lb

OVEN TEMPERATURES

Celsius °C	Fahrenheit °F	Gas Mark
110°C	225°F	¼
120°C	250°F	½
140°C	275°F	1
150°C	300°F	2
160°C	325°F	3
180°C	350°F	4
190°C	375°F	5
200°C	400°F	6
220°C	425°F	7
230°C	450°F	8
240°C	475°F	9

The Low-Carb Companion

APPENDICES

The Low-Carb Companion

ACKNOWLEDGEMENTS

As I near the end of this journey of writing my first book and getting it to a state fit for publication, I want to recognise a number of people for their invaluable contributions. Recognition goes first to my mentor and my personal hero, Professor Tim Noakes, for his inspiration from the beginning and for his continued dedicated efforts in raising awareness of the links between nutrition and health. He has done me a great honour in writing the foreword to this book. My deep gratitude goes next to my family for their unwavering support in thought, word and deed throughout. I would like to acknowledge Linda, my clinic program co-ordinator, for all her hard work in keeping our patients on track and our education programs in motion. I owe a huge thank you to all my patients and friends who have pursued a low-carb, real-food lifestyle with knowledge and faith and who have enjoyed a positive outcome. Their participation reinforced my resolve to write a book that will inform and reach many more people than we can possibly engage with directly. I am indebted to Lucy for her 'evangelic' support of the low-carb movement, her photography and invaluable assistance with online platforms for education and communication. I am grateful to Annie, proofreader and copy-editor extraordinaire, for her many hours of work in getting the manuscript to a publishable level, and to Danielle, for her deft skills at formatting and design, making this book look like a book.

LIST OF WORKS CITED

Abramson, J.D., HG Rosenberg, N Jewell, JM Wright. 'Should People At Low Risk of Cardiovascular Disease Take a Statin?' *BMJ* 2013; 347:f6123 doi: 10.1136/bmj.f6123. Print.

Academy of Nutrition and Dietetics. Comments on the Scientific Report of the 2015 Dietary Guidelines Advisory Committee. May 2015. *http://www.eatrightpro.org/resource/advocacy/take-action/regulatory-comments/dgac-scientific-report*

Accurso, A, et al. 'Dietary Carbohydrate Restriction In Type 2 Diabetes Mellitus And Metabolic Syndrome: Time For A Critical Appraisal'. *Nutrition & Metabolism 2008*, 5:9. Print.

Acharya, T, et al. 'Statin Use and the Risk of Kidney Disease With Long Term Follow-Up (8.4-Year Study)'. *American Journal of Cardiology* 2015. DOI: http://dx.doi.org/10.1016/j.amjcard.2015.11.031

Anderson, KM, W Castelli, D Levy. 'Cholesterol And Mortality. 30 Years Of Follow-Up From The Framingham Study'. *JAMA* 1987, 257:2176-2180. Print.

Astrup, A, et al. 'The Role Of Reducing Intakes Of Saturated Fat In The Prevention Of Cardiovascular Disease: Where Does The Evidence Stand In 2010'? *Am J Clin Nutr* 2011, 93(4):684-688. Print.

Avena, N, et al. 'Evidence For Sugar Addiction: Behavioural And Neurochemical Effects Of Intermittent, Excessive Sugar Intake'. *Neuroscience & Behavioral Reviews* 2008, 32(1):20-29. Print.

List Of Works Cited

Baar, K, S McGee. 'Optimizing Training Adaptations By Manipulating Glycogen'. *European Journal of Sport Science* 2008, 8:97-106. Print.

Bantle, JP, et al. Position Statement of the ADA. *Diabetes Care* 2008, 31 suppl A.

Basu, S, P Yoffe, N Hills, RH Lustig. 'The Relationship Of Sugar To Population-Level Diabetes Prevalence: An Econometric Analysis Of Repeated Cross-Sectional Data'. *PLoS One* 2013, 8: e57873. Print.

Bazzano, LA, et al. 'Effects of Low-Carbohydrate and Low-Fat Diets, A Randomized Trial'. *Ann Int Med* 2014, 161:309-318. Print.

Bell, K. Clinical Application of the Food Insulin Index to Diabetes Mellitus. Sept 2014 *http://ses.library.usyd.edu.au/handle/2123/11945*.

Brehm, BJ, RJ Seeley, SR Daniels, DA D'Alessio. 'A Randomized Trial Comparing A Very Low-carbohydrate Diet And A Calorie-Restricted Low Fat Diet On Body Weight And Cardiovascular Risk Factors In Healthy Women'. *J Clin Endocrinol Metab* 2003, 8(4):1617-23. DOI: *http://dx.doi.org/10.1210/jc.2002-021480*.

Bril, F, et al. 'Hepatic Steatosis and Insulin Resistance, But Not Steatohepatitis, Promote Atherogenic Dyslipidemia in NAFLD'. *JCEM* 2015, 101(2). DOI: http://dx.doi.org/10.1210/jc.2015-3111

Burke, LM, et al. 'Carbohydrate For Training And Competition'. *Jnl of Sports Sciences* 2011, 29 (Suppl 1), S17-S27. Print.

Carpender, D. *200 Low-Carb, High-Fat Recipes*. Fair Winds Press, 2014. Print.

Chowdhury, R, Warnakula S, Kunutsor S, et al. 'Association Of Dietary, Circulating, And Supplement Fatty Acids With Coronary Risk: A Systematic Review And Meta-Analysis'. *Ann Intern Med* 2014; 160(6): 398-406. Print.

Christofferson, T. *Tripping Over the Truth: The Metabolic Theory of Cancer*. CreateSpace Independent Publishing Platform. 2014. Print

Covey, S. *The 7 Habits of Highly Effective People*. DC Books, 2005. Print.

Crofts, C, et al. 'Hyperinsulinemia: A Unifying Theory Of Chronic Disease?' *Diabesity* 2015; 1 (4): 34-43 DOI: 10.15562/diabesity.2015.19

Culver, AL., et al. 'Statin Use And Risk Of Diabetes Mellitus In Postmenopausal Women In The Women's Health Initiative'. *Arch Intern Med* 2012, Jan 23, 172(2):144-52. Print.

Davidson's Principles & Practice of Medicine. 22nd ed. Churchill Livingstone, 2014. Print.

Davis, PG, S Phinney. 'Differential Effects Of Two Very Low Calorie Diets On Aerobic And Anaerobic Performance'. *Int. J. Obes.* 1990; 14(9):779-87. Print.

Davis, W. *Wheat Belly*. Harper Thorsons, 2014. Print.

Diamond, DM, U Ravnskov. 'How Statistical Deception Created The Appearance That Statins Are Safe And Effective In Primary And Secondary Prevention Of Cardiovascular Disease.' *Expert Rev Clin Pharmacol* 2015 Mar;8(2):201-10. DOI: 10.1586/17512433.2015.1012494. Epub 2015 Feb 12.

Dias, CB, R Garg, LG Wood, ML Garg. 'Saturated Fat Consumption May Not Be The Main Cause Of Increased Blood Lipid Levels'. *Med Hypotheses*. 2014;82(2):187-95. Print.

Dietary Guidelines Advisory Committee; Scientific Report Of The 2015 Dietary Guidelines Advisory Committee. 2015; *http://www.health.gov/dietaryguidelines/2015-scientific-report.*

DiNicolantonio, J. 'The Cardiometabolic Consequences Of Replacing Saturated Fats With Carbohydrates Or Ω-6 Polyunsaturated Fats: Do The Dietary Guidelines Have It Wrong'? *Open Heart* 2014; 1(1). Print.

DiNicolantonio, J, et al. 'The Evidence For Saturated Fat And For Sugar Related To Coronary Heart Disease.' *Prog Cardiovasc Dis* 2015. DOI.org/10.1016/j.pcad.2015.11.006

Distiller, LA. 'Why Do Some Patients With Type 1 Diabetes Live So Long'? *World J Diabetes* 2014, 5(3): 282–287. DOI:10.4239/wjd.v5.i3.282.

Edmond, JA, et al. 'Risk Of Breast Cancer Recurrence Associated With Carbohydrate Intake And Tissue Expression Of IGFI Receptor'. *Cancer Epidemiology Biomarkers & Prevention*, 2014, DOI: 10.1158/1055-9965.EPI-13-1218.

Estruch, R, E Ros, J Salas-Salvadó, et al., PREDIMED Study Investigators. Primary Prevention Of Cardiovascular Disease With A Mediterranean Diet. *N Engl J Med* 2013, 368(14):1279-1290. Print.

Feinman, R, et al. 'Dietary Carbohydrate Restriction As The First Approach In Diabetes Management: Critical Review And Evidence Base'. *Nutrition* 2015, 31:1-13. Print.

Fettke, G. Nutrition And Cancer – Time To Rethink. *Presentation To The Old Mutual Health Convention*. Cape Town. February, 2015.

Forslund, M. Low-Carb Living For Families. *Struik Lifestyle*, 2013.

Frieden, T, D. Berwick. 'The "Million Hearts" Initiative – Preventing Heart Attacks And Strokes'. *N Engl J Med*. 29, 2011. Print.

Fung, J. Novel Management Of Diabetes And Insulin Resistance. *Presentation To The Old Mutual Health Convention*. Cape Town. February, 2015.

Gearhardt, A, et al. 'Binge Eating Disorder and Food Addiction'. *Curr Drug Abuse Rev* 2011, 4(3): 201–207. Print.

Goldacre, B. Bad Science. *Fourth Estate*, 2009. Print.

Gow, M, et al. 'Impact of Dietary Macronutrient Distribution on BMI and Cardiometabolic Outcomes in Overweight and Obese Children and Adolescents: a Systematic Review'. *Nutrition Reviews* 2014, 72(7): 453-70. Print.

Grundy, Scott M. 'Gamma-Glutamyl Transferase. Another Biomarker for Metabolic Syndrome And Cardiovascular Risk.' *Arteriosclerosis, Thrombosis, and Vascular Biology*. 2007; 27: 4-7doi: 10.1161/01.ATV.0000253905.13219.4b. Print.

Hanak, V, et al. 'Accuracy of the triglyceride to high-density lipoprotein cholesterol ratio for prediction of the low-density lipoprotein phenotype B.' *Am J Cardiol*. 2004 Jul 15;94(2):219-22.

Harcombe, Z, J Baker, SM Cooper, et al. 'Evidence From Randomised Controlled Trials Did Not Support The Introduction Of Dietary Fat

List Of Works Cited

Guidelines In 1977 And 1983: A Systematic Review And Meta-Analysis'. *Open Heart* 2015;2:e000196. Print.

Harcombe, Z. The Obesity Epidemic. Columbus Publishing, 2010. Print.

Hite, AH, et al. 'Low-Carbohydrate Diet Review: Shifting The Paradigm'. *Nutr Clin Pract* 2011, 26:300-308. Print.

Hoenselaar, R. 'Saturated Fat And Cardiovascular Disease: The Discrepancy Between The Scientific Literature And Dietary Advice'. *Nutrition.* 2012;28(2):118-23. Print.

Holt, SH, JC Miller, P Petocz. 'An Insulin Index Of Foods: The Insulin Demand Generated By 1000-Kj Portions Of Common Foods'. *Am J Clin Nutr* 1997, 66(5):1264-1276. Print.

Hooper, L, et al. 'Reduced Or Modified Dietary Fat For Preventing Cardiovascular Disease.' *Cochrane Database Syst Rev*. 2011 Jul 6;(7):CD002137. Print.

Howard, B, L Van Horn, J Hsia, et al. 'Low-Fat Dietary Pattern And Risk Of Cardiovascular Disease: The Women's Health Initiative Randomized Controlled Dietary Modification Trial'. *JAMA* 2006;295:655–66. Print.

Hu, FB, VS Malik. 'Sugar-Sweetened Beverages And Risk Of Obesity And Type 2 Diabetes: Epidemiologic Evidence'. *Physiology & Behaviour* 2010, 100(1):47-54. Print.

Imamura, F, et al. 'Consumption Of Sugar Sweetened Beverages, Artificially Sweetened Beverages, And Fruit Juice And Incidence Of Type 2 Diabetes: Systematic Review, Meta-Analysis, And Estimation Of Population Attributable Fraction'. *BMJ* 2015;351:h3576, DOI: 10.1136/bmj.h3576.

Jackson, SE, F Johnson, H Croker, J Wardle. 'Weight Perceptions In A Population Sample Of English Adolescents: Cause For Celebration Or Concern'? *Int J Obes (Lond)*. 2015 Oct;39(10):1488-93. DOI: 10.1038/ijo.2015.126

Jakobsen, MU, et al. 'Major Types of Dietary Fat and Risk of Coronary Heart Disease: A Pooled Analysis of 11 Cohort Studies', *Am J Clin Nutr* 2009;89(5):1425-32. Print.

Keith, L. *The Vegetarian Myth: Food, Justice, and Sustainability*. PM Press, 2009. Print.

Kendall, M. Food Insulin Index. *https://optimisingnutrition.wordpress.com*

Kendrick, M. *The Great Cholesterol Con*. John Blake Publishing, 2007. Print.

Khaw, KT, et al. 'Association Of Haemoglobin A1c With Cardiovascular Disease And Mortality In Adults: The European Prospective Investigation Into Cancer In Norfolk'. *Ann Intern Med* 2004, 141:413-420. Print.

Klement, RJ, U Kämmerer. 'Is There A Role For Carbohydrate Restriction In The Treatment And Prevention Of Cancer'? *Nutrition & Metabolism* 2011, 8:75. Print.

Kuipers, et al. 'Saturated Fat, Carbohydrates And Cardiovascular Disease'. *Neth J Med*. 2011 Sep;69(9):372-8. Print.

Le Fanu, J. *The Rise and Fall of Modern Medicine*. Great Britain: Abacus, 2000. Print.

Lose It Magazine. Vol 4, Media 24 Publishing, 2014. Print.

List Of Works Cited

Lose It Magazine. Vols 5,6,7. Media 24 Publishing, 2015. Print.

Lucan, SC, J DiNicolantonio. 'How Calorie-Focused Thinking About Obesity And Related Diseases May Mislead And Harm Public Health. An Alternative'. *Public Health Nutr* 2015, 18(4):571-81. DOI: 10.1017/S1368980014002559.

Lustig, R. *Fat Chance: Beating the Odds Against Sugar, Processed Food, Obesity and Disease*. Hudson Street Press, 2012. Print.

Lustig, R, LA Schmidt, CD Brindis. 'The Toxic Truth About Sugar'. *Nature*. February 2012, 482(27). Print.

Malhotra, A. 'Saturated Fat Is Not The Major Issue'. *BMJ* 2013; 347. Print.

Malik, VS, Hu FB. 'Sweeteners and Risk of Obesity and Type 2 Diabetes: The Role of Sugar-Sweetened Beverages'. *Curr Diab Rep*. 2012 Jan 31. [Epub ahead of print].

Malik, VS, et al. 'Sugar-Sweetened Beverages And Risk Of Metabolic Syndrome And Type 2 Diabetes: A Meta-Analysis'. *Diabetes Care* 2010 Nov:33(11):2477-83. DOI: 10.2337/dc10-1079. Epub 2010 Aug 6.

Mascitelli, L, et al. 'The Epidemic Of Nonmelanoma Skin Cancer And The Widespread Use Of Statins'. *Dermato-Endocrinology* 2010, 2:1, 37-38. DOI: 10.4161/derm.2.1.12128.

Mensink, RP, PL Zock, AD Kester, MB Katan. 'Effects Of Dietary Fatty Acids And Carbohydrates On The Ratio Of Serum Total To HDL Cholesterol And On Serum Lipids And Apolipoproteins: A Meta-Analysis Of 60 Controlled Trials'. *Am J Clin Nutr* 2003, 77(5):1146-1155. Print.

Meule, A. 'How Prevalent is "Food Addiction"'? *Front Psychiatry* 2011, 2:61. DOI:10.3389/fpsyt.2011.00061.

Minger, D. *http://rawfoodsos.com/2010/09/02/the-china-study-wheat-and-heart-disease.*

Moss, M. *Salt Sugar Fat: How The Food Giants Hooked Us*. Random House, 2013. Print.

Mozaffarian, D. 'Dietary and Policy Priorities for Cardiovascular Disease, Diabetes, and Obesity. A Comprehensive Review.' *Circulation* 2016;133:187-225. DOI: 10.1161/CIRCULATIONAHA.115. 018585.

Mozaffarian, D, D Ludwig. The 2015 US Dietary Guidelines Lifting the Ban on Total Dietary Fat, *JAMA* 2015, 313(24). Print.

Mozaffarian, D. 'Diverging Global Trends In Heart Disease And Type 2 Diabetes: The Role Of Carbohydrates And Saturated Fats'. *Lancet Diabetes Endocrinol* 2015 Published Online June 29, 2015 *http://dx.doi.org/10.1016/S2213-8587(15)00208-9.*

Nagourney, R. *Outliving Cancer*. Laguna Beach: Basic Health Publications, 2013. Print.

Nielsen, JV, C Gando, E Joensson, C Paulsson. 'Low-carbohydrate Diet In Type 1 Diabetes, Long-Term Improvement And Adherence: A Clinical Audit'. *Diabetol Metab Syndr* 2012, 4(1):23. DOI:10.1186/1758-5996-4-23.

Noakes, T, SA Creed, D Grier, J Proudfoot. *The Real Meal Revolution*. Quivertree Publications, 2013. Print.

List Of Works Cited

Noakes, T, M Vlismas. *Challenging Beliefs*. Cape Town: Zebra Press, 2012. Print.

Noakes, T, S Phinney, JS Volek. 'Low-Carbohydrate Diets For Athletes: What Evidence'? *Br J Sports Med* 2014, 48:1077-1078. Print.

Noakes, T. *Lore of Running* 4th Edition. Southern Africa: Oxford University Press, 2001. Print.

Okuyama, H, et al. 'Statins Simulate Atherosclerosis And Heart Failure: Pharmacological Mechanisms.' *Expert Rev Clin Pharmacol* 2015 Mar;8(2):189-99. DOI: 10.1586/17512433.2015.1011125. Epub 2015 Feb 6.

Paoli, A., A. Bianco, K Grimaldi. 'The Ketogenic Diet And Sport: A Possible Marriage'? *Exerc. Sport Sci. Rev.* 2015; 43(3):153-162. Print.

Paoli, A, K Grimaldi, D D'Agostino, et al. 'Ketogenic Diet Does Not Affect Strength Performance In Elite Artistic Gymnasts'. *J. Int. Soc. Sports Nutr.* 2012; 9(1):34. Print.

Paoli, A, A Rubini, JS Volek, KA Grimaldi. 'Beyond Weight Loss: A Review Of The Therapeutic Uses Of Very-Low-Carbohydrate (Ketogenic) Diets'. *European Journal of Clinical Nutrition* 2013, 67: 789–796. Print.

Pavlova, NN, CB Thompson. 'The Emerging Hallmarks of Cancer Metabolism.' Cell *Metabolism* 2016. 23(1):27-47. DOI.org/10.1016/j.cmet.2015.12.006.

Perlmutter, D, K Loberg. *Grain Brain*. Yellow Kite Books, 2014. Print.

Phinney, S. 'Ketogenic Diets And Physical Performance'. *Nutrition & Metabolism* 2004, 1:2 DOI:10.1186/1743-7075-1-2.

Puaschitz, NG, E Strand, TM Norekvål, et al. 'Dietary Intake Of Saturated Fat Is Not Associated With Risk Of Coronary Events Or Mortality In Patients With Established Coronary Artery Disease'. *J Nutr.* 2015;145(2):299-305.

Ramsden, CE, D Zamora, B Leelarthaepin, et al. 'Use Of Dietary Linoleic Acid For Secondary Prevention Of Coronary Heart Disease And Death: Evaluation Of Recovered Data From The Sydney Diet Heart Study And Updated Meta-Analysis'. *BMJ.* 2013;346:e870. Print.

Rauch, JT, et al. 'The Effects Of Ketogenic Dieting on Skeletal Muscle And Fat Mass.' *Journal of the International Society of Sports Nutrition* 2014;11(1):1-1.

Ravnskov, U. *Ignore the Awkward: How the Cholesterol Myths are Kept Alive.* CreateSpace Independent Publishing Platform, 2010. Print.

Reaven, G, et al. 'Insulin Resistance and Coronary Heart Disease in Nondiabetic Individuals'. *Arteriosclerosis, Thrombosis, and Vascular Biology* 2012, 32:1754-1759. Print.

Reynierse, I, *Low-carb is Lekker*. Struik Lifestyle, 2015.

Romaguera, D, et al. 'The InterAct Consortium. Consumption Of Sweet Beverages And Type 2 Diabetes Incidence In European Adults: Results From EPIC-Interact'. *Diabetologia*, 2013 DOI: 10.1007/s00125-013-2899-8.

List Of Works Cited

Santos, FL, et al. 'Systematic Review And Meta-Analysis Of Clinical Trials Of The Effects Of Low-carbohydrate Diets On Cardiovascular Risk Factors'. *Obes Rev.* 2012 Nov;13(11):1048-66. Print.

Schofield, G, et al. 'Very Low-Carbohydrate Diets In The Management Of Diabetes Revisited'. *NZMJ* 2016;129(1432).

Schulte, EM, N Avena, A Gearhardt. 'Which Foods May Be Addictive? The Roles of Processing, Fat Content, and Glycemic Load'. *PLoS One* Feb 18, 2015 DOI: 10.1371/journal.pone.0117959.

Schwingshackl, L, G Hoffmann. 'Dietary Fatty Acids In The Secondary Prevention Of Coronary Heart Disease: A Systematic Review, Meta-Analysis And Meta-Regression'. *BMJ Open* 2014; 4(4). Print.

Scientific Report of the 2015 Dietary Guidelines Advisory Committee (DGAC Report). *http://www.health.gov/dietaryguidelines/2015-scientific-report.* February 23, 2015.

Servan-Schreiber, D. Anticancer: *A New Way of Life*. Penguin Books, 2011. Print.

Shai, I, et al. 'Weight Loss With A Low-Carbohydrate, Mediterranean, Or A Low-Fat Diet'. *N Engl J Med* 2008, 359(3):229-241. DOI: 10.1056/NEJMoa0708681.

Shulman, G. 'Ectopic Fat in Insulin Resistance, Dyslipidemia and Cardiometabolic Disease'. *N Engl J Med* 2014, 371:1131-41. DOI: 10.1056/NEJMra1011035.

Silva, J. 'The Effects Of Very High Fat, Very Low Carbohydrate Diets On Safety, Blood Lipid Profile, And Anabolic Hormone Status.' *Journal of the International Society of Sports Nutrition* 2014; 11(1):1-1

Siri-Tarino, et al. 'Meta-Analysis Of Prospective Cohort Studies Evaluating The Association Of Saturated Fat With Cardiovascular Disease'. *Am J Clin Nutr.* 91, 2010b. Print.

Siri-Tarino, et al. 'Saturated Fat, Carbohydrate And Cardiovascular Disease'. *Am J Clin Nutr.* 91, 2010a. Print.

Smith, RN, et al. 'A Low Glycaemic-Load Diet Improves Symptoms In Acne Vulgaris Patients: A Randomised Controlled Trial'. *American Journal of Clinical Nutrition* 2007, 86:107-115. Print.

Sondike, SB, et al. 'Effects of a Low-carbohydrate Diet on Weight Loss and Cardiovascular Risk Factor in Overweight Adolescents'. *The Journal of Paediatrics* 2003, 142(3): 253-8. Print.

Steinvil, A, et al. 'The association of higher levels of within-normal-limits liver enzymes and the prevalence of the metabolic syndrome'. *Cardiovascular Diabetology* 2010, 9:30. Print.

Steven, S, et al. 'Weight Loss Decreases Excess Pancreatic Triacylglycerol Specifically in Type 2 Diabetes'. *Diabetes Care*. Published online before print December 1, 2015, DOI: 10.2337/dc15-0750.

Stevenson, K, F Cowdell. 'Acne And Diet: A Review Of The Latest Evidence'. *Dermatological Nursing* 2013, 12(2):28-34. Print.

Taubes, G. *The Diet Delusion*. Vermilion, 2007. Print.

Taubes, G. 'The Science Of Obesity: What Do We Really Know About What Makes Us Fat? An essay by Gary Taubes'. 2013. *BMJ*, 346;f1050.

Taubes, G. *Why We Get Fat and What To Do About It*. Alfred A. Knopf Publishers, 2011. Print.

Taylor, R. 'Type 2 Diabetes: Etiology and Reversibility'. *Diabetes Care*. 2013 Apr; 36(4):1047-55. DOI:10.2337/dc12-1805.

Taylor, RS, et al. 'Reduced Dietary Salt For The Prevention Of Cardiovascular Disease (Review)'. *The Cochrane Collaboration and published in The Cochrane Library* 2011, Issue 7. Print.

Teicholz, N. *The Big Fat Surprise*. Scribe Publications, 2014. Print.

Tóth, C, Z Clemens. 'Type 1 Diabetes Mellitus Successfully Managed With The Paleolithic Ketogenic Diet'. *Int J Case Rep Images* 2014;5 (10):699–703. Print.

Tröhler, U. 'James Lind And Scurvy: 1747 To 1795. *JLL Bulletin* 2003: Commentaries On The History Of Treatment Evaluation, 2003 *(http://www.jameslindlibrary.org/articles/james-lind-and-scurvy-1747-to-1795/)*.

Vannice, G, H Rasmussen. 'Position Of The Academy Of Nutrition And Dietetics: Dietary Fatty Acids For Healthy Adults'. *Journal Of The Academy Of Nutrition & Dietetics* 2014, 114(1):136-153. Print.

Varona, V. *Nature's Cancer-Fighting Foods*. Perigee Books, 2014.

Veech, RL. 'The Therapeutic Implications Of Ketone Bodies: The Effects Of Ketone Bodies In Pathological Conditions: Ketosis, Ketogenic Diet, Redox States, Insulin Resistance, And Mitochondrial Metabolism'. *Prostaglandins Leukot. Essent. Fatty Acids.* 2004; 70(3):309-19. Print.

Volek, J, et al. 'Body Compostion And Hormonal Responses To A Carbohydrate-Restricted Diet.' *Metabolism* 2002; 51(7):864-870

Volek, J, et al. 'Dietary Carbohydrate Restriction Induces A Unique Metabolic State Positively Affecting Atherogenic Dyslipidaemia, Fatty Acid Partitioning And Metabolic Syndrome'. *Prog Lipid Res* 2008, 47(5):307-318. Print.

Volek, J, S Phinney. 'A New Look at Carbohydrate-Restricted Diets: Separating Fact From Fiction'. *Nutrition Today* 2013, 48(2):53-93. Print.

Volek, J, S Phinney. *The Art and Science of Low-carbohydrate Living*. Beyond Obesity LLC, 2012. Print.

Volek, J, et al. 'Carbohydrate Restriction Has A More Favourable Impact On The Metabolic Syndrome Than A Low Fat Diet'. *Lipids 2009* Apr; 44(4):297-309. Print.

Volek, J, S Phinney. *The Art and Science of Low-carbohydrate Performance*. Beyond Obesity LLC, 2012. Print.

Westman, E, S Phinney, J Volek. *New Atkins New You*. Fireside Publishing, 2010. Print.

Westman, E. et al. 'Low-Carbohydrate Nutrition And Metabolism'. *Am J Clin Nutr* 2007 Aug, 86(2):276-84. Print.

westonprice.org/health-topics/studies-showing-adverse-effects-of-isoflavones-1950-2010

Whybrow, S, et al. 'The Effect Of An Incremental Increase In Exercise On Appetite, Eating Behaviour And Energy Balance In Lean Men And Women Feeding Ad Libitum'. *Brit Jnl of Nutr* 2008, 100(5), 1109 15. Print.

List Of Works Cited

Williams, PG. 'Nutritional Composition Of Red Meat'. *Nutrition & Dietetics* 2007, 64(Supplement 4), S113-S119. Print.

Wu, S, et al. 'Substantial contribution of extrinsic risk factors to cancer development'. *Nature* (2015) DOI:10.1038/nature16166.

Yang, Q, et al. 'Added Sugar Intake And Cardiovascular Diseases Mortality Among US Adults'. *JAMA Internal Medicine*, 2014; DOI: 10.1001/jamainternmed.2013.13563.

Yudkin, J. 'Diet And Coronary Thrombosis Hypothesis And Fact'. *Lancet* 1957, 273:155-162. Print.

Zajac, A, S Poprzecki, A Maszczyk, M Czuba, M Michalczyk, G Zydek. 'The Effects Of A Ketogenic Diet On Exercise Metabolism And Physical Performance In Off-Road Cyclists'. *Nutrients*. 2014; 6(7):2493-508. Print.

www.authoritynutrition.com

www.cancerresearchuk.org

www.carbsmart.com

www.dietdoctor.com

www.eatingacademy.com

www.intensivedietarymanagement.com

www.nutritiondata.self.com

www.optimisingnutrition.wordpress.com

www.realmealrevolution.com

www.thenoakesfoundation.org

List Of Works Cited

INDEX

A

Acne, 123, 157
Adenosine triphosphate (ATP), 75, 188, 193, 195, 230, 240
Adiponectin, 87, 228
Advanced glycation end-products (AGEs), 50, 103, 213, 219-220, 228-229
Alcohol, 141, 147, 209-210
Almonds, 127, 132, 135, 143, 155, 185
Alzheimer's dementia, 50, 80, 88, 123, 165, 229
Amino acids, 147, 171, 198, 209, 215, 229, 234, 242
   children and, 155
   essential, 67
   protein and, 65
   sport and, 201
Ancestors' diet, 42
Appetite, 38, 47, 55, 66, 79, 81, 89-91, 146, 156, 172, 206, 214, 239
Arteries, 30, 218, 229-230, 232
   inflammation and, 87, 220
Artificial sweeteners, 125, 127, 129, 131, 144, 154, 214
Atherogenic dyslipidaemia, 103, 115, 118, 164-165, 230, 237, 240

Atherosclerosis, 104-105, 230
   diabetes and, 167
Atkins diet, 122
Avocado, 56, 58, 61, 68, 106, 124, 126, 132, 134, 145, 153-155, 156, 182, 185, 215
Avocado oil, 63, 127, 141, 143, 212

B

Bacon, 124, 126, 156, 182, 185
Banting, 122, 218, 230
Beef, 60-61, 69, 72, 126, 134, 141, 145, 153, 155-156, 182, 185, 215, 244
Belly fat, 29, 36-37, 79-80, 86-88, 90, 93, 243
   cancer and, 88
   diabetes and, 164, 167-168, 176
   heart disease and, 103
   leptin and, 91-92
   metabolic syndrome and, 103
Blood lipids, 95, 98-99, 103, 115-116, 228, 239
Blood pressure, 29-30, 32, 36, 38, 50, 80, 210, 230, 236, 240
   diabetes and, 168-169, 176

Index

heart disease and, 103, 115
low-carb and, 158
obesity and, 88
salt and, 218
Blood sugar (blood glucose), 29, 33, 38, 46-48, 50, 79, 91-92, 103, 158, 213, 234-237, 240
  cancer and, 187-189
  diabetes and, 162, 164-165, 168-171, 173-179
  glycation and, 228
  heart disease and, 115, 118,
Blood tests, 37, 105, 140, 164
  health profile, 33
  lipids, 116
Body fat, 46, 54, 79, 86-93, 200, 203, 241
  sites, 87, 203, 244-245 see also belly fat
Body mass index (BMI), 32, 88, 167, 231, 241
Brain, 54, 66, 97, 117, 155, 158, 221, 229, 238-239, 244-245
  Alzheimer's and, 50
  appetite and, 37, 47, 55, 81, 83, 91-92
  diabetes and, 169, 171
  ketones and, 171, 196, 198, 208
Bread, 28, 44, 46-47, 49, 124, 128, 138, 144, 157, 177, 183, 206, 214, 216, 220
Bread low-carb, 144, 154, 156
Breast cancer, *see cancer*
Breast milk, 57, 152-153, 211
Butter, 56, 60-62, 124, 127, 134

C

Calories, 79, 156, 178, 180, 184, 195, 245
  from carbs, 43
  from fats, 54-55
  obesity and, 88
  sugar and, 114
  restriction of, 89
  weight and, 90, 207
Cancer, 36, 38, 58, 75, 80, 123, 165, 186-191, 213-214, 217, 231, 237, 241-242
  breast, 87-88, 187-188, 190, 217
  cholesterol and, 102, 105
  colon-rectal, 88, 165, 207
  prostate, 123
Canola oil, 56, 62, 129
Carbohydrates, 28-31, 36-42, 78-85, 89, 153, 193, 202, 231
  cancer and, 189-191
  diabetes and, 162-181
  heart disease and, 106, 108, 111-114, 230
  macronutrient, 43-53
  metabolism, 245
  refined, 47, 75, 243
  weight loss and, 146-147
Carbohydrate-intolerance, 230-231
Cardiovascular disease, *see heart disease*
Cereals, 28, 44, 47, 69, 92, 124, 128, 138, 144, 154, 206, 216, 236
Children, 75, 152-158, 216
  ADHD and, 228
  low-carb and, 160, 163, 186, 211

obesity and, 92-93
Cholesterol, 30, 33, 75, 94-119, 198, 229, 231, 244
  dietary, 57, 211
  Familial hypercholesterolemia, 233
  lipoproteins and, 236-239, 246
Chylomicrons, 100, 231, 239
Cigarette smoking, 23, 88, 103, 115, 187
Coconut oil, 56-57, 127, 134, 139, 141, 143, 153, 184, 203, 212
  fat content of, 59, 61
  smoking point of, 62-63
Coeliac disease, 123, 187, 231
Coffee, 28, 127, 139, 144, 214
Colon cancer, see cancer
Constipation, 208
Cooking oils, 58, 143
  smoking points of, 62-63
Corn, 115, 128, 139, 142, 153, 167, 183, 234-236, 241, see also high-fructose corn syrup
Coronary heart disease, see heart disease
Cravings, 29, 31, 37, 47, 49, 208, 214

D

Dairy products, 46, 48, 56-57, 59, 65, 67-69, 95, 124, 127, 130, 132, 139-140, 146, 159, 184-185, 206, 209, 215, 217, 238, 242-243
  children and, 154-155
  low-fat and, 125, 129

Dementia, see Alzheimer's dementia
Dental caries, 194
Diabesity, 163
Diabetes type 1, 174-185
Diabetes type 2, 26, 29, 36-38, 75, 87-88, 92, 113, 116, 162-173, 228-230, 232, 234-235, 239-240, 242-244
  carbs and, 83
  cancer and, 187
  heart disease and, 103-104, 106, 115
  insulin and, 80, 166, 237
  ketogenic diet and, 238
  low-carb diet and, 91, 123, 145-146, 158
Dietary guidelines, 26, 42-43, 83, 98-99, 107-108, 113, 163, 232
Diet-heart hypothesis, 94
DNA, see genes

E

Eggs, 46, 56-58, 60-61, 65, 69-72, 153-159, 215, 241, 243
  cholesterol and, 95, 97, 269
Energy, 37-38, 65, 75, 81, 91, 146, 169, 171, 188-189, 206-208, 219, 230-231, 240
  fat and, 54-57, 172, 233, 238
  sport and, 193-203
  sugar and, 40-48, 79, 89, 235
Epilepsy, 123, 132
Essential fatty acids, 55, 58, 60, 109, 202, 212

Index

omega-3 and, 58, 217, 241
omega-6 and, 58, 213, 241
Exercise, 30, 37, 243
  diabetes and, 168
  the athlete and, 192-203
  weight loss and, 79, 81, 90-91, 93, 207

F

Fasting, 146-147, 171, 238, 241
Fat, dietary, 26, 42, 54-56, 58-59, 61, 86, 94-95, 107, 135, 195, 206, 208, 211-212, 219, 231, 233
  cancer and, 187
  calories and, 55, 207
  diabetes and, 163-165, 168-169, 171, 174-176
  insulin and, 179
  low-fat and, 26, 37, 43, 55, 75, 88-91, 93, 99-101, 107-108, 113, 125, 129, 139, 207
  metabolism and, 209
  obesity and, 88
  trans-fats and, 187
  triglycerides and, *see triglycerides*
Fats, monounsaturated, 55-56, 58-59, 61-62, 106, 240
Fats, polyunsaturated, 55-56, 58-59, 61, 103, 213, 236, 242
Fats, saturated, 56-57, 61, 153, 197, 211, 243
  cholesterol, LDL and, 97-98, 174, 211, 231
  heart disease and, 94-114, 118
  obesity and, see obesity
Fat-soluble vitamins, 54, 68
Fatty acids, *see essential fatty acids*
Fermented foods, 48, 159
Fibre, 48, 70, 135, 231, 233, 243
Fish and Fish oils, 56, 58, 67-69, 75, 124, 126, 129, 139, 154-155, 159, 185, 217, 241
Flour, 46, 70-71, 74, 86, 124, 127-128, 139, 144, 153, 157, 220, 235
Framingham Heart Study, 102
Free radicals, 50, 103, 189, 233
Friedewald, William (equation), 211, 233
Fructose, 28, 44-46, 50, 53, 129, 142, 144, 147, 154, 189, 212, 219-220, 234, *see also high fructose corn syrup*
  heart disease and, 103, 115, 167
  hypertension and, 218
  triglycerides and, 48
Fruit juices, 44, 47, 49, 92, 125, 128-129, 139, 143-144, 158, 206
Fruits, 38, 44, 46, 48, 68-69, 91, 126-132, 139, 141, 143, 145, 147, 154, 159, 185, 215
Fung, Jason, 22, 165, 174, 176, 222

G

Gall bladder, 123, 212, 234
Gamma-glutamyl transferase (GGT), 33, 164
Genes, 50, 79, 163, 186, 189, 234

Gluconeogenesis, 66, 147, 171-172, 196, 209, 234
Glucose, 45-46, 48-50, 66, 79, 103, 129, 142, 147, 169, 171, 177, 208-209, 220, 228, 230, 234-236, 238, 244, *see also blood sugar*
   athletes and, 193-196
   cancer and, 188-190
Glucotoxicity, 164, 176, 234
Gluten, 128, 154-155, 169, 231, 234
Gluten-free, 38, 128, 139, 144, 155, 159
Glycaemic index (GI), 46-47, 111, 234
Glycaemic load (GL), 220, 235
Glycation, 50, 99, 235
Glycogen, 46, 193-203, 235
Good Calories, Bad Calories (Gary Taubes), 222
Grains, 24, 38, 44, 46, 48, 58, 69-70, 91, 128, 140, 154-155, 159, 213, 235, 242-243
Gut biome (gut bacteria), 159, 179, 214

H

Haemoglobin A1c (HbA1c), 33, 50, 115-116, 198, 235
Harcombe, Zoe, 22, 71, 74, 134
Heart attacks, *see heart disease*
Heart disease, 36, 94-119, 123, 158, 232
   carbs and, 52
   cholesterol and, 174, 211, 233
   diabetes and, 165, 176

   inflammation and, 228-229
   lipoproteins and, 240
   saturated fat and, 54
   statins and, 104
   sugar and, 50, 214
   triglycerides and, 54, 100-101, 230, 240
High-fructose corn syrup, 44-46, 48-50, 115, 142, 153, 167, 219, 241
High protein diet, 67, 141
High-density lipoprotein (HDL), *see lipoproteins*
Honey, 28, 129, 131, 133, 139, 142, 144, 154, 162, 184, 212, 234
Hunger, 37, 47, 66, 81, 89, 91, 145, 207-208, 215, 219
Hydrogenated oils, *see vegetable oil*
Hypercholesterolemia, *see cholesterol*
Hyperglycaemia, 175, 188, 236-237
Hyperinsulinemia, 83, 116, 167, 188, 236, 240
Hypertension, 92, 123, 165, 176, 213, 228, 230, 232, 236
Hyperuricaemia, 50, 236
Hypoglycemia, 170-171, 236

I

Infant formula, 153
Inflammation, 58, 80, 82, 164, 235-236, 243, 245-246
   arteries and, 50, 87, 103, 115, 118, 220
   heart disease and, 228-229

Index

cancer and, 190-191
Insulin, 29, 33, 38, 46, 55, 66, 80, 91, 147, 182-185, 230, 237, 242, *see also insulin resistance*
   blood sugar and, 75, 158
   body fat and, 48, 91, 207
   cancer and, 188-189, 191
   carbs and, 47, 118, 213, 231
   diabetes and, 162-181, 232
   exercise and, 197-198, 200
   heart disease and, 103-104, 115, 118, 218
   hyperinsulinaemia, 83, 116, 236, 240
   hunger and, 206, 214
   obesity and, 146
   therapy and, 171, 210, 234, 240
Insulin index, 177-183, 233
Insulin like growth factor (IGF-1), 167, 188-191, 237
Insulin resistance (IR), 26, 36, 39, 47, 50, 78-84, 87, 89, 92-93, 158, 164, 219-220, 228, 237, 240-241, 243-245
Inuit, 75
Irritable bowel syndrome (IBS), 123

K

Kendall, Marty, 177-178, 180
Ketoacidosis, 171, 216, 238
Ketogenic diet, 92, 95, 97, 122-123, 132, 209, 212, 245
   athletes and, 192, 195-197, 200-202
   diabetes and, 168-191
Ketones, 55, 171-172, 189, 195-198, 209, 238, 241
Ketosis, 55, 159, 170-171, 190, 216, 241
Keys, Ancel, 94, 114
Kidney disease, 50, 105, 165, 175-176, 215, 217

L

Lactose, 142, 146, 169, 212, 238
Lard, 55-56, 61-62, 124, 127, 134, 141, 143, 184, 213, 262-263
LDL, *see low density lipoproteins*
Legumes, 128, 135, 154
Leptin, 87, 91-93, 239
Lind, James, 22
Lipids, *see cholesterol, lipoproteins and triglycerides*
Lipolysis, 79, 172, 239
Lipoproteins, 95-106, 231, 237, 239
   HDL, 29, 33, 112, 117, 165, 176, 198, 211, 230, 236, 240
   heart disease and, 116-117
   LDL, 33, 109-110, 113, 115, 117, 165, 211, 229-230, 238
   VLDL, 219, 229-230, 233, 246
Liver, 47-48, 66, 95-96, 101-102, 105, 196, 212, 219, 231, 234, 237-240, 245
   glycogen and, 46, 193-194, 235
   non-alcoholic fatty liver disease (NAFLD), 84, 123, 164-165, 168, 240-241, 244

Low-calorie diets, 37, 89
Low-carbohydrate nutrition, 122-136, 138-148
Low-density lipoprotein (LDL), *see lipoproteins*
Low-fat diets, *see fat, dietary (low-fat)*
Lustig, Robert, 22, 43, 50, 224

M

Macronutrients, 40-43, 70-71, 135, 152, 158, 193, 240
Malhotra, Aseem, 22, 109
Margarine, 28, 55-56, 58, 64, 118, 125, 129, 139, 143, 219, 236
Metabolic syndrome, 21, 29, 75, 80, 87-88, 123, 158, 214, 224-225, 230, 237, 240, 244
   diabetes and, 164, 167, 176
   heart disease and, 103, 115-116
Metabolism, 35, 75, 89, 91, 101, 207, 209, 219, 223-225, 228, 230, 240
   cancer and, 186-189
Metformin, 170, 240
Micronutrients, 243, *see also Vitamins, Minerals*
Milk, 38, 49, 59, 61-62, 68-74, 127-132, 134, 139, 143-146, 154, 182-184, 238, 242
Minger, Denise, 52
Minerals, 40-41, 43, 68-76, 152, 158, 179, 192, 197, 202

Monounsaturated fat, *see fat, monounsaturated*
Mozaffarian, Dariush, 48, 91, 106-107, 225
Muscle glycogen, *see glycogen*
Muscles, 46, 55, 78, 157, 237-238, 246
   sports nutrition and, 193-199, 202-203

N

Net carbs, 133
Noakes, Tim, 19, 22, 25, 222
Non-alcoholic fatty liver disease (NAFLD), *see liver*
Nut butters, 125, 127, 132, 139, 144, 155, 203
Nutritional ketosis, *see ketosis*
Nuts, 38, 46, 48, 56, 58, 65, 68-69, 72, 91, 202, 240, 242
   children and, 154-158
   insulinogenic and, 184-185
   low-carb and, 124, 127-129, 131-132, 139, 141, 143-146, 215, 219
   macronutrient composition of, 135

O

Obesity, 21-22, 26, 29, 36, 86-93, 123, 132, 145, 215, 241, 244-245
   belly fat and, *see belly fat*
   cancer and, 187
   causes of, 39, 54, 64, 113, 243
   diabetes and, 163, 167

Index

insulin and, 237
metabolism and, 78-84, 240
sugar and, 50, 220
Oils, *see fats*
Olive oil, 61-63
Oxidation, 57, 99, 198, 213, 229, 241
    fat oxidation in exercise and, 194, 196, 200

P

Paleo diet, 122, 242
Pancreas, 46-47, 78, 162, 164, 168, 230, 232, 234, 237, 242
Peanuts, 127, 132, 135, 143, 145, 154, 158, 182, 185, 215
Phinney, Stephen D., 19, 22, 192, 196-197, 199-200, 222-223, 226
Polycystic ovary syndrome (PCOS), 123, 219
Polyunsaturated fat, *see fat, polyunsaturated*
Pre-diabetes, *see metabolic syndrome*
Pregnancy, 37, 79, 159-160, 231
    diabetes and, 158, 162, 167, 232, 234
Processed foods, 49, 70, 89, 115, 136, 140, 152, 158, 168, 211, 214, 217, 219, 236, 242, 245
    real foods vs. processed foods, 134
Proteins, 42, 70, 72, 160, 172, 206-209, 212-213, 215, 217, 219, 228-229, 234-235, 242-243, 245
    athlete and, 157, 192, 196-200, 202
    diabetes and, 170-171, 175, 177, 179-181
    macronutrient, 40-41, 65-67, 134-135, 153, 155, 159, 240
    weight gain and, 144, 146-147

R

Recipes, 251
    Beef, 319
    Bread, 393
    Broths & Soups, 253
    Conversion Tables, 461
    Cupcakes, Cakes & Cookies, 421
    Desserts, 433
    Eggs, 271
    Fish, 287
    Lamb, 337
    Pancakes & Muffins, 413
    Pizza, Quiches & Pasta, 401
    Pork, 345
    Poultry, 299
    Salad Dressings, Sauces, Marinades & Rubs, 371
    Sides, Salads & Vegetables, 353
    Smoothies & Shakes, 441
    Snacks & Miscellaneous, 447
Red wine, 139, 210, 243
Refined carbohydrates, *see carbohydrates*
Rice, 28, 44, 46-47, 74, 124, 128, 139, 143, 155, 183, 206, 213, 216, 220, 243

S

Salt, 49, 199, 208, 218, 243
Saturated fat, *see fat, saturated*
Scurvy, 22, 74-75
Seed oils, *see vegetable oil*
Semmelweis, Ignaz, 23
Seven Countries Study, 94, 114
Soft drinks, *see sugar sweetened beverages*
Soya (soy) products, 48, 59, 125, 129, 131, 139, 153, 216-217, 237, 241
Sports nutrition, 192-203
Starch, 38, 43-44, 47, 91, 107, 123, 125, 139-140, 145, 159, 178-179, 206, 213, 216, 220, 231, 244
Statins, 26, 29, 104-105, 117, 167-168, 244
Sucrose, *see sugar*
Sugar, 38, 43-53, 55, 70-71, 74, 78-84, 86, 89, 91-92, 123, 125, 129, 136, 138-140, 147, 184, 194, 199, 202, 206-207, 209-211, 214-216, 218-219, 230-231, 234, 236, 238-239
   addiction, 29-31, 220, 224
   cancer and, 188-189, 191
   children and, 152-158
   diabetes and, 166-168, 178
   heart disease and, 94, 103, 107, 114-115, 118
   other names, 142
Sugar sweetened beverages, 28, 31, 44, 47, 53, 92, 129, 139, 144, 156, 210
   dental caries and, 194
   diabetes and, 163

Supplements, 75, 99, 157, 196-197, 217-218
Stevia, *see sweeteners*
Sweeteners, 125, 127, 129, 133, 139, 144, 154, 212, 214

T

Taylor, Roy, 164, 224
Teicholz, Nina, 113, 222
Thermic effect of food, 172, 245
Tooth decay, *see dental caries*
Trans-fats, 38, 55-56, 58, 63-64, 103, 111, 118, 245
Triglycerides, 29-30, 33, 235, 245
   fat and, 54, 228, 233, 244
   heart disease and, 101, 116, 230
   lipoproteins and, 237-239, 246
   metabolic syndrome and, 240
Twelve (12) steps to weight loss, 146

V

Vegetable oils, 28, 56, 58-60, 64, 91, 129, 139, 143, 213, 228
   cancer and, 189
   heart disease and, 103, 118
   hydrogenated, 56, 236
   smoking points, 62-63
Vegetarians, 65, 72, 74, 215
Very low density lipoprotein (VLDL), *see lipoproteins*

Index

Visceral fat, *see belly fat*
Vitamin C, 22, 69, 71, 74-75, 217
Vitamins, 40-41, 43, 54, 68-76, 97, 152, 179, 201, 212, 217
VO2max, 196-200, 246
Volek, Jeff, 19, 22, 194, 200, 203, 222-223, 225-226

W

Waist circumference, 32, 88, 187
Warburg, Otto, 188
   Warburg effect, 188-189
Weaning, 153
Weight loss, 37, 52-54, 66, 207-209, 212, 218
   alcohol and, 210
   diabetes and, 164, 169-170
   exercise and, 90-93, 207
   in sport, 198, 200-203
   low-carb and, 38, 64, 108, 122-136, 138-148, 172, 217, 230
Westman, Eric, 19, 22, 169-170, 222-223
Wheat, 44, 47, 52, 89, 128, 134, 138, 143-144, 155, 169, 183, 187, 213, 220, 231, 234-235
WHO (World Health Organisation), 86, 187

X

Xylitol, *see sweeteners*

Y

Yudkin, John, 114

The Low-Carb Companion

Proofreading and editing by Ann Beattie
Email: annrothrockbeattie@gmail.com

Ann Beattie
Proofreading and Copy Editing

Book design and layout by Danielle Demblon
Email: dansdem@gmail.com

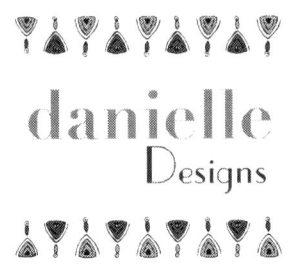

danielle Designs

Author photograph by Lucy Broderick

Printed in Great Britain
by Amazon